The Challenges of MRI

SCIENCES

Image, Field Director – Laure Blanc-Féraud

Imagery in Life Sciences, Subject Head – Françoise Peyrin

The Challenges of MRI

Techniques and Quantitative Methods for Health

Coordinated by
Hélène Ratiney
Olivier Beuf

iSTE

WILEY

First published 2024 in Great Britain and the United States by ISTE Ltd and John Wiley & Sons, Inc.

ISTE Ltd
27-37 St George's Road
London SW19 4EU
UK

www.iste.co.uk

John Wiley & Sons, Inc.
111 River Street
Hoboken, NJ 07030
USA

www.wiley.com

Library of Congress Control Number: 2023943624

British Library Cataloguing-in-Publication Data
A CIP record for this book is available from the British Library
ISBN 978-1-78945-113-9

ERC code:
LS7 Applied Medical Technologies, Diagnostics, Therapies and Public Health
LS7_1 Imaging for medical diagnosis

Contents

Introduction

Hélène RATINEY and Olivier BEUF
CREATIS, CNRS, Inserm, INSA Lyon, Université Claude Bernard Lyon 1, France

Since its inception in 1973, magnetic resonance imaging has experienced remarkable technological and methodological advancements. Magnetic resonance imaging (MRI) has reached a certain level of maturity, as well as complexity, where several expertise domains merge: biology, medicine, physical chemistry, physics and computer science. A great number of publications on this topic are aimed at the medical world (radiologists, radiographers), while others describe the physics of MRI and target a wider public, including scientists, from the master level to senior researchers. The present work seeks to cover the techniques and methods considered promising for the future of MRI. These approaches provide data way beyond the anatomical structure, including functional, hemodynamic, structural, biomechanical or even biochemical information. Retrieving each of these kinds of data requires understanding and describing a physical phenomenon and putting this knowledge into practice by drawing upon the areas of engineering and, in particular, signal and image processing.

This work thus strives to describe the practical implementation of a great variety of techniques by recalling the underlying physics and by giving details of the modelization and analysis that enable acquisition strategies and retrieval informations. The authors approached the challenge of providing in each chapter the keys to a general overview of a technique or domain by following summarized formulations and citing bibliographic references considered the most relevant. Indeed, each chapter's topic could be covered in a separate book in order to completely satisfy the authors' pedagogic goal. Whether the reader is a master's or

The Challenges of MRI,
coordinated by Hélène RATINEY and Olivier BEUF. © ISTE Ltd 2024.

doctoral student, a researcher in medical imaging or a staff member at a university hospital, they will find in this work the information necessary for understanding multiparametric MRI and today's challenges in the field of MRI.

In the first four chapters, this work covers the fundamental notions and principles, deemed useful in MRI, in a brief but sometimes new way. Chapter 1 describes the basics of an MRI scan and the related instrumentation signal chain while introducing the notion of quantification. A special overview is dedicated to the radiofrequency coils used for the excitation and reception of MRI signals in Chapter 2. In Chapter 3, the main acceleration techniques for fast imaging are described along with citations of the most recent methods. Chapter 4 covers the basics of diffusion MRI. Chapters 5–8 are dedicated to a group of MRI techniques for probing or characterizing tissues and organs in vivo. These include functional imaging (Chapter 5), vascular imaging (Chapter 6), quantitative elastography imaging (Chapter 7), magnetization transfer and ultra-short echo-time imaging (Chapter 8), in vivo nuclear magnetic resonance (NMR) spectroscopy and chemical exchange saturation transfer (CEST) imaging (Chapter 9). Chapter 10 presents some novel methods which provide multiple parameters using a single sequence by combining fast acquisition techniques and advanced data processing. Finally, the last two chapters cover a broader overview by describing the state-of-the-art techniques and challenges in interventional MRI in Chapter 11 and ultra-high-field MRI in Chapter 12.

All the co-authors are members of the French Society for Magnetic Resonance in Biology and Medicine (Société française de résonance magnétique en biologie et médecine – SFRMBM) and this work represents an educational contribution of this community stemming from and disseminating for scientific research.

1

MRI Principles, Hardware Components and Quantification

Hervé SAINT-JALMES[1], Hélène RATINEY[2] and Olivier BEUF[2]

[1] LTSI, Inserm, Université de Rennes, France

[2] CREATIS, CNRS, Inserm, INSA Lyon, Université Claude Bernard Lyon 1, France

1.1. Introduction

The demonstration of the nuclear magnetic resonance (NMR) phenomenon in condensed matter in 1946 (Bloch 1946; Purcell et al. 1946) certainly stems from significant progress accrued during the previous decade and in particular during the war with the development of radars and radiofrequency technology. Today, a similar consideration can be made for magnetic resonance imaging (MRI), where technological progress contributes significantly to the improvement of measurement instrumentation and therefore to the quality of signal and images produced by these devices. Such progress paves the way for imaging techniques that are not exclusively qualitative but also quantitative.

This introductory chapter concisely describes MRI principles and the main components of an MRI scanner, in particular those responsible for the generation of magnetic fields and signal acquisition.

Schematically, several steps are required to obtain a localized spectrum or an image (see Figure 1.1):

For a color version of all the figures in this chapter, see www.iste.co.uk/ratiney-beuf/challenges.zip.

The Challenges of MRI,
coordinated by Hélène RATINEY and Olivier BEUF.

1) the system of spins in a sample must reach thermal equilibrium, which leads to a macroscopic magnetization M_0 being produced in the presence of a static polarization field B_0;

2) the equilibrium of the macroscopic magnetization is perturbed by tilting the M_0 vector away from its equilibrium position by means of a radiofrequency magnetic field B_1;

3) spatial encoding is performed using magnetic field gradients;

4) the system's response following the perturbation is observed by gathering the MR signal by means of a radiofrequency coil;

5) the spectrum or image is reconstructed and quantitative parameters are extracted.

In the following, we will focus on recalling the physical principles of MRI along with the associated technological solutions and their implementation (Saint-Jalmes 2022) up to a general overview of quantitative MRI approaches that are amply presented in this book.

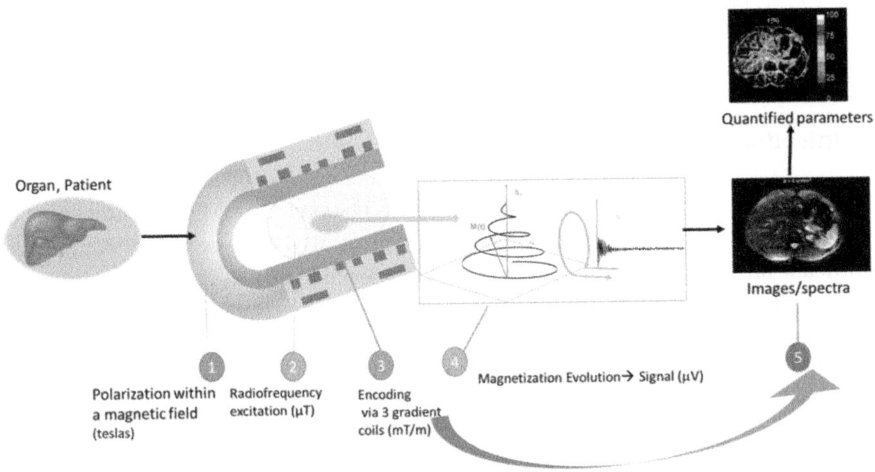

Figure 1.1. *Sequence of four key steps of an MRI scan of an organ, with a fifth step of image/spectrum reconstruction and extraction of quantified parameters*

In NMR and MRI, the denomination of magnetic field ***B*** is commonly used. From a physical point of view, ***B*** is a fundamental quantity, similar to the electric field ***E*** in electrostatics (Gié et al. 1976). In the past, the mathematical analogy between vectors ***E*** and ***H*** led to ***H*** being called the magnetic field, with ***B*** being then referred to as magnetic induction. The latter term will not be used in this work, although it is still widely used.

1.2. Macroscopic magnetization and static magnetic field B_0

1.2.1. *Nuclear magnetization*

NMR makes use of the magnetic properties of nuclei having a non-zero spin $\hbar \boldsymbol{I}$. Among nuclei with such a feature, the most commonly studied are the hydrogen nucleus (^1H or proton), phosphorus-31 (^{31}P), sodium-23 (^{23}Na), fluorine-19 (^{19}F) and carbon-13 (^{13}C) (see Chapter 9). In a nucleus with a spin number I (integer or half-integer), the magnetic nuclear moment $\boldsymbol{\mu}$ is aligned with the spin moment, such that $\boldsymbol{\mu} = \gamma\hbar\boldsymbol{I}$, where γ, called the gyromagnetic ratio, is a characteristic constant of the nucleus of interest and $\hbar$ is the reduced Planck's constant $h/2\pi$ with $h = 6.62 \times 10^{-34}$ J.s.

Whenever a sample with a large number N of identical nuclei having spin number I is subjected to a magnetic field $\boldsymbol{B_0}$, it possesses a resulting magnetization vector $\boldsymbol{M_0}$ according to the Boltzmann equation:

$$\boldsymbol{M_0} = \frac{N\gamma^2\hbar^2 I(I+1)}{3k_B T}\boldsymbol{B_0} \quad [1.1]$$

where k_B is the Boltzmann constant (k_B = 1.38 × 10^{-23} $J.K^{-1}$) and T the absolute temperature. At thermal equilibrium, the macroscopic magnetization $\boldsymbol{M_0}$ has only one longitudinal component oriented along $\boldsymbol{B_0}$, which can be expressed as $\boldsymbol{M_0} = \chi_0 \boldsymbol{B_0}$, where χ_0 is the nuclear magnetic susceptibility. This nuclear magnetization, the evolution of which is inversely proportional to temperature T, is extremely small (typically of 4.8 pA/m for 1 mm^3 of water at 1.5 T and T = 300 K) (Abragam 1961).

1.2.2. *Magnet*

An MRI system is similar to a chain: the weakest component determines the final performance of the entire system. In this regard, a significant role is played by the magnet as its choice and features directly influence image quality together with the purchase and operations costs of an MRI device.

1.2.3. *Roles and orders of magnitude*

The static magnetic field is employed both for polarizing the sample and imposing the frequency of excitation and signal acquisition. These two aspects determine the specifications and constraints of the magnet. In the remainder of this chapter, we shall limit ourselves to the description of devices for clinical imaging; nevertheless, most of the arguments are largely transposable to preclinical imaging (i.e. imaging used in animal model studies).

1.2.3.1. *Field strength*

Performing medical MRI scans at fields lower than a tenth of a tesla seems difficult since the field should be sufficiently high in order to produce an image with an acceptable spatial resolution within a reasonable acquisition time. Indeed, the lower the field, the lower the signal is, and therefore the signal-to-noise ratio (S/N) is low.

By increasing the field strength, S/N is increased and therefore the spatial resolution and/or the scan time is reduced (a trade-off between the two always exists). However, the higher the field, the more challenges arise related to the propagation of radiofrequency waves and safety aspects (see Chapter 12). Furthermore, the cost of a magnet and that of the entire MRI scanner increase significantly with field strength. Thus, magnets with fields higher than 3 T are seldom encountered in clinical routine, with ultra-high-field magnets nowadays typically built to satisfy research needs. Finally, regulations (2013/35/UE) describe the minimal safety indications for the staff exposed to magnetic fields.

1.2.3.2. *Volume of interest, spatial uniformity and temporal stability*

The strong magnetic field (between a few tenths of a tesla and a few teslas) has to be induced over a volume of interest (e.g. tens of liters in clinical imaging) while allowing the scanned body to access the center of the magnetic field region.

In order to produce a spatially well-resolved image or a fine spectrum, the magnet's B_0 field must be as uniform (or homogeneous) as possible over the volume of interest. For whole-body imaging, uniformity of the order of a part per million over volumes of several tens of liters is sought. As an example, in a field of 1.5 T, 1 ppm corresponds to a tiny field variation of 1.5 μT. At the same time, extremely high stability of the field, of the order of 0.1 ppm, is expected over the duration of an exam (between 30 min and 1 h).

1.2.4. *Technical approaches*

To create such a magnetic field, several approaches are available. One of these consists of using the magnetic energy stored in a permanently magnetized material, a magnet. Magnetic fields of the order of tenths of a tesla can be created using ferrites or NdFeB. The shape of the magnet and/or polar ferromagnetic parts can channel the magnetic flux for a uniform distribution inside the region of interest. The undeniable advantage of this approach is the absence of energy sources. On the other hand, the magnet's mass is considerable (e.g. about ten tons for a field of 0.3 T). In addition, the field intensity in such magnets varies noticeably with temperature (typically 0.1 %/°C). The race toward higher fields has certainly made this approach marginal, although it offers several advantages.

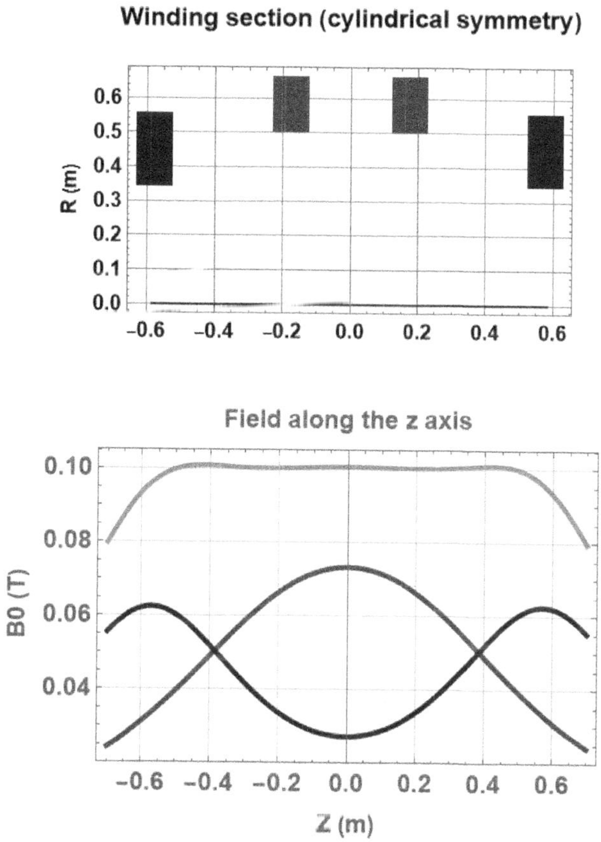

Figure 1.2. *Magnet with two pairs of coils (axisymmetric around the z-axis) and representation of the magnetic fields created along the symmetry axis of the magnet. The two red coils create a strong field at the center of the magnet, together with a significant second-order component (red curve). When the blue pair of coils are added, despite being less efficient, they produce a negative second-order component (blue curve) which can compensate for the imperfection and provide a uniform field (green curve)*

The most widely employed approach consists of a constant direct current flowing in a conducting or superconducting material. The superconducting approach is unavoidable for creating strong fields used for clinical imaging.

The design of the first MRI magnets was based on the pioneering work by Garrett in the 1950s. Garrett was the first person to solve the magnet design problem (Garrett 1951) by expressing the field distribution in the form of zonal harmonics. For this series, the goal consists of canceling as many components as possible up to the 12th, 16th or even 20th order via compensations between different coils, such that only the constant component B_0 remains dominant. This principle is illustrated in Figure 1.2.

1.2.4.1. *Physical size (imaging volume, length, diameter)*

The scanned volume with a uniform field has to be sufficiently large to accommodate the body part to be scanned. In practice, the magnet volume has to be larger than that, since patient access must be possible in a magnet for medical imaging. Patient comfort is an additional challenge. A typical imaging volume in clinical systems is a sphere or an ellipsoid of about 45–55 cm in diameter. The minimum length of the magnet is constrained by the field homogeneity requirement. However, from a patient's point of view, a shorter magnet is better, since the claustrophobic feeling during an imaging scan can be consequently reduced. Typically, the magnets employed in clinical systems have a minimum total length (i.e. including the cryostat) between 150 cm for a 1.5 T field and about 300 cm for 7 T. At the same time, the diameter of the magnet has to be as large as possible for patient access. On the other hand, for a given performance, the cost of the magnet and its footprint increase very rapidly with its diameter.

1.2.4.2. *Installation site requirements*

Among other constraints, the magnet has to meet its siting requirements, taking into consideration aspects such as the footprint, mass and shielding. One of the main concerns is the magnet's fringe field: although the magnetic field targets the center of the magnet (e.g. for a value of 1.5 T), it extends beyond the magnet's boundaries, which may cause problems in a hospital environment. For security reasons, the location of the 0.5 mT or 5-gauss (1 T = 10,000 G) line is considered. This field limit was defined in the early days of MRI to guarantee the safe operation of cardiac stimulators. Any access to the area where B_0 is higher than 0.5 mT must be controlled and notified by panels, such as ones that read "Caution – strong magnetic field". Thus, there is a need to shield the magnet to restrict this "0.5 mT area" as much as possible. This is an important aspect in practice because the hospital obviously seeks to use the smallest rooms possible. The fringe field in a non-shielded 1.5 T magnet extends in three spatial directions up to about ±10 m along the field direction and ±7 m in the other directions; this means that a 300 m^2 room is required to site the magnet, which is not very realistic. Therefore, some kind of shielding is inevitably necessary. The shielding can be passive or active.

The first possible idea for shielding for fringe field suppression is to add iron beams. However, the magnet mass increases significantly and an accurate calculation of the magnetic field becomes very challenging due to the strongly nonlinear behavior of the materials.

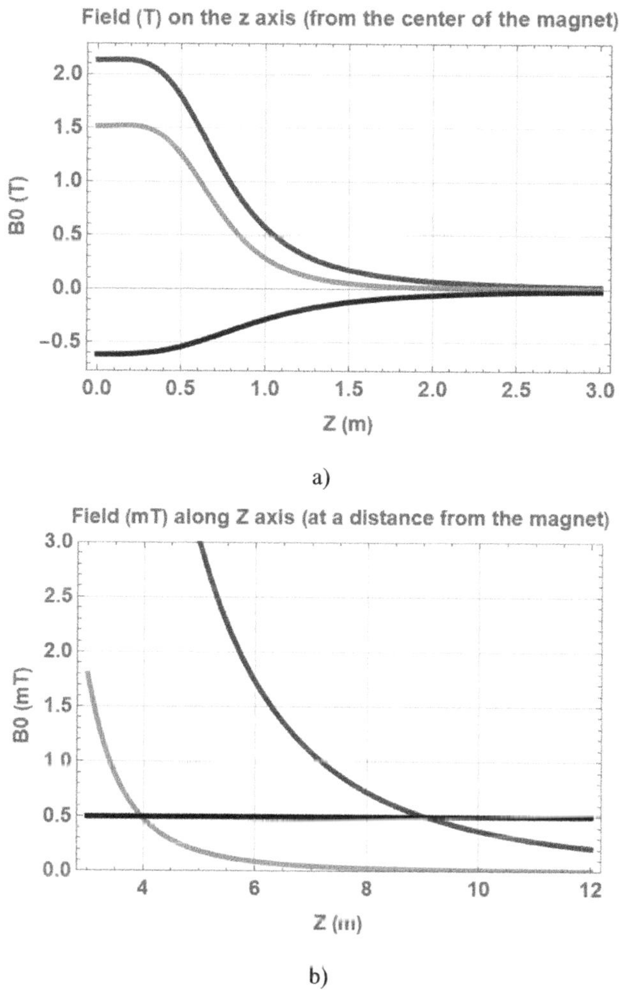

Figure 1.3. *The field produced by the coils is the strongest at the center of the magnet (red curve a), but it is also strong outside the magnet (red curve b)*

COMMENT ON FIGURE 1.3.– *The 0.5 mT line (straight black curve, b) is located at 9 m from the center of the magnet. If coils with opposite currents are added, the field strength at the center is reduced (blue curve, a), but the resulting field (green curve, b) makes the 0.5 mT line located 4 m from the magnet center. For that, in this example, a 2 T field and an opposing 0.5 T field have to be produced to obtain a 1.5 T field at the magnet center.*

Active shielding was introduced at the end of the 1980s. In this approach, shielding coils with a diameter larger than the main magnet carry a current with the opposite orientation with respect to the main magnet coils' current. The effect of such a configuration on the fringe field is shown in Figure 1.3. In this way, the field produced outside the magnet (fringe field) is significantly reduced. This approach increases the magnet cost not only because of a larger number of coils but also because the field produced by the main magnet coils is reduced at the center of the scanner by the shielding coils. Consequently, the number of turns of the main magnet coils has to be increased to compensate for the significant decrease in field strength at the magnet center. The magnet complexity increases and the design process becomes longer since minimizing the 0.5 mT area introduces an additional constraint to the optimization process. Nevertheless, active shielding also has great advantages, being a solution that is lightweight and not dependent on the environment of the magnet.

1.2.4.3. *Costs*

The fabrication and operation costs of a magnet are high. These costs are related to the magnetic energy E_s stored in the magnet. In general, for resistive and superconducting magnets, $E_s \sim B_0^2 V$, where V is the accessible patient volume. Therefore, increasing the field B_0 or increasing the volume corresponds to increasing the magnetic energy, and thus an increase in costs, even though the latter consequence is indirect. For example, by increasing the field from 0.3 T to 1.5 T, the required energy is multiplied by 25 and reaches several MJ in a 1.5 T magnet for clinical imaging use.

1.2.4.4. *Typical superconducting magnet for MRI*

A typical magnet for a clinical MRI scanner creates a magnetic field of 1.5 T or 3 T. For such field values, the only possible technology today consists of superconductors. Once a wire made of NbTi is immersed in liquid helium at 4.2 K, this wire does not oppose any resistance to current flow, at least if critical current density and maximum field values along the wire are not reached. Hence, the entire coil has to be drowned in liquid helium, which requires a volume of the order of a thousand liters. Additionally, due to the temperature gradient between the helium and the magnet's outside, rather elaborate cryostats have to be used to limit helium leakage as much as possible. Currently, a cryo-cooling system employing a cold head can avoid wasting helium, which is a non-renewable and expensive element; however, the operation of such systems requires electrical power. In the vast majority of MRI scanners, the magnet has a cylindrical shape, which is motivated by the constraints described earlier: homogeneity over the volume of interest, patient access to the region with a homogeneous field and costs minimization. Patient access is achieved via a tunnel of 60 or 70 cm in diameter. Today, the typical length of the magnet is between 150 cm and 200 cm for these field strengths (1.5 T and 3.0 T). This leads to coils built following a cylindrical shape of about 1 m in diameter. In a superconducting magnet, the magnetic field inside the coil wires has to be evaluated, as well as the magnetic forces between them. The main constraints are thus an acceptable current density within the wire and reasonable geometrical size and position of the coils inside the magnet. All the primary coils are located on the same support; otherwise, the cryogenic system becomes too large to be practical and/or the supporting mechanical structure becomes too complex. For this reason, the radii of the various coils should not differ too much (a few percent). An integer number of turns is defined for each coil, enabling all the magnet coils to be connected in series. The magnet includes a dozen coils, plus active shielding. A typical example of such a structure providing a homogeneity of 1 ppm over a spherical volume of 50 cm in diameter is given in Figure 1.4.

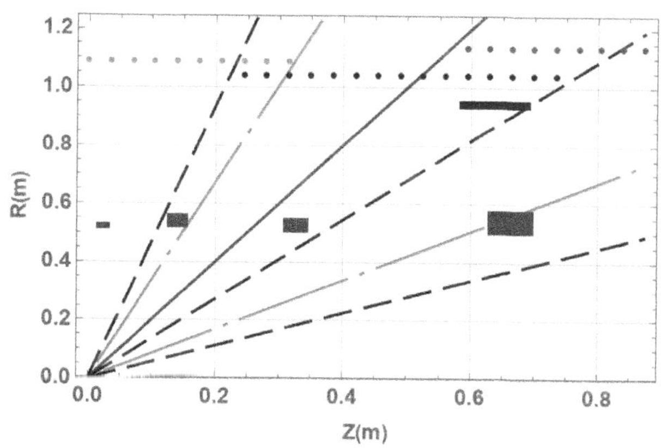

Figure 1.4. *Example of a magnet structure for clinical MRI with a field of 1.5 T*

COMMENT ON FIGURE 1.4.– *The figure employs a quadrant representation: the magnet is symmetrical with respect to the vertical axis, and the cylindrical coils with axial symmetry around the Z-axis are represented by their red and blue sections. The magnet is composed of four coil pairs (red sections) wired on a cylinder and one pair of coils (blue sections with an opposing field, see Figure 1.3) that significantly reduces the extension of the 0.5 mT line. Magnet optimization is performed globally and we can observe that the reduced coordinate of the coils (Z/R) reduces the z harmonics of the field. The zeros of the latter are represented in red for the second order, in green for the fourth order and in blue for the sixth order.*

Once an appropriate architecture is defined, the other elements required for the magnetic system design have to be considered for the construction of the magnet. In a superconducting magnet, once the magnetic forces acting between the different magnet coils have been evaluated during the mechanical drawing phase, the mechanical tools and the support structure must be designed so that they minimize the coil movements during the magnet's cooling down and later when the magnet's field is ramped up. For instance, a magnet designed for a 1 ppm homogeneity can present a variation of the magnetic field of the order of hundreds of ppm once built. The best achievable values one can hope to get after assembly are of the order of 300–400 ppm. This variation can be partially compensated by using dedicated coils (*shim coils*) inserted into the magnet or via calibrated ferromagnetic parts placed with great precision around the internal surface of the magnet. However, compensating for a variation greater than ~2,000 ppm is impossible. Therefore, it is worth taking into account the influence of these variations during the design of a magnet such that, once built, it will be relatively close to the desired performance and sufficiently adjustable.

1.2.4.5. *Compensation or "shim" coils*

Once the magnet is ramped to the target field, the adjustments described above are usually insufficient for reaching a target homogeneity. Approximatley 10 supplementary compensation coils are added for that purpose. The main role of these coils conveying low currents (of the order of a few amperes) is dynamic field correction, an approach that is particularly useful for localized spectroscopy studies (Juchem and De Graaf 2017).

1.2.5. *Novel technologies*

Many new directions are being explored in addition to the development of ultra-high-field magnets. One of these consists of the development of magnets that employ no or very little helium. Indeed, this gas is non-renewable and its cost has increased significantly over the last decades. MRI is actually one of the main consumers of this resource. Permanent magnets are interesting in this sense for creating fields of a few tenths of tesla (see section 1.2.4) and, additionally, they do not require electrical power. For superconducting approaches, the implementation of NbTi coils cooling via conduction from a cold source in a cryocooler is reaching the market after many technological challenges (vibration minimization, helium-storing thermal buffers with a volume of tens of liters, etc.) have been solved, at least partially. These approaches are more feasible at low to medium fields (≤1.5 T) and many manufacturers offer these kinds of systems with magnetic fields between 0.55 and 1.5 T. Compared with NbTi, cooling is significantly simpler for superconducting materials with a high critical temperature (39 K for MgB_2, over 90 K for mixed oxides of barium, copper and rare-earth elements). However, several limiting aspects remain: above all, the material cost, but also the manufacturing cost of long-length wires required in MRI and the production of controlled systems for transitioning between the superconducting and the conducting states (Parizh et al. 2017). In recent years, such magnets based on MgB_2 or mixed oxides of barium, copper and rare-earth elements have been appearing on the market. Of course, all things being equal, using lower fields considerably simplifies manufacturing and reduces the cost of the magnet. Several researchers have seemingly rediscovered a medical and economic interest in magnetic fields of a few tenths of tesla (Campbell-Washburn et al. 2019). The decrease in S/N in such scanners is compensated by, without any particular order, a decrease in power deposited in the patient and acoustic noise, a very notable reduction of image artifacts, such as those of susceptibility, a larger inner diameter of the scanner (Marques et al. 2019), interventional imaging possibilities, etc.

1.3. Description of the magnetization evolution

In general, understanding NMR phenomena requires quantum physics formulations, but most of these phenomena can still be explained using classical descriptions. In particular, the Bloch model describes the classical fundamentals of most MRI scans.

The evolution of the nuclear magnetization $\boldsymbol{M}$ in the presence of a magnetic field $\boldsymbol{B}$ is described by the phenomenological Bloch equations:

$$\frac{d\mathbf{M}}{dt} = \gamma\mathbf{M} \wedge \mathbf{B} - \frac{M_x\mathbf{i}+M_y\mathbf{j}}{T_2} + \frac{M_0-M_z}{T_1}\mathbf{k} \quad [1.2]$$

where M_x, M_y, M_z are the components of $\boldsymbol{M}$ in an orthonormal reference frame of unit vectors $\boldsymbol{i}, \boldsymbol{j}, \boldsymbol{k}$. T_1 and T_2 are the two characteristic time constants of the recovery of the magnetization $\boldsymbol{M}$ to its equilibrium position $\boldsymbol{M_0}$ aligned with $\boldsymbol{k}$ and the decay of the magnetization components perpendicular to this direction, respectively.

During excitation, the magnetic field $\boldsymbol{B}$ in equation [1.2] corresponds to the static magnetic field $\boldsymbol{B_0}$ – which is the origin of the macroscopic magnetization as described above – plus a radiofrequency field $\boldsymbol{B_1}$, generally of lower amplitude, which temporarily tilts the magnetization vector. During signal detection, $\boldsymbol{B}$ is composed only of the static field $\boldsymbol{B_0}$. The first term in the Bloch equation describes the rotation of the nuclear magnetization around the magnetic field direction. During excitation, we consider the rotation around the effective field given by B_0 plus B_1 (the latter modulated in amplitude and/or frequency). During signal reception, the macroscopic magnetization motion consists of a precession around $\boldsymbol{B_0}$ with an angular frequency ω, called Larmor frequency, such that $\boldsymbol{\omega_0} = -\gamma\boldsymbol{B_0}$. The other two terms describe the relaxation phenomena with phenomenologically introduced time constants T_1 and T_2. Without going into details about their cause, these terms are related to the interaction of nuclear magnetic moments with their environment and to their individual evolution in the presence of an external perturbation. The evolution of the transverse magnetization component $\boldsymbol{M_{xy}}$ is due to inter-spin dephasing. Its characteristic time T_2 is thus called the transverse or spin–spin relaxation time. The evolution of the longitudinal component $\boldsymbol{M_z}$ is characterized by T_1, the spin-lattice relaxation time. This longitudinal relaxation corresponds to the energy exchange between the spins contributing to the magnetization and the surrounding lattice in order to return to thermal equilibrium. In general, the radiofrequency field B_1 is applied with a short duration with respect to T_1 (of the order of milliseconds) such that the terms with T_1 and T_2 in equation [1.2] are neglected during excitation. During signal reception, equation [1.2] can be solved to obtain the formulas of the evolution of magnetization components over time:

$$M_{xy}(t) = M_{xy}(0)e^{-t/T_2} \quad [1.3]$$

$$M_z(t) = M_z(0)e^{-t/T_1} + M_0\left(1 - e^{-t/T_1}\right) \quad [1.4]$$

where $M_{xy}(0)$ and $M_z(0)$ are the transverse and longitudinal magnetization component values at the initial time, while M_0 is the magnetization value at thermodynamic equilibrium.

1.4. Excitation: perturbing the magnetization

1.4.1. *Principle*

The spins system is perturbed by applying a rotating field B_1 perpendicularly to B_0. This radiofrequency field with an angular frequency ω is generated by an alternating current circulating within a coil. If the magnetic field B_1 oscillates at the Larmor angular frequency ($\omega_0 = \gamma B_0$), the magnetization is tilted from its equilibrium position and starts precessing around B_1 at the angular frequency $\omega_1 = \gamma B_1$, with such a motion being superposed to the precession around B_0. This synchronization between the characteristic frequency of the spins system and the RF pulse frequency is denoted by the term "resonance" and corresponds to a perturbation of nuclear magnetization. For an RF pulse with a constant amplitude B_1 and duration τ, the tilting or "flip" angle α (in radians) is $\alpha = \gamma B_1 \tau$.

The magnetization tilting RF pulse gives rise to a transverse component of the magnetization vector, as the latter starts rotating at the angular frequency ω_0 around B_0 and induces a measurable electromotive force (emf) in a coil. The decay of the transverse magnetization to equilibrium is observed as a free induction decay signal (FID). In sections 1.5 and 1.7, we shall see how the magnetization relaxation to equilibrium can be modulated to obtain information on spatial localization or tissue composition.

1.4.2. *Transmit coil*

The B_1 field is created via a current oscillating at the Larmor frequency in a coil. This magnetic field pulse, with a duration of the order of milliseconds, has a very low amplitude of only a few μT. In clinical imaging, this field is produced by a large transmit coil (about 70 cm in diameter and 50 cm in length). Although the field amplitude is low, the same cannot be said about the required power and typically radiofrequency amplifiers of several tens of kW power this coil (see Chapter 2). The power deposited inside the patient by this radiofrequency emission is non-negligible and it grows rapidly with frequency and hence with B_0 field strength (see Chapter 2). To limit the dissipated power, quadrature excitation is favored. Moreover, at high frequencies (e.g. >100 MHz for a whole body) and thus at high fields, the electrical properties of biologic tissue (permittivity and resistivity) cause significant inhomogeneity of the excitation performed by a single coil. To tackle this problem, a set of transmit coils with signals of different amplitude and phase are implemented (see Chapter 12), similar to the coil arrays used for several years to improve the reception of the NMR signal.

1.4.3. *Radiofrequency signal reception*

Once the B_1 field has tipped the magnetization to the transverse plane, the magnetization's relaxation to equilibrium via a rotating motion at the Larmor frequency produces a magnetic flux variation, which can be measured by a radiofrequency detector. In its simplest version, this can be done once again via a coil, which is placed perpendicularly to the direction of the B_0 field. The flux variation generates an alternating voltage in the coil, which is then amplified and demodulated (see Chapter 2). The induced voltage is particularly low, typically of the order of μV, hence the need for amplifying and maximizing the signal with respect to undesired noise in the reception signal chain.

Signal reception can be performed with the same coil that is used for transmission. However, the requirements for these two steps are different. Often, a separate coil with an important feature of high uniformity of the RF field B_1 is used for transmission, and a second coil or probe for the reception, where the main requirement is a high sensitivity and high S/N (see Chapter 2). For a surface coil, these properties increase with decreasing diameter of the coil. A significant improvement in image quality, without reducing the imaging field of view, has been enabled by the introduction of phased arrays (Rœmer et al. 1990), where multiple surface coils collaborate to measure the signal simultaneously.

Various acquisition strategies dedicated to the simultaneous scanning of small animals have been developed starting from this approach (Beuf et al. 2006). While the first coils were designed on rigid support structures and were dedicated to limited anatomical regions, the need for patient comfort and continuity among anatomical regions (e.g. head-neck-spine, thorax-abdomen) spurred the manufacturers to develop flexible and lightweight coils, which can be placed on the patient and around different anatomical regions. The latest evolution in this sense is represented by blanket-like coils called AIR (*adaptive imaging receive*). Today's development efforts are oriented toward coils with flexible conductors (McGee et al. 2018) or with extensible ones (Port et al. 2020), which can be worn close to the body like garments, or even coils based on micro-electro-mechanical systems (MEMS) capable of modifying the loops' geometry or changing the frequency to acquire the signal at different frequencies sequentially (Raki et al. 2020). Doing away with the cable connecting the coils to the receiving system is another development path explored in recent years, which however still encounters challenges due to constraints of power supply and noise level which affect the images (Byron et al. 2017). Intermediate approaches based on optical transmission have been developed to get rid of safety concerns (Memis et al. 2008; Saniour et al. 2017). In preclinical settings, coils cooled down to very low temperatures (*Cryocoils*) using helium gas (of the order of 30–35 K) and dedicated to small-animal imaging have provided significant gains in S/N, on average of the order of 3 for magnetic fields between 4.7 T and 11.7 T (Darasse and Ginefri 2003).

1.5. Spatial localization in MRI

1.5.1. *Principle*

We will now tackle the principles of encoding an NMR image performed using gradients of magnetic fields in a rather succinct way. An understanding of these notions is required for the following chapters.

MRI consists of measuring an NMR signal coming from "volume elements" (voxels) in a sample. An image is obtained by discriminating between the signals coming from different voxels. To spatially differentiate these signals, linear variations of the magnetic field, called gradients, are superposed to the static field B_0 along the three spatial directions (Lauterbur 1973). The magnetization's resonance frequency will thus be related to its location. For each point (x, y, z), the magnetic field is given by $B(x,y,z) = B_0 + G_x x + G_y y + G_z z$ (B_0 is oriented along O_z by convention) and is characterized by an angular frequency $\omega(x,y,z) = \omega_0 + \gamma$ $(G_x x + G_y y + G_z z)$. Since it is impossible to localize the signal in several directions simultaneously, the Fourier transform imaging method (Kumar 1975) consists of applying gradients in three steps: a selective excitation of a slice (or a volume), a phase encoding and a frequency encoding in the selected plane.

1.5.1.1. *Selective slice excitation*

For two-dimensional scans, a slice of the sample volume has to be acquired. The slice selection is performed by applying a frequency-selective excitation in the presence of a gradient field perpendicular to the desired slice. By performing the excitation via an RF pulse with limited spectral bandwidth (BW_{RF} in Figure 1.5), only the magnetizations whose frequency is within such bandwidth are excited. The position of the slice plane is determined by the excitation frequency ($\nu = \omega / 2\pi$). The thickness of the slice depends on the applied slice gradient value for a given pulse shape and duration. The most commonly used pulse shapes are the sinc and Gaussian shapes.

Typically, once the slice selection has been performed, a "refocusing" gradient has to be applied because the magnetizations inside the slice have been dephased (e.g. in the case of a sinc or Gaussian pulse). Afterward, the encoding of the imaging plane is performed by applying a phase gradient and a readout gradient, which are necessary for phase encoding and frequency encoding, respectively.

1.5.1.2. *Phase encoding*

The phase gradient is applied with a fixed duration τ and its amplitude is incremented at each new RF pulse. Supposing that the gradient is applied along the direction O_x, the magnetization dephasing θ at the coordinate x is given by $\theta = \gamma G_x x \tau$.

1.5.1.3. *Frequency encoding*

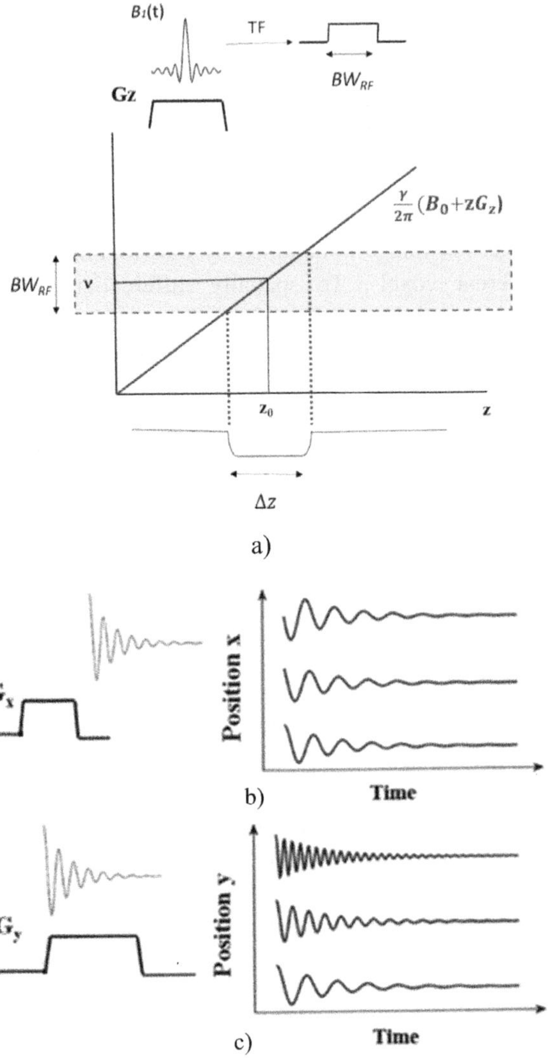

Figure 1.5. *Principles of spatial encoding in MRI: (a) selection of a slice with a thickness Δz and bandwidth BW_{RF} of the pulse (here, a sinc); (b) phase encoding; (c) frequency encoding*

The readout gradient with constant amplitude is applied for the entire duration of signal acquisition. If the gradient is applied in the direction O_y with an amplitude G_y, the angular frequency of the magnetization's precession at a coordinate y is given by $\omega = \gamma G_y y$.

1.5.1.4. *Image and Fourier space*

In an imaging scan based on bi-dimensional Fourier transform (2DFT), the signal acquired at a time t is proportional to

$$S(G_x,t) = \iint_{xy} \rho(x,y,p_{x,y}) e^{j\gamma G_x x\tau} e^{j\gamma G_y yt} dxdy$$

where $\rho(x,y,p_{x,y})$ is the spatial distribution of the image contrast and is related to the proton density in the excited slice. ρ depends on the spatially varying parameters $p_{x,y}$ that are related to phenomena such as diffusion and perfusion and to relaxation times, which will provide a signal weighting according to the timing of the pulse sequence.

By defining the variables $k_x = \gamma G_x \tau$ and $k_y = \gamma G_y t$, the signal can be expressed as:

$$S(k_x,k_y) = \iint_{xy} \rho(x,y,p_{x,y}) e^{jk_x x} e^{jk_y y} dxdy \qquad [1.5]$$

This is a formula of a 2D Fourier transform with respect to x and y variables. The inverse Fourier transform with respect to k_x and k_y variables represents the image of the spatial distribution of the protons in the selected plane. The space of k_x and k_y variables is called the reciprocal or Fourier space and it represents the spatial frequencies of the image. In an imaging scan, k_x and k_y coordinates do not depend on the considered source point (sample), therefore the representation in the reciprocal space (the space where data acquisition is performed) is quite suitable for describing the signal sampling for most imaging sequences.

The k_x and k_y variables are the reciprocal of x and y variables, respectively, and the Fourier transform properties define the relations between the respective spaces. The field of view (FOV) of an image along the O_x axis is given by $\mathrm{FOV}_x = \dfrac{2\pi}{\delta k_x}$, where δk_x is the separation between two consecutive values of the k_x variable. The pixel width is given by $\Delta x = \dfrac{2\pi}{\Delta k_x}$, where Δk_x is the separation between the maximum and minimum acquired spatial frequencies. Analogous relationships can be derived for O_y and O_z axes.

The description presented here corresponds to acquiring the Fourier/reciprocal space (commonly called k-space) in a Cartesian way. Other trajectories are possible, the most common among which cover the k-space along radial or spiral trajectories (see Chapter 3).

1.5.2. *Magnetic field gradients*

In order to perform the spatial encoding of information, additional magnetic fields have to be superposed to the main static magnetic field. These auxiliary magnetic fields, oriented along the axis of the main magnetic field, vary linearly with position along the three Cartesian axes. The methods for designing gradient coils are similar to those for the main magnet, although the constraints are different. Linearity performance (correspondence between spatial coordinate and additional field) should be high, but not necessarily better than 1%. In addition, fast imaging methods require a very quick variation of strong magnetic field gradients. Therefore, the goal is to maximize the gradient produced by a unit of injected current *Ga* while minimizing the coil inductance *L*. An example of a longitudinal gradient coil is given in Figure 1.6. The set of three coils constitutes the gradients insert.

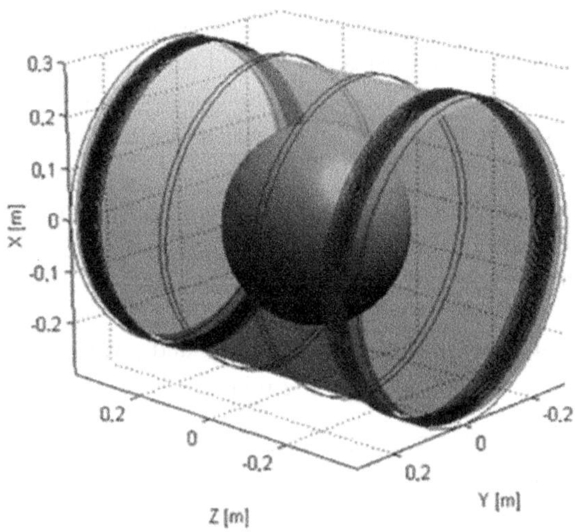

Figure 1.6. *The gradient coil dB_0/dz is located on a cylindrical surface. The turn distribution creates a very linear gradient while minimizing the power required for its control*

The amplifiers for these three gradient coils must be very powerful (several tens of kVA) to meet today's requirements of producing gradient amplitudes of several tens of mT/m (between 20 and 80 mT/m) with ramp times (for rise or descent) of hundreds of μs, which means slew rates of amplitude divided by ramp time of the order of 200 T/m/s. Besides these technological limitations, one must consider physiological limits as well: too fast gradient variations may cause peripheral neurostimulations and muscular fibrillations. Finally, the rapid switching of high currents in these coils inside the static magnetic field produces Laplace forces. Such forces lead to coil vibrations that generate acoustic noise, whose level increases with magnetic field strength.

1.5.2.1. *Eddy currents and their mitigation*

An additional constraint has to be considered in particular for integrating gradient coils with magnetic fields varying outside the gradient insert. The currents induced by these fields in the adjacent conducting structures due to gradient switching will produce additional undesired fields, whose spatial and temporal variations will perturb image encoding. Similar to active shielding for superconducting magnets, coils with an opposite current flow are then added to the gradient insert. The optimization of the entire coil set is performed by adding a minimization criterion for the fringe field created in the adjacent conducting structures. For a given amplitude and switching time, the required power is increased by more than 50%. Moreover, the remaining eddy current effects are minimized via a technique of *preemphasis* of the currents injected into the gradient coils. It should be noted that the latter kind of compensation is global and does not take into account the spatial dependence of the fields due to eddy currents.

1.6. Signal-to-noise ratio notion in MRI

The quality of an MRI is partially determined by *S/N*. Without considering a specific imaging technique, *S/N* of an MR at a given field B_0 can be expressed as:

$$S/B \propto {D_{acq}}^{1/2} \cdot (T_r/T_R)^{1/2} \cdot \Delta V \cdot S(\text{Tissue, Method}) \qquad [1.6]$$

where D_{acq} is the total image acquisition duration, ΔV is the elementary volume (voxel), T_r is the signal readout time, T_R is the sequence repetition time, and S (Tissue, Method) is a function that depends on tissue characteristics (proton density, T_1, T_2, etc.) and on the employed imaging sequence (flip angle, delays between pulses, etc.).

For example, in the case of imaging with a Cartesian Fourier-encoded space and frequency encoding in one of the directions and phase encoding in the others (in a 2D or 3D case), $D_{acq} = N_p \cdot NA \cdot T_R$, where N_p is the total number of phase-encoding steps and NA is the number of accumulations. Signal readout time is defined as $T_r = N \cdot t_e$ with N the number of points along the readout direction and t_e the sampling period. Spectral bandwidth per pixel (Hz/Px) is then $\delta f = 1/T_r$. The S/N for an image with "phase-frequency" encoding can then be expressed as:

$$S/B \propto \delta f^{-1/2} \cdot (NA \cdot N_p)^{1/2} \cdot \Delta V \cdot S(\text{Tissue, Method}) \qquad [1.7]$$

Reducing the voxel size by two in all of the three spatial directions will lead to a decrease in S/N by a factor of 8. This reduction can be compensated by increasing the number of accumulations NA at the price of a 64-fold longer scan time, which is quite significant and rarely feasible.

1.7. Useful signal and information

1.7.1. *A "complex" signal in a mathematical and bio-physical sense*

The NMR signal measured by a magnetic flux detector is obtained after the steps of amplification, demodulation, sampling and digitization via analog or digital converters. The magnetization rotation will correspond to an oscillating signal characterized by amplitude, frequencies and phases in the form of complex values. In MRI, the main oscillating component is the one related to water, but as soon as other molecules are considered (e.g. for differentiating water and fat, and for spectroscopy in general), a combination of oscillating components must be taken into account.

Thus, the complex signal acquired in the transverse plane, without any gradient encoding, and after demodulation is directly related to magnetization:

$$S(t) \propto M_x(t) + iM_y(t) = M_+(0)\exp(i\phi)\exp(i\gamma\Delta Bt)\exp(-\frac{t}{T_2^*}) \qquad [1.8]$$

The decay of this signal is characterized by the apparent relaxation time T_2*. The irreversible part of this decay has a characteristic time constant T_2, called transverse or spin-spin relaxation time. The other contribution to T_2* is related to the inhomogeneities of the magnetic field B_0. The signal is complex with one term varying with phase ϕ and one varying with angular frequency $\gamma\Delta B$, both of which express the magnetization's phase differences with respect to a vector rotating at a resonant frequency ν_0.

The most commonly displayed type of image is a magnitude image, which shows a contrast between tissues that is mainly due to their intrinsic properties, such as proton density, T_1 and T_2 or T_2* relaxation times, or diffusion. In a phase image, the useful information depends on:

– the position of the radiofrequency coil with respect to the signal source;

– the difference in local resonance frequencies due to variations of magnetic susceptibility in tissues or blood oxygenation rate;

– the time evolution of the phase of the magnetization vector and the phase difference between different isochromats[1]. Indeed, the resonant frequency does not only depend on the applied B_0 field, but also on the electronic environment of a given nucleus (the chemical shift notion, see Chapter 9).

Although harder to analyze, phase images contain valuable information for many applications. Some examples include field mapping for the geometric correction of echoplanar images or for the compensation of magnetic field inhomogeneities (*shim*), thermometry, blood flow measurement, image weighting, elastography, differentiation and mapping of water and fat.

1.7.2. *From qualitative to quantitative*

The MR signal provides us with an anatomical image, obtained by means of magnetic field gradients, similar to a "photograph" of the inside of a human body. However, it should be remembered that an MRI system is first of all an instrument for measuring a signal, which combines several types of information on the tissues, cells and molecules where the magnetic moments producing the signal are located.

Being a physical measurement, signal modeling can be used in MRI to provide quantitative parameters representing a physical, physiological or biological phenomenon. A property is called quantitative when its estimated values belong to a graduated scale and can be used for rigorous comparisons.

1.7.2.1. *MRI richness*

The goal of MR signal quantification is to extract quantitative information from the acquired signal regarding a tissue property. This approach is not biased by a

1 Isochromat: a set of spins resonating at the same frequency.

measurement system's transfer function (gain, spatial inhomogeneity in reception, etc.), which makes it possible to establish reference values (characterizing a healthy subject or a given pathology), to facilitate multicenter studies, or simply to objectively compare two scans. Thus, MRI quantification applications include conventional diagnostic imaging, functional imaging and interventional imaging. MRI's power consists of providing parameters on morphology, structure, biomechanics, hemodynamics and biochemistry at the same time. For such purposes, several types of MR sequences can be used and acquisitions can focus on a single localized voxel or a group of voxels.

Type of information	Parametric property/effects	Chapters
Perfusion	Blood flow and volume, etc./relaxivity, susceptibility	4, 6
Diffusion	ADC (apparent diffusion coefficient), pseudo perfusion	4, 5, 12
Connectivity	Connectivity indexes, functional networks, white matter bundles	5
Fat/iron	Fat fraction, T_1, T_2, T_2*	10
Metabolism	CEST contrast, metabolites/electrolytes concentration, pH	9, 12
Temperature	T_1, T_2, M_0, ν_0	11
Magnetic property	Magnetic susceptibility χ	10
Biomechanics	Shear modulus, viscosity	7
Semi-solid composition	Magnetization transfer, T_{1D}	8

Table 1.1. *Overview of the variety of acquisitions and parameters available in MRI that will be described in detail in this book*

Since its early days, MRI has involved quantitative and parametric approaches (Orthendahl et al. 1984). Mapping of relaxation times or diffusion parameters has been proposed along with anatomical images "weighted" by the T_1, T_2 relaxation and diffusion. Usually, this requires varying some acquisition parameters (flip angle, delays, gradient amplitudes, etc.) sequentially, which leads to longer acquisition times. Therefore, whenever parameters have to be obtained, it will be necessary to use faster acquisitions and make compromises (see Chapters 3 and 10). By developing knowledge on what affects the information gathered via the MR signal in biological tissue and on the technical aspects acting on the macroscopic magnetization (magnet, gradient, radiofrequency fields), a large number of MRI sequences have been developed to obtain different parameters of interest for the analysis of healthy and pathological living tissue or to perform interventional imaging. Table 1.1 lists most of them and where they will be tackled in the following chapters of this book.

1.7.2.2. *Challenges*

For any quantitative MRI measurement, the goal is to objectively compare the conditions of a subject during a longitudinal follow-up of a patients/subjects population. Clearly, these parameters will be relevant only if they can be linked to a biological effect. The quest for objectivity and specificity is carried out not without difficulty and is always a relevant topic of research and development.

Below are the main challenges regarding quantitative MRI techniques:

– Obtaining useful information as quickly as possible, without artifacts and with an optimized S/N per unit of time. Moreover, a single parameter is often insufficient to describe a physiological or pathological tissue state. Therefore, the maximum amount of useful and complementary information per unit of time is sought.

– Taking into account all confounding factors which can bias the measurement or the parameters of interest.

– Establishing the conditions for a reliable, robust and as precise a parametric estimation as possible. To address these challenges, deep knowledge of the signal acquisition and processing chain used in MRI is necessary and requires expertise in several domains.

1.8. Conclusion

The techniques based on the magnetic resonance phenomenon used to probe, characterize and scan a body non-invasively appeared during the 1970s. In other words, the concepts, methods and technologies related to today's MRI have reached a clear maturity resulting from several innovations and know-how accumulated over many years. The generation of researchers that bore witness to the birth of MRI and the Internet is now passing the baton to the next generation. The techniques have diversified and the applications too. Upcoming is a new era for the development of these techniques, which will have to address the expectations and challenges of research and clinical routine settings without disposing of "fundamental" and methodological research, and will have to include – in a controlled way – the so-called "computational" research. Indeed, the advances in applied mathematics and computer science together with the growth of computing power will certainly have a great impact on future innovations. Nonetheless, by briefly providing the MRI basics, this chapter has presented the hardware components without which no measurement would be possible. Indeed, progress regarding the instrumentation has been the most significant contributor to the remarkable improvement in image quality, while the development of NMR methods has highlighted the richness of NMR signal information, as presented in the following chapters of this book.

1.9. Acknowledgments

The authors warmly thank Christophe Barles, Fraser Robb, Florence Delmas and Tim Wokrina for sharing non-confidential technical data.

1.10. References

Abragam, A. (1961). *The Principles of Nuclear Magnetism*. Oxford University Press, Oxford.

Beuf, O., Jaillon, F., Saint-Jalmes, H. (2006). Small animal MRI: Signal to noise ratio comparison at 7T and 1.5T with multiple-animal acquisition strategies. *Magn. Reson. Mater. Phy.*, 19(4), 202–208.

Bloch, F. (1946). Nuclear induction. *Physical Review*, 70(7/8), 460.

Byron, K., Robb, F., Stang, P., Vasanawala, S., Pauly, J., Scott, G. (2017). An RF-gated wireless power transfer system for wireless MRI receive arrays. *Concepts Magn. Reson. Part B Magn. Reson. Eng.*, 47(4), 21360.

Campbell-Washburn, A.E., Ramasawmy, R., Restivo, M.C., Bhattacharya, I., Basar, B., Herzka, D.A., Balaban, R.S. (2019). Opportunities in interventional and diagnostic imaging by using high-performance low-field-strength MRI. *Radiology*, 293(2), 384–393.

Darrasse, L. and Ginefri, J.C. (2003). Perspectives with cryogenic RF probes in biomedical MRI. *Biochimie*, 85(9), 915–937.

Garrett, M.W. (1951). Axially symmetric systems for generating and measuring magnetic fields. *Journal of Applied Physics*, 22(9), 1091–1107.

Gié, H. and Sarmant, J.P. (1976). *Électricité : 2e année*. J.B. Baillière, Paris.

Juchem, C. and de Graaf, R.A. (2017). B_0 magnetic field homogeneity and shimming for in vivo magnetic resonance spectroscopy. *Analytical Biochemistry*, 529, 17–29.

Kumar, A. and Welti, D. (1975). RR Ernst NMR Fourier zeugmatography. *J. Magn. Reson.*, 18, 69–83.

Lauterbur, P.C. (1973). Image formation by induced local interactions: Examples employing NMR. *Nature*, 242, 190–191.

Marques, J.P., Simonis, F.F., Webb, A.G. (2019). Low-field MRI: An MR physics perspective. *Journal of Magnetic Resonance Imaging*, 49(6), 1528–1542.

McGee, K.P., Stormont, R.S., Lindsay, S.A., Taracila, V., Savitskij, D., Robb, F., Witte, R.J., Kaufmann, T.J., Huston, J., Riederer, S.J. et al. (2018). Characterization and evaluation of a flexible MRI receive coil array for radiation therapy MR treatment planning using highly decoupled RF circuits. *Phys. Med. Biol.*, 63.

Memis, O.G., Eryaman, Y., Ayturn, O., Atalar, E. (2008). Miniaturized fiber-optic transmission system for MRI signals. *Magn. Reson. Med.*, 59(1), 165–173.

Ortendahl, D.A., Hylton, N., Kaufman, L., Watts, J.C., Crooks, L.E., Mills, C.M., Stark, D.D. (1984). Analytical tools for magnetic resonance imaging. *Radiology*, 153(2), 479–488.

Parizh, M., Lvovsky, Y., Sumption, M. (2016). Conductors for commercial MRI magnets beyond NbTi: Requirements and challenges. *Superconductor Science and Technology*, 30(1), 014007.

Port, A., Luechinger, R., Albisetti, L., Varga, M., Marjanovic, J., Reber, J., Brunner, D.O., Pruessmann, K.P. (2020). Detector clothes for MRI: A wearable array receiver based on liquid metal in elastic tubes. *Scientific Reports*, 10, 8844.

Purcell, E.M., Torrey, H.C., Pound, R.V. (1946). Resonance absorption by nuclear magnetic moments in a solid. *Phys. Rev.*, 69, 37–38.

Raki, H., Tse Ve Koon, K., Souchay, H., Lambert, S., Robb, F., Beuf, O. (2020). Serial and parallel active decoupling characterization using RF MEMS switches for receiver endoluminal coils at 1.5 T. *IEEE Sensors Journal*, 20(18), 10511–10520.

Rœmer, P.B., Edelstein, W.A., Hayes, C.E., Souza, S.P., Mueller, O.M. (1990). The NMR phased array. *Magn. Reson. Med.*, 16, 192–225.

Saint-Jalmes, H. (2022). Instrumentation en imaging par résonance magnétique. Critères de choix et implantation d'un équipement. *EMC – Radiologie et imagerie médicale – Principes et techniques – Radioprotection*, 35(209), 1–20.

Saniour, I., Ayde, R., Perrier, A.L., Gaborit, G., Duvillaret, L., Sablong, R., Beuf, O. (2017). Active optical-based detuning circuit for receiver endoluminal coil. *Biomed. Phys. Eng. Express*, 3(2).

2

Radiofrequency Coils: Theoretical Principles and Practical Guidelines

Aimé LABBÉ and Marie POIRIER-QUINOT

BIOMAPS, CNRS, Inserm, CEA, Université Paris-Saclay, France

A radiofrequency (RF) antenna is most fundamentally a resonant circuit designed to transmit and sense energy in the form of electromagnetic radiation. Nevertheless, in practice, the term "antenna" includes devices with completely opposite design goals. Under the same label, we can find radio broadcasting towers, which are rectilinear structures up to hundreds of meters tall, sensitive to the electric component of the electromagnetic fields and designed to emit energy in all directions to cover as wide an area as possible. On the other hand, the same term can be associated with MRI coils, which can have a loop shape of a few centimeters in diameter, are sensitive to the magnetic field component and aimed at concentrating the wave energy in a small volume and minimizing the radiated power far from the device.

In addition to these functional differences, an RF coil can also be considered from several different points of view. For an MRI researcher, an RF coil is, above all, a tool for inducing (transmitting) and then collecting (receiving) a magnetic resonance signal that is required to obtain an MR image, without regard for the detailed functioning of the detector (Figure 2.1(a)). For an electronic engineer, an RF coil is an electric circuit composed of various electronic components: conducting wires, capacitors, diodes, etc., whose behavior is described by electrical circuit theory (Figure 2.1(b)). According to Maxwell's equations, an antenna is a source of a magnetic RF field

The Challenges of MRI,
coordinated by Hélène RATINEY and Olivier BEUF.

with a desired spatial distribution that is determined by the detector's construction and properties (Figure 2.1(c)).

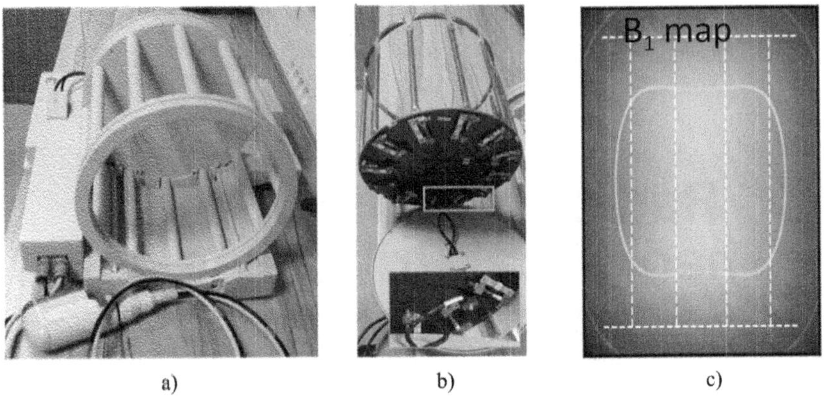

Figure 2.1. *Example of a "birdcage" RF coil. For color version of this figure, see www.iste.co.uk/ratiney-beuf/challenges.zip*

COMMENT ON FIGURE 2.1.– *The coil structure is visible in (a) with (b) conducting wires and various electronic components, which can be modeled as an equivalent electrical circuit and generate (c) a magnetic RF field* B_1.

In this chapter, the MRI antenna, which will be interchangeably referred to as sensor, detector and coil, will be presented to an audience of researchers from the point of view of an electronic engineer. Therefore, the chapter's goal is to provide a general understanding of the fundamental concepts regarding RF coils. After recalling some fundamental notions of resonant circuits implemented in MRI, we will consider the RF coil as a generator of an RF magnetic field B_1. Afterward, we will see how an RF coil is used in transmission first and in reception later, together with the main considerations involved in the design and characterization of coils for these two operation modes. In addition, we will tackle the decoupling challenges and safety issues regarding RF coils used in MRI. Finally, more advanced topics and recent developments of RF coils for some applications, in particular for high and low magnetic fields, will be presented.

2.1. Coil as an electrical resonant circuit

2.1.1. *Basic concepts*

An RF coil can be modeled as a closed circuit composed of impedances with a reactive part made up of an inductance L_c in henry (H) and a capacitance C_c in farad (F) and a resistive component R_{eq} in ohm (Ω) related to the losses in the circuit, in particular due to the coil resistance R_c and the sample load R_s, as schematically represented in Figure 2.2. In this circuit, energy is alternately stored as electric energy in the capacitance and as magnetic energy in the inductance. The energy emitted by the RF coil originates from the coil's inductance, whose value is determined by the geometry of the coil's conducting wire. If assembled correctly, such a circuit can generate or detect an RF magnetic field B_1 oscillating at a characteristic frequency ω_0, which is defined as:

$$\omega_0^2 = \frac{1}{L_a C_a} \qquad [2.1]$$

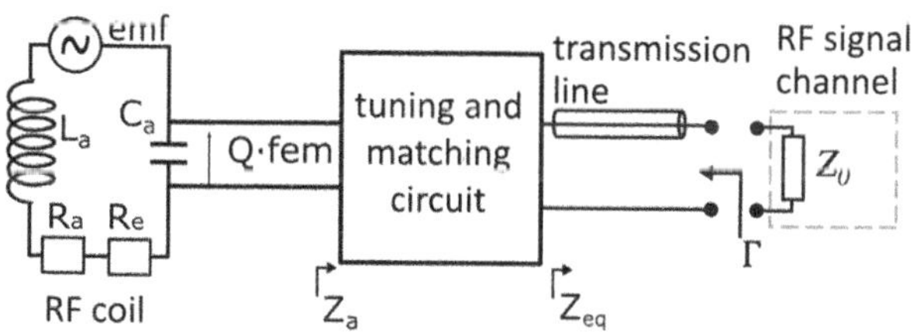

Figure 2.2. *Equivalent circuit of an RF coil*

COMMENT ON FIGURE 2.2.– *The equivalent model of an RF coil in which the NMR signal induces an emf voltage is represented on the left of the reflection coefficient Γ; L_c, C_c and R_c are the main components of the coil, while R_s is the load resistance of the sample. $Q \cdot fem$ is the voltage across the capacitance, with Q being the quality factor. The RF coil presents an impedance Z_c in input to the variable circuit used for frequency tuning and impedance matching to the RF signal channel with impedance Z_0. Z_{eq} is the impedance of the RF coil seen from the output of the matching circuit.*

For an efficient coil, the angular frequency ω_0 must be equal to the Larmor frequency:

$$\omega_0 = \gamma B_0 \qquad [2.2]$$

where we recall that B_0 is the static magnetic field strength and γ is the gyromagnetic ratio, a coefficient that depends on the considered nucleus. For most clinical studies focusing on MRI of protons ^1H, this frequency corresponds to a resonant frequency $\nu_0 = \omega_0/2\pi$ of 64 MHz at 1.5 T and 128 MHz at 3 T, which are both in the range of RF waves (between a few kHz and a few GHz).

Besides its resonant frequency, the coil is also characterized by its spectral bandwidth $\Delta\omega$, that is, the range of frequencies in which the coil can efficiently transmit or receive an RF signal[1], which defines the quality factor Q of the coil:

$$Q = \frac{\omega_0}{\Delta\omega} = \frac{\omega_0 L}{R} \qquad [2.3]$$

From theory, the quality factor can be interpreted as the ratio between the energy stored for each cycle in the resonator ($\propto \omega_0 L$) and the power dissipated by its resistance ($\propto R$). In practice, when an NMR signal induces a voltage emf in volts (V) in the coil, the voltage across the capacitance C_c will be $Q \cdot$ emf (see Figure 2.2).

2.1.2. *Coil tuning and matching*

Since the coil is part of the RF signal channel of an MRI system, in addition to frequency tuning, it is also often necessary to perform the coil's impedance matching[2]. The goal of this step is to optimize the power transmission between a source and a load. When an MRI coil is used in transmission, the matching condition ensures that the amplitude of the B_1 field produced by the coil is maximized; in reception, impedance matching optimizes the power transmission of the NMR signal[3]. Since the impedance is intrinsically complex, a coil is said to be matched when its impedance Z_c is transformed into an equivalent impedance Z_{eq} thanks to a transformation circuit, which we call the tuning and matching circuit (see Figure 2.2). Additionally, $Z_{eq} = Z_0^*$, where Z_0^* is the complex conjugate of the characteristic impedance of the RF signal channel in the MRI system. Most often, Z_0 is purely resistive, for example, $Z_0 = R_0 = 50\ \Omega$.

In practice, frequency tuning and impedance matching are generally linked and both are done via a matching circuit. The design of such a circuit can be more or less complex (Mispelter et al. 2015), but in general it involves (1) discrete reactive (capacitive and sometimes inductive) components of fixed value, carefully chosen after analyzing the coil's electrical circuit (they provide an approximate starting coil

1 The coil's bandwidth $\Delta\omega$ should not be confused with the signal bandwidth in transmission and reception. In most cases, $\Delta\omega$ is much larger than these signal bandwidths.

2 Sometimes called power matching in literature.

3 Ideally, one would seek maximum voltage transmission by connecting the coil directly to a high-impedance input of a preamplifier. In a classical configuration, the coil is located far from the preamplifier and the two are connected via a coaxial cable with a characteristic impedance $Z_0 = 50\ \Omega$. To avoid signal reflection phenomena, the input of the preamplifier and the coil must be matched to Z_0.

matching), as well as (2) variable components allowing for fine tuning and matching adjustments.

Often, coil matching operations and characterization measurements are performed by means of a vector network analyzer. This instrument measures the frequency dependence of the coil's reflection coefficient Γ:

$$\Gamma(\omega) = \rho(\omega)e^{i\phi(\omega)} \quad [2.4]$$

where ρ and ϕ are the norm and phase of the reflection coefficient, respectively. To obtain this parameter, once the analyzer is connected to the coil via a port with a characteristic impedance Z_0, the instrument sends an incident RF voltage V_{inc} toward the coil and measures the reflected wave V_{ref} at the same port. The ratio of these two quantities defines the reflection coefficient Γ, which is also called S_{11} in literature. Supposing that $Z_0 = R_0$ is real, it is possible to express a relation between Γ and the equivalent impedance Z_{eq} of the coil and its matching circuit:

$$\Gamma(\omega) = \frac{V_{ref}(\omega)}{V_{inc}(\omega)} = \frac{Z_{eq}(\omega) - R_0}{Z_{eq}(\omega) + R_0} \quad [2.5]$$

Typically, for a tuned and matched coil, the reflection coefficient Γ exhibits the shapes shown in Figure 2.3. Close to the resonant frequency, that is, when $|\omega - \omega_0| \leq \Delta\omega$, $Z_{eq} \approx R_0$ and the reflection coefficient tends to zero, which corresponds to the incident wave being entirely transmitted. On the other hand, for $|\omega - \omega_0| \gg \Delta\omega$, Z_{eq} is completely unmatched and the incident wave will be entirely reflected with $\rho = 1$ (or 0 dB in Figure 2.3(a)) and a phase opposition $\phi = \pm\pi$. The coil tuning and matching operations consist of adjusting the variable parameters of the tuning and matching circuit such that the modulus ρ is minimized and its phase ϕ is canceled out at $\omega = \omega_0$, which is equivalent to canceling out the reactive part of Z_{eq} (i.e. Z_{eq} becomes purely real) and achieving $Z_{eq} = R_0$.

From the modulus $\rho(\omega)$, it is possible to measure the coil's bandwidth $\Delta\omega$ and to calculate from its value the quality factor Q. Under the hypothesis of a tuned and matched coil, the bandwidth corresponds to the width at half-peak of the resonant response $\rho(\omega)$. If $\rho(\omega)$ is displayed in dB (which is generally the case), then $\Delta\omega$ corresponds to the width at –3 dB with respect to the baseline of $\rho(\omega)$, as shown in Figure 2.3(a). The use of a network analyzer is rather common for characterizing these electrical properties. The precision of this method mostly depends on the instrument's quality, in particular on its calibration, and care taken in choosing its settings for each measurement.

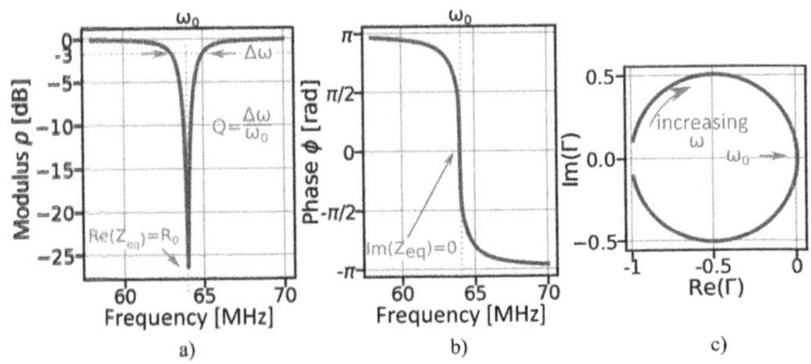

Figure 2.3. *Frequency dependence of the (a) modulus ρ and (b) phase ϕ of the reflection coefficient $\Gamma = \rho \exp(i\phi)$. c) Real and imaginary components of Γ for different frequencies*

From the point of view of signal reception, the issue of tuning and matching is more critical than for transmission.

Indeed, in receive operation, the weak free induction signal of the coil has to reach the input of a low-noise preamplifier in an optimal way. As an example of the orders of magnitude, in the case of a 40 mm^3 volume of water at 1 T, the amplitude of the electromotive force induced in a five-turn solenoid coil, 4 mm in diameter and 1 mm long, is of the order of 100 μV.

2.2. Coil as a source of a magnetic RF field

In the context of an MRI scan, the RF coil is coupled to the patient via its magnetic field. Therefore, understanding the properties of the B_1 field is fundamental for choosing a coil for a desired application. Let us remind you that a magnetic field is a vector field with an amplitude and orientation that potentially vary in space and over time. The behavior of electromagnetic fields is fully described by Maxwell equations. In practice, some parameters have a greater effect than others on the properties of this field.

The first and foremost influencing aspect is the geometry of the coil used to generate the magnetic field $\mathbf{B}_1$ because this field is produced by the circulation of an electrical current with an intensity I in amperes (A) within the conducting wire of the coil. In MRI, a few common geometry shapes are encountered, some examples of which are presented in Figure 2.4. Usually, they are classified into two categories: (1) volume coils and (2) surface coils, depending on whether the coil is positioned around or on the patient, respectively. The choice of the type of coil is restricted by the geometrical constraints of an MR scan and by the orientation of the RF field B_1

generated by the coil, which has to remain perpendicular to B_0 in order to be useful. In addition, Figure 2.4 compares the transverse component of the magnetic field $B_{1,xy}$ per unit current I produced by a volume coil and a surface coil. Volume coils mostly create homogeneous magnetic fields, which is not the case with surface coils. On the other hand, a surface coil provides a higher amplitude of the magnetic field, as shown in Figure 2.4. To give an estimation, for a given current, a surface coil of 23 mm produces magnetic fields a hundred times stronger than a volume coil of 600 mm in diameter.

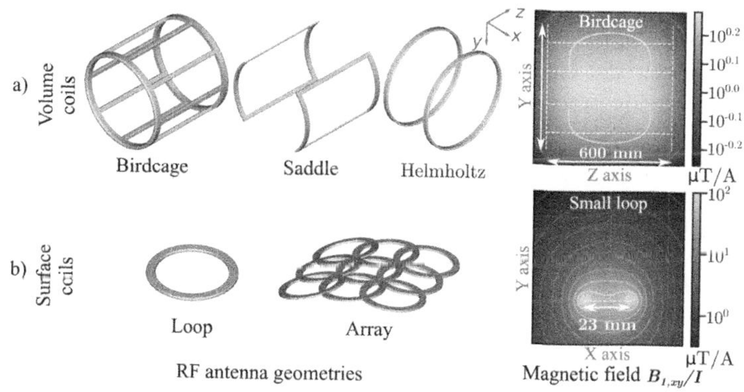

Figure 2.4. *Volume and surface coils. For a color version of this figure, see www.iste.co.uk/ratiney-beuf/challenges.zip*

COMMENT ON FIGURE 2.4.– *(a) Main RF coil geometries used in MRI. Here, the B_0 field is oriented along the z-axis and the B_1 field is produced along the x-axis for the volume coils and along the y-axis for the surface coils. (b) Comparison of the transverse components $B_{1,xy}/I$ of the magnetic field created by a volume coil and a surface coil. The variation between two isolines corresponds to dividing the amplitude of $B_{1,xy}/I$ by a factor of two. The white dashed lines indicate the projection of the coil's geometry on the field map.*

A second important aspect is the *wavelength* λ in meters (m) of the magnetic signal produced or received by the coil:

$$\lambda = \frac{c}{\nu} \tag{2.6}$$

where $\nu = \omega/(2\pi)$ is the frequency in hertz (Hz) and $c = (\mu\epsilon)^{-1/2}$ is the wave propagation speed in a medium, which depends on the medium's magnetic permeability μ and electric permittivity ϵ. Table 2.1 provides values of wavelengths for a few important media in MRI at 1.5 T and 3 T. The wavelength affects the propagation of a signal by modifying its phase in space and potentially distorting the magnetic field. In the coil's conducting metal, propagation effects modify the current distribution in the wires. In tissues, where the wavelength is typically 10 times shorter than in air, this can lead to interference phenomena that can locally increase the magnetic field amplitude, as shown in Figure 2.5, and represent a potential safety risk by increasing the local specific absorption rate (SAR). The challenges of safety related to RF coils will be described in more detail in section 2.6. These effects become critical whenever the dimensions of the cables and imaging volume are not negligible with respect to the wavelength, which is the case of high frequencies, that is, at high static magnetic field B_0. In practice, propagation effects can be ignored when the characteristic lengths of a system are shorter than $\lambda/10$. Approaches for reducing or removing propagation effects will be presented in section 2.6.2.

Frequency (B_0)	Air	Coaxial cable	Brain
64 MHz (1.5 T)	4.7 m	3.1 m	0.50 m
128 MHz (3 T)	2.3 m	1.5 m	0.25 m

Table 2.1. *Wavelength λ in different propagation media*

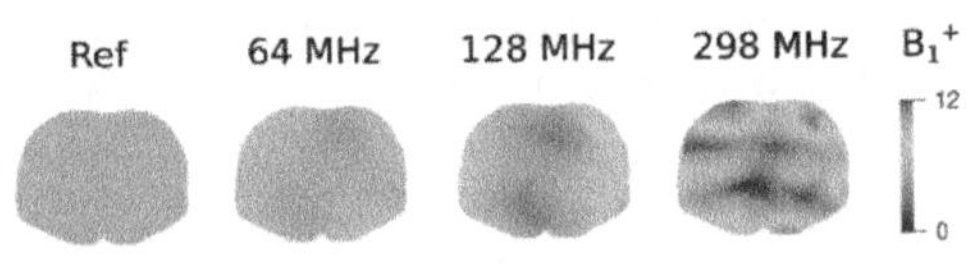

Figure 2.5. *Maps of local variations of the magnetic field B_1 in a human abdomen at three different operating frequencies. A reference with a homogeneous magnetic field is provided. Figure inspired by the works of Cloos et al. 2016, under the license CC BY 4.0. For a color version of this figure, see www.iste.co.uk/ratiney-beuf/challenges.zip*

Finally, the tissue electric conductivity σ_e in siemens per meter ($S{\cdot}m^{-1}$) can also modify the magnetic field. As a response to an incident alternating magnetic field, eddy currents are created in conductive tissues. In turn, these currents induce a magnetic field that opposes the incident magnetic field. As a result, the magnetic field cannot efficiently penetrate into the tissues and remains confined to the surface with a characteristic depth δ, called the skin depth. While these effects are not critical at intermediate magnetic fields, they can become problematic at higher fields. For example, considering the electric properties of muscle at 1.5 T (intermediate field) and at 11.7 T (ultra-high field) (Gabriel et al. 1996), the skin depth of the RF wave changes from 20 to 7 cm at the respective fields. Skin depth will be discussed in more detail in section 2.4.1.

2.2.1. *Polarization and B_1^+ and B_1^- fields*

The concept of polarization is employed to describe the temporal evolution of the amplitude and orientation of the magnetic field $\mathbf{B}_1$ produced by the coil. Two limit cases can be considered: the linear and circular polarizations, as depicted in Table 2.2. In the case of linear polarization, the wave vector is periodic in time, while its orientation is constant (up to a sign). On the other hand, circularly polarized waves have a constant modulus while their orientation rotates in a plane. In between these two cases are the "elliptical" polarizations.

<table>
<tr><th>Type of description</th><th>Linear polarization</th><th>Circular polarization</th></tr>
<tr><td>Schematic representation
$\mathrm{B}_1(t) = B_x(t)\mathrm{x} + B_y(t)\mathrm{y}$</td><td>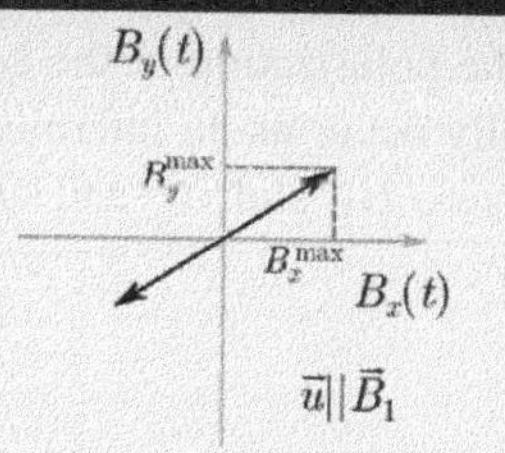

$B_1^2 = (B_x^{max})^2 + (B_y^{max})^2$</td><td>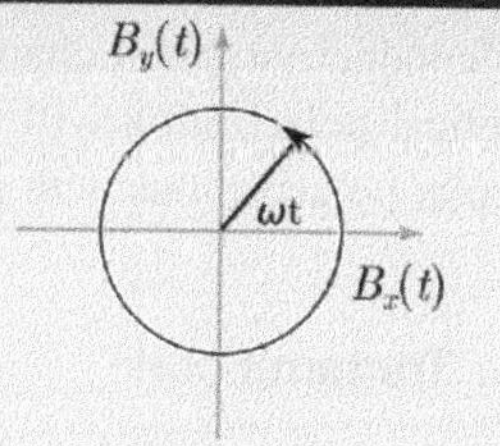

$B_1^2 = B_x^2 + B_y^2$</td></tr>
<tr><td>Decomposition into linear polarizations</td><td>$(B_x^{max}\mathbf{x} + B_y^{max}\mathbf{y})\cos(\omega t) = [B_1 \cos(\omega t)]\,\mathbf{u}$</td><td>$B_1 \cos(\omega t)\mathbf{x} + B_1 \sin(\omega t)\mathbf{y}$</td></tr>
<tr><td>Decomposition into circular polarizations</td><td>$B_1^+ e^{i\omega t} + B_1^- e^{-i\omega t}$
with $B_1^+ = B_1^- = B_1/2$</td><td>$B_1^+ e^{i\omega t}$
with $B_1^+ = B_1$ ($B_1^- = 0$)</td></tr>
</table>

Table 2.2. *Description of linear and circular polarizations*

Another useful representation considers the polarization of $\mathbf{B}_1$ with its components B_1^+ and B_1^-, which are two circularly polarized waves rotating in opposite directions with angular frequencies $+\omega$ and $-\omega$ (Hoult 2000). In practice, the importance of this distinction lies in the fact that the B_1^+ component of the transmit coil is the only one actually contributing to the flipping of the magnetization during transmission. On the other hand, the B_1^- component contributes to the undesired increase in power deposited in the tissues, and thus to the increase in the SAR. In the case of a linearly polarized coil, half of the RF power is lost via the B_1^- component. Therefore, such a configuration has a relatively low efficiency in MRI. For circularly polarized coils, all the RF power of the coil field is useful and conveyed via the B_1^+ component. In the same way, since the magnetic resonance signal is circularly polarized, half of its power is also lost when it is acquired using linearly polarized coils.

Initially, most MRI coils emit waves with linear polarization. To obtain a circular polarization, one requires a coil or a combination of coils that produces two orthogonal components of the magnetic field (along $\mathbf{x}$ and $\mathbf{y}$) phase-shifted by $\pi/2$, one with respect to the other. The coil is said to be used in quadrature. Circular polarization is typically found in volume coils. In particular, "birdcage" coils are specifically designed for such a purpose. When powered at a single point, a birdcage coil produces a linearly polarized B_1 field, which becomes circularly polarized when two input points are controlled in quadrature.

Finally, anything that is capable of modifying the amplitude and phase of the wave in space, that is, coil geometry, propagation effects, as well as tissue shape and conductivity, will change the polarization of the coil's field. In such conditions, elliptical polarization will usually occur as an intermediate case between linear and circular polarizations with non-zero B_1^+ and B_1^- and such that $B_1^+ \neq B_1^-$.

2.3. Transmit coil

In MRI, the RF coils are recruited for two roles: generating (transmission) and acquiring (reception) the magnetic resonance signal. Using two separate coils for transmission and reception is a very common configuration in clinical imaging. Such an approach offers the possibility of separately designing two optimized circuits that fulfill their respective role.

During transmission, the magnetic field B_1 with a frequency ν_0 created by an RF coil flips the nuclear spins of the scanned subject to the transverse plane. The magnetization flip angle α (in radians) is:

$$\alpha(\mathbf{r}) = \gamma B_1(\mathbf{r})\tau \qquad [2.7]$$

where $\mathbf{r}$ is the spatial position and τ the duration of the RF pulse. The flipped magnetization will then induce a free-precession signal proportional to its transverse component, i.e. $\sin\alpha(\mathbf{r})$.

As a result, the first property of a transmit coil is the homogeneity of the generated magnetic field over a given region of interest (ROI). In this condition, the subtle differences in image contrast will be unambiguously related to tissue type and not to spatial variations of the flip angle $\alpha(\mathbf{r})$. As an example, Figure 2.6 shows two images of a homogeneous 2 mL sample of water obtained with a 16 mm diameter surface coil employed in transmit–receive mode. The structures observed inside the sample in Figure 2.6(b) are B_1 inhomogeneity artifacts, also called B_1 artifacts. However, by selecting more suitable acquisition parameters, such as a smaller flip angle, it is possible to reduce the effect of B_1 inhomogeneities (Figure 2.6(a)).

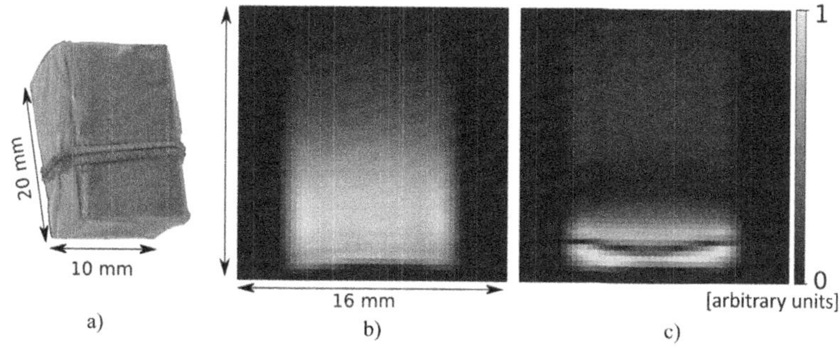

Figure 2.6. *Transverse slice of (a) a homogeneous 2 mL sample of water showing artifacts of B_1 field inhomogeneity, with (b) moderate intensity and (c) high intensity, measured with the same surface coil used in transmit–receive. For a color version of this figure, see www.iste.co.uk/ratiney-beuf/challenges.zip*

A homogeneous RF field is fundamental for a great number of MRI approaches, such as the addition of saturation steps to MRI sequences for suppressing the signal from fat, or in the case of moving organs. A homogeneous B_1 is also preferable for "quantitative" imaging scans providing a map of a physical parameter over a ROI, such as tissue relaxation times T_1 and T_2. Performing an acquisition of B_1 distribution, called "B_1^+-mapping" in literature, can be additionally used to compensate for inhomogeneities.

In practice, most often the transmit coil is implemented in the form of a volume coil (Figure 2.4) connected and properly adapted to the transmit signal channel of the MRI system. To flip the magnetization in a short time ($\tau \sim 1$ ms), the RF coil has to generate a magnetic field of the order of a few 10 μT, which implies currents reaching several tens of amperes for the volume coils used in clinical scanners. For this reason, the transmit signal channel includes a high-power amplifier. The great power required increases with operating frequency ($\propto \nu_0$), that is, with the strength of the static field B_0, with the coil's radius ($\propto r^4$ for a volume coil), and with the amplitude of the RF field ($\propto B_1^2$), which calls for a suitable designing of the amplifier. For example, the power employed in a clinical 1.5 T scanner is of the order of tens of kilowatts.

The use of a surface coil for transmitting is justified in certain applications. When SAR becomes a limiting factor, a transmit surface coil reduces the heating of the ROI. Such an aspect, related to SAR but also to the decreased wavelength as described above, becomes particularly important at ultra-high fields ($B_0 \geq 7$ T). Moreover, specific, more exotic applications employ custom and in-house-made instrumentation, which is the case when the observed nucleus differs from ^1H (multinuclear imaging[4]). In such cases, it may be necessary to design a single coil in order to reduce the costs and development time and thus favor the reception properties of the coil.

2.4. Receive coil

2.4.1. *Sensitivity factor*

The most useful criterion for evaluating the performance of a receive coil is the sensitivity factor S_{RF} (Darrasse and Ginefri 2003):

$$S_{\mathrm{RF}}(\mathbf{r}) = \frac{\omega\left(\frac{B_{1,xy}(\mathbf{r})}{I}\right)}{\sqrt{4k_B\left[R_c(T_c)T_c + R_s(T_s)T_s\right]}} \qquad [2.8]$$

where k_B is Boltzmann's constant and T_c and T_s, in kelvin (K), are the operating temperatures of the coil and sample (or patient), respectively.

The sensitivity factor describes the coil's contribution to the signal-to-noise ratio (SNR) in an MRI scan. The numerator term represents the electromotive force induced in the coil per unit magnetic moment. This is an equivalent description of the Faraday effect using the reciprocity theorem[5] (Hoult and Lauterbur 1979). On the other hand, the denominator corresponds to the noise voltage measured across the detector per unit bandwidth (V·Hz$^{1/2}$). This noise includes two main contributions, both of thermal origin: (1) the electrical noise resulting from the intrinsic coil's resistance R_c and (2) the magnetic noise coming from the sample and modeled in the coil circuit as an impedance of load R_s (see Figure 2.2), with the two contributions weighted by the respective temperatures T_c and T_s. The second noise source is irreducible since it originates from the same region producing the NMR signal. An MRI scan can also be affected by other sources of noise and losses, in particular, the environmental RF noise detected by the coil and the dielectric losses due to electrical coupling between

4 In multinuclear imaging, coils can have two resonances: ν_{1H} for localizing and homogenizing the B_0 field, with the other frequency ν_X tuned for the nucleus of interest X.

5 The reciprocity theorem can be used to invert the roles of source and detector for the calculation of the NMR signal induced in the coil by the precessing magnetic moment. In other words, the calculation of the NMR signal amplitude can be done by considering the magnetic field that would be generated by the coil if a current were to flow in it. This approach usually turns out to be simpler and more fundamental than considering the magnetic field produced by the magnetization of the sample or patient.

the coil and the patient. Nevertheless, the impact of these noise sources can be reduced by using electromagnetic shields (e.g. a Faraday cage) or by carefully designing the detector (e.g. distributing the capacitance) respectively. Therefore, they do not appear in the equation of the coil's sensitivity factor.

To approach the sensitivity factor in a more tangible way and describe its constraints and scaling behavior, let us consider S_{RF} in the case of a loop with radius a made of copper wire with a cylindrical section and a surface πr^2, centered at $\mathbf{r}_0 = (0, 0, 0)$, whose normal vector to the surface is oriented along y, as represented schematically in Figure 2.7. In practice, $a \gg r$ is usually considered.

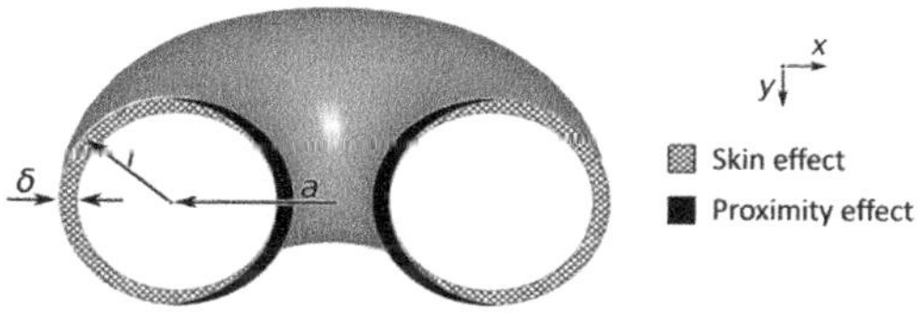

Figure 2.7. *Schematic representation of the skin and proximity effects in a transverse section of a loop coil of radius a made of wire with a cross-section πr^2. Overall, the effective cross-section where the current actually flows is much smaller than the conductor's cross-section*

First of all, the magnetic field per unit current B_1/I generated on the loop's axis along y is described by:

$$\frac{B_1}{I}(y) = \mu_0 \frac{a^2}{(a^2 + y^2)^{3/2}} \propto \frac{1}{a} \qquad [2.9]$$

In the proximity of the loop, the B_1/I ratio decreases following $1/a$ with increasing loop radius.

The loop's resistance R_c is governed by the following equation:

$$R_c(T_c) = \frac{\rho_c(T_c)a}{r} \frac{\xi}{\delta(T_c)} \qquad [2.10]$$

where ρ_c is the conductor's resistivity ($\rho_{\text{Cu}} = 17 \times 10^9$ Ω·m for copper at room temperature), δ is the skin depth and $\xi \geq 1$ is the proximity factor. In practice, resistivity decreases almost linearly with decreasing temperature in metals such as copper. Below a certain temperature, it tends to an asymptotic value defined by the residual resistivity ratio (RRR). This value depends on the quality of the crystal lattice and its imperfections (Matula 1979). Skin and proximity effects are illustrated in Figure 2.7. They occur only at RF regimes. Skin effect refers to the RF current's tendency to flow within a small depth from the surface of the material, with a characteristic depth δ that decreases with increasing frequency:

$$\delta(T_c) = \sqrt{\frac{2}{\rho_c(T_c)\mu\omega}} \qquad [2.11]$$

where μ is the magnetic permeability of the material ($\mu \approx \mu_0$ for copper). Typically, at 64 MHz (1.5 T), $\delta = 8.15\ \mu$m for copper, which considerably reduces the effective section ($2\pi r\delta$) where the current flows with respect to a direct-current regime (πr^2), which noticeably increases the coil's resistance. Furthermore, the proximity effect consists of the current's tendency to flow along a path that minimizes the coil's inductance. This effect depends on the frequency and on the coil's geometric factor a/r. For a loop coil, the consequence of the proximity effect is a concentration of the current on the inner part of the loop, leading once again to higher electrical resistance of the coil. In literature, ξ has been estimated to be between 3 and 6 (Hoult and Lauterbur 1979). For a constant a/r ratio, R_c does not depend on a and:

$$R_c \propto \omega^{1/2} \qquad [2.12]$$

In the following, losses due to the sample are considered. By reciprocity, the load impedance R_e corresponds to the resistance to the eddy current flow inside the sample. These current would be induced by the B_1 field of the receive coil if the latter was used for transmission (Macovski 1996; Suits et al. 1998). For a surface coil:

$$R_s = C\sigma_s \frac{\mu_0^2\omega^2 a^3}{3} \propto \omega^2 a^3 \qquad [2.13]$$

where $C \sim 1$ is the coil's filling factor and σ_s is the electrical conductivity of the sample[6]. Thus, the magnetic sample noise occurs only in conducting samples. In the case of volume coils, the dependence will be $R_s \propto \omega^2 a^4$.

2.4.2. *Noise regimes*

In the following, we will consider the behavior of the RF sensitivity factor S_{RF} as a function of the coil radius a and frequency ν. Two loss regimes can be distinguished,

6 According to theory, conductivity σ and resistivity ρ are related via the equation $\sigma = 1/\rho$.

depending on whether the dominant noise is coming from the coil ($R_c T_c > R_s T_s$) or from the sample ($R_c T_c < R_s T_s$):

$$S_{\mathrm{RF}} \propto \begin{cases} \omega^{3/4} a^{-1} & \text{if} \quad R_c T_c > R_s T_s \\ a^{-5/2} & \text{if} \quad R_c T_c < R_s T_s \end{cases} \qquad [2.14]$$

These equations tell us that (1) frequency does not contribute to the coil's sensitivity when S_{RF} is dominated by sample noise and that (2) reducing the detector size corresponds to increased sensitivity, especially when sample noise dominates.

The noise regimes and function plots are presented in Figure 2.8. In Figure 2.8(a), the transition between two noise regimes is shown for three different media: pure non-conductive water, muscle and salty water (a medium that conducts well). Figure 2.8(b) shows the sensitivity factor S_{RF} in muscle as a function of frequency for two circular surface coils of radius 2.5 cm and 3.25 cm. It highlights the saturation of S_{RF} at high frequencies. The plateau is reached faster for greater coil diameters and its value is higher for smaller coil sizes. For muscle tissue, Figure 2.8(c) also shows S_{RF} as a function of the radius for the frequencies of 15.8 MHz and 64 MHz. It highlights the two loss regimes, one constrained by the coil noise (following a^{-1} for smaller coils), and the one dominated by the sample noise (following $a^{-2.5}$).

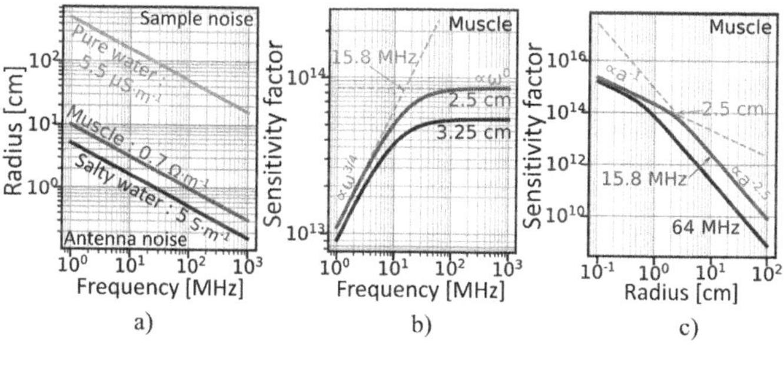

Figure 2.8. *Noise regimes and plots as a function of frequency and coil radius for different media or tissues. For a color version of this figure, see www.iste.co.uk/ratiney-beuf/challenges.zip*

COMMENT ON FIGURE 2.8.– *(a) Transitions between the two noise regimes for three different conducting media. Interpretation: considering a surface coil of radius* a *and resonant frequency* $\nu = \omega/2\pi$ *used for scanning a tissue of conductivity* σ_s *and the corresponding straight line on the plot, whenever* (ν, a) *is below the line, the noise is dominated by the coil (and vice versa, noise is sample-dominated above the line). Sensitivity factor* S_{RF} *(in* $\mathrm{A}^{-1}\mathrm{m}^{-2}\mathrm{s}^{-1/2}$*) and its function plots (b) over frequency (at a constant radius) and (c) over size (at a constant frequency) for muscle imaging.*

For a given application, it is imperative to choose the dimensions of the receive coil such that its field-of-view will correspond to the volume to be scanned. This is the main reason for the multitude of detectors provided with an MRI scanner. Indeed, using a small detector on the body surface for acquiring a shallow-depth and well-localized region is much more convenient than employing a large detector that encompasses the entire body. In general, as a take-home message, a surface coil is more efficient for scanning regions close to the surface at a maximum depth between one radius and one diameter of the loop coil.

To tackle the problem of a reduced field-of-view covered by small-sized coils, it is possible to combine several small independent coils in order to cover a larger field-of-view with the benefit of high sensitivity of each small coil (Roemer et al. 1990): this is called a coil array.

In practice, almost all clinical receive coils are arrays of coils. They can have different geometries, depending on the targeted application, such as cylindrical shape for brain or knee imaging or planar coils for the spine. Currently, commercial coil arrays include up to 74 elements and coil arrays in scientific research reach up to 128 elements (Schmitt et al. 2008). In addition to the sensitivity advantage provided by a coil array, its usage enables accelerated acquisitions based on parallel imaging techniques (Sodickson and Manning 1997; Pruessmann et al. 1999; Griswold et al. 2002).

Finally, when sensitivity is lacking and the ROI is sufficiently small for the noise to be dominated by the receive coil noise, it is still possible to increase the sensitivity factor by decreasing the detector's temperature T_c (equation [2.8]).

This approach decreases the electrical resistivity ρ_c of the conducting material and the coil's thermal noise. Typically, using cryogenic detectors commercialized for preclinical imaging or NMR spectroscopy improves SNR by a factor between 3 and 5. In the case of poorly conducting samples, the usage of superconducting materials instead of copper can improve the detection limit by increasing SNR by a factor of 16 (Labbé et al. 2021).

2.5. Decoupling

The problem of decoupling in MRI arises when two RF coils with the same resonant frequency ν_0 are magnetically coupled, that is, positioned one close to the other, for example, a transmit and a receive coil or two elements in a coil array. A split of the resonant frequency of the coupled coils is observed, and therefore the signal at the initial resonance frequency is rejected, as shown in Figure 2.9. In the case of decoupling between a transmit coil and a receive one, the current induced via mutual inductance becomes amplified due to the resonance effect, which can perturb the homogeneity of the B_1 RF field seen by the sample (as presented in Figure 2.6), constitute a risk for the reception signal channel which is not designed for the high voltages of a transmit pulse[7] and lead, in the worst case, to localized hot spots inside the body, with a consequent safety risk for the patient. To avoid such coupling issues, the various receiving elements must be magnetically isolated from each another. Decoupling can be achieved in several ways.

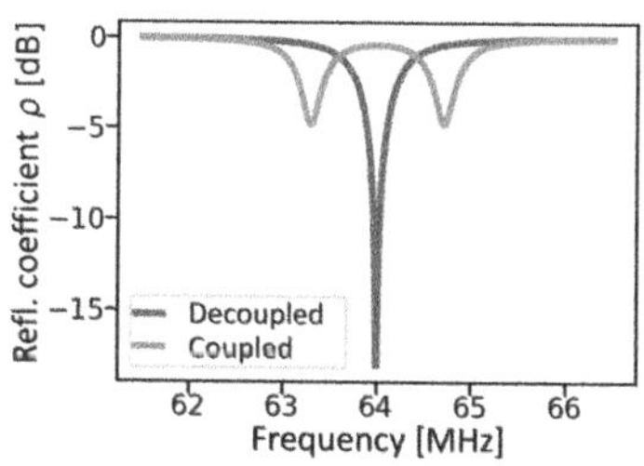

Figure 2.9. *Frequency response of the reflection coefficient modulus ρ for two coupled and uncoupled coils. For a color version of this figure, see www.iste.co.uk/ratiney-beuf/challenges.zip*

To decouple transmit and receive coils, most approaches are based on the use of *positive intrinsic negative* (PIN) diodes. Depending on the voltage across the diode, this device behaves either as an open circuit (zero current), thus disabling the coil, or as a closed circuit that activates the coil at the required moment. The diodes can be powered directly by the current flowing in the coil (passive decoupling) or polarized via an external circuit synchronized with the MRI sequence (active decoupling). Figure 2.10a illustrates an example of an active-decoupling circuit based on a diode. An alternative to this approach consists of replacing the diodes with micro-electromechanical systems (MEMS), which are used to modify the current flow in the coil (Raki et al. 2020).

In the case of coil array elements, the decoupling must allow the different elements to remain simultaneously active. One approach is based on the cancellation of the mutual inductance between two neighboring array elements. Geometric decoupling, shown in Figure 2.10(b), can be obtained by partially overlapping two adjacent elements of the array such that their mutual inductance is canceled out

7 Typically, a difference of about six orders of magnitude is observed for the RF power between a transmit pulse and a received signal, which corresponds to three orders of magnitude of difference between the B_1 field employed during transmission (10 μT) and the one generated by the sample during signal reception ($\sim$ 6 nT at 1.5 T).

(Roemer et al. 1990). Other methods achieve the same result by employing inductors (Adriany et al. 2008), capacitors (Avdievich 2011) or even decoupling annexes or shielding rings shared between array elements (Frass-Kriegl et al. 2016; Hosseinnezhadian et al. 2018).

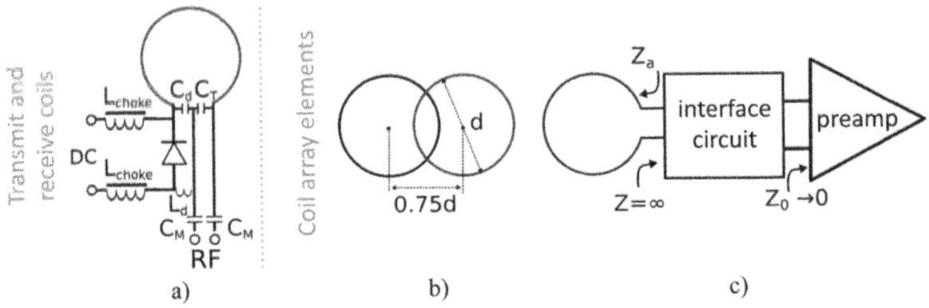

Figure 2.10. *(a) Example of active decoupling implementation based on a diode. (b) Geometric decoupling where the mutual inductance between the two coils is canceled out. (c) Preamplifier decoupling. For a color version of this figure, see www.iste.co.uk/ratiney-beuf/challenges.zip*

However, this approach is physically impossible for more than three or four elements and the coupling between non-adjacent elements has to be removed via complementary methods. For this, another almost systematic approach is to block current flow in the coils by means of an interfacing circuit and a preamplifier with low input impedance (Figure 2.10(c)) (Roemer et al. 1990). The principle of this approach relies on the transformation of the preamplifier's input impedance Z_0 into high impedance performed by the interface circuit. The loop coil behaves in such a case as an open circuit and any magnetic signal (originated from NMR relaxation or neighboring coil coupling) does not induce any current. The electromotive force induced in the coil loop is transformed into a current signal by the interface circuit, which is then acquired by the preamplifier. As an analogy, the array elements are still capable of hearing each other (non-zero induced voltage), but they become muted (zero current). As a result, the array is still sensitive to the MRI signal, however, the cross-talk between the array elements that caused the resonance frequency splitting does not happen any more.

2.6. RF coil and safety

Until now, we have considered the RF coil as a generator or receiver of the magnetic RF field $\mathbf{B}_1$, but it is equally important to take into account the fact that this circuit is also a source of an electric field $\mathbf{E}$. Indeed, any magnetic field $\mathbf{B}_1(t)$ that varies in time creates an electric field $\mathbf{E}(t)$ (Lenz–Faraday law). The eddy currents induced in the tissues by this electric field lead to energy deposition in the body, which can represent a risk for the patient.

2.6.1. *Specific absorption rate and temperature*

To quantify this risk, the notion of SAR is introduced (Collins and Wang 2011). SAR is a measure of the energy flux deposited inside tissues exposed to electromagnetic radiation. Formally, it is defined as the ratio between the average volumetric power dissipated in tissue and the volumetric density ρ_m of the latter:

$$\mathrm{SAR} = \frac{1}{2}\frac{\sigma_s E^2}{\rho_m} \propto \omega^2 B_1^2 \quad \left[\mathrm{W} \cdot \mathrm{kg}^{-1}\right] \qquad [2.15]$$

In practice, rather than SAR, an important quantity is the local heating dT/dt caused by SAR:

$$\frac{dT}{dt} = \frac{\mathrm{SAR}}{C_s} \qquad [2.16]$$

where C_s is the specific caloric capacity of the tissue (in J·kg^{-1}·K^{-1}).

The International Electrotechnical Commission (IEC) has imposed strict regulations regarding the maximum allowed temperature and SAR in human tissue. In particular, these safety directives limit the local heating to 39°C while maintaining the average temperature variation in the body below 0.5°C (IEC 60601-2-33:2010 standard). With regard to SAR, the International Commission on Non-Ionizing Radiation (ICNIRP) recommends never exceeding 2 W/kg in the head and 4 W/kg in the rest of the body for SAR averaged over a volume corresponding to 10 g for at most 6 min (Fiedler et al. 2018).

In practice, SAR is difficult to determine. On the one hand, it cannot be measured in any direct way during an MRI scan. On the other hand, SAR can vary greatly from one patient to another. In fact, in section 2.2, we have seen that the local value of $\mathbf{B}_1$ field is strongly related to electromagnetic wave propagation phenomena inside the patient (see Figure 2.5). As a result, SAR does not depend only on the morphology and spatial variations of dielectric properties in a patient, but it can also vary by orders of magnitude depending on the tissue (Gabriel et al. 1996), as well as on the operating frequency. Therefore, it has to be systematically calculated at the beginning of each MRI scan and for each MRI sequence. To do that, MRI system manufacturers employ numerical patient models, advanced numerical calculation methods and a certain amount of conservative hypotheses, that is, considering the worst case possible. This ensures that no patient will be exposed to higher RF energy than the authorized limits.

2.6.2. *Transmission and safety*

Another source of electric fields, and thus of heating, is the cabling used to connect the detectors to the imaging system. In normal usage contexts, a coaxial cable carries only the "differential-mode" currents, and electric and magnetic fields are confined inside the electrically shielded cable. Nevertheless, this shielding is not perfect and the coaxial cable can sense a part of the signal emitted by the transmit coil. The cable behaves as a dipolar coil with a stationary wave propagating within. A "common-mode" current is then induced, with the position of its maxima along the wire that depends on the wavelength and thus on the frequency. Two issues arise in such a situation. First, undesired cross-talk between cables can perturb the NMR signal integrity and cause imaging artifacts. Second, and most importantly, local heating occurs in correspondence to the current maxima, which can lead to burns on the patient's body.

Various solutions have been proposed to reduce electromagnetic coupling between the transmit coil and the cables located in the MRI system environment. Their main idea consists of blocking the common-mode current, that is, to make sure that no current flows on the external shielding of the coaxial cable. This can be achieved via a local interruption of the circuit by means of very high impedances, for example, (1) traps (Harrison et al. 1987; Peterson et al. 2003) and (2) "baluns"[8] (Murphy-Boesch and Koretsky 1983) that are seen as a high impedance by the common-mode current, (3) ferrites (Ladd and Quick 2000) or (4) transformers (Weiss et al. 2005).

2.7. Advanced topics and coil challenges

Until now, we have described the general challenges related to RF coils in MRI in terms of performance, sensitivity and safety. At this point, we would like to touch on more specific challenges related to some applications that have experienced recent developments in research.

One important research direction is concerned with MRI coil ergonomics, which means lighter detectors, easier use by the technicians and more safety and comfort for the patient. A good example is represented by flexible receive coils, which adapt their geometry to the different patient shapes and sizes. Such coils are directly integrated into garments (gloves, caps, socks, kneepads, etc.) worn by the patient during MRI scans and they can be fabricated as self-resonant multi-gap transmission lines using, for example, commercial non-magnetic coaxial cables (Zhang et al. 2018) or

8 Balun stands for BALanced UNbalanced.

screen-printed ultra-flexible cables (Corea et al. 2016). These solutions are affordable and have an additional advantage of a considerable gain in sensitivity due to a closer fit to the patient's body. Flexible coils can be particularly useful in pediatric MR imaging, an application for which standard coils are usually not suitable.

Optical or wireless technology for signal transmission is another way of improving the detectors' ergonomics (Nohava et al. 2020). With this approach, the NMR signal is digitized closer to the detection loop and information transmission is performed via optical or hyper-frequency (e.g. Wi-Fi) chains that do not interfere with the NMR signal. In this way, the operator's coil handling is simplified. Furthermore, since the number of detectors in coil arrays keeps increasing, it is important to remember that their cabling is a whole challenge in itself: its electromagnetic compatibility with MRI scans has to be guaranteed while keeping its weight and space occupation at a minimum. By getting rid of cables, wireless coils avoid these design issues and provide comfort, safety and ease of use.

Another challenge concerns the correction of magnetic field inhomogeneities due to propagation phenomena in tissues. This problem is typical in high-field (> 3 T) and ultra-high field (UHF ≥ 7 T) imaging scanners, which are more and more developed for clinical MRI applications. One solution can be achieved by parallel transmit coils, that is, transmit coil arrays, where each element can be controlled in an independent way. The magnetic field generated in this way is a linear combination of the fields produced by each element. As a result, it is possible to produce an excitation field B_1 optimized for each patient's morphology by carefully setting the amplitude and phase of the RF fields produced by each array element. As an alternative, the same goal can be achieved via passive dielectric elements in a volume coil (Webb et al. 2011) or metamaterials (Hurshkainen et al. 2016) with controlled electric and magnetic properties. These different approaches have become standard ways to homogenize excitation fields B_1 and additionally limit the local SAR.

On the other hand, it is also possible to perform MRI at low (≤ 1 T) and ultra-low (≤ 4 mT) magnetic fields (Sarracanie and Salameh 2020). Reducing the main field strength is mainly motivated by low-cost MRI opportunities, which could improve the access to MRI and develop relaxometry methods using field cycling (Broche et al. 2019), in addition to offering useful advantages for interventional MRI. However, this approach faces great technological challenges related to the low sensitivity of MRI scans, with a consequent infinitesimal nuclear spin polarization at low fields and insufficient RF coil sensitivity at the corresponding frequencies. At ultra-low fields, classical coils measuring temporal variations of the magnetic flux (Faraday law) have to be replaced by magnetometers measuring the magnetic field value directly. Most scans at ultra-low fields employ superconducting quantum interference devices (SQUIDs) (Espy et al. 2015), that is, superconducting devices that make use of quantum interference phenomena. Other approaches are also possible, such as using detectors based on the giant magnetoresistance phenomenon (Sergeeva-Chollet et al. 2011).

2.8. Conclusion

In this chapter, we presented an overview of RF coils used in MRI. First of all, we discussed the fundamental concepts of tuning and impedance matching a coil as an electronic circuit, followed by a description of the main parameters determining the magnetic field B_1 created by an RF coil. A coil used for transmission has to produce a magnetic field B_1 with as much homogeneity as possible. Consequently, most transmit coils are volume coils. In reception, the sensitivity factor of the detector has to be maximized over a given ROI, often by using single surface coils or arrays of such coils. This has brought us to discuss the source of reception noise in MRI and to distinguish two regimes where either the electric noise of the coil or the magnetic noise from the sample dominates. The importance of these notions lies in their constraints in regard to the design of receive coils. Additionally, we presented the challenge of decoupling in MRI. The latter can cause imaging artifacts, as well as pose significant safety risks. Several approaches tackle either the coupling between transmit and receive coils or the coupling between two elements of a coil array. Subsequently, we went into safety notions related to RF coils in depth, in particular at high frequencies. These risks can be controlled by following regulations that restrict the SAR and heating in tissues as well as by ensuring correct electromagnetic compatibility of coaxial cables used for transmitting MRI signals.

Finally, this chapter briefly touched on today's challenges in the development of new generations of RF coils. Specifically, these include challenges related to high fields, where propagating effects and high SAR can be addressed using coil arrays or metamaterials; challenges related to ergonomics tackled by the development of flexible or wireless coils; and challenges of low fields, where classical coils can be replaced by ultra-sensitive magnetometers.

2.9. References

Adriany, G., Van de Moortele, P.F., Ritter, J., Moeller, S., Auerbach, E.J., Akgün, C., Snyder, C.J., Vaughan, T., Uğurbil, K. (2008). A geometrically adjustable 16-channel transmit/receive transmission line array for improved RF efficiency and parallel imaging performance at 7 Tesla. *Magn. Reson. Med.*, 59, 590–597.

Avdievich, N.I. (2011). Transceiver-phased arrays for human brain studies at 7 T. *Appl. Magn. Reson.*, 41, 483–506.

Broche, L.M., Ross, P.J., Davies, G.R., MacLeod, M.J., Lurie, D.J. (2019). A whole-body fast field-cycling scanner for clinical molecular imaging studies. *Sci. Rep.*, 9, 10402.

Cloos, M.A., Knoll, F., Zhao, T., Block, K.T., Bruno, M., Wiggins, G.C., Sodickson, D.K. (2016). Multiparametric imaging with heterogeneous radiofrequency fields. *Nat. Commun.*, 7, 12445.

Collins, C.M. and Wang, Z. (2011). Calculation of radiofrequency electromagnetic fields and their effects in MRI of human subjects. *Magn. Reson. Med.*, 65(5), 1470–1482.

Corea, J.R., Flynn, A.M., Lechêne, B., Scott, G., Reed, G.D., Shin, P.J., Lustig, M., Arias, A.C. (2016). Screen-printed flexible MRI receive coils. *Nat. Commun.*, 7, 10839.

Darrasse, L. and Ginefri, J.C. (2003). Perspectives with cryogenic RF probes in biomedical MRI. *Biochimie*, 85(9), 915–937.

Espy, M.A., Magnelind, P.E., Matlashov, A.N., Newman, S.G., Sandin, H.J., Schultz, L.J., Sedillo, R., Urbaitis, A.V., Volegov, P.L. (2015). Progress toward a deployable SQUID-based ultra-low field MRI system for anatomical imaging. *IEEE Transactions on Applied Superconductivity*, 25(3), 1–5.

Fiedler, T.M., Ladd, M.E., Bitz, A.K. (2018). SAR simulations & safety. *NeuroImage*, 168, 33–58.

Frass-Kriegl, R., Laistler, E., Hosseinnezhadian, S., Schmid, A.I., Moser, E., Poirier-Quinot, M., Darrasse, L., Ginefri, J.C. (2016). Multi-turn multi-gap transmission line resonators – Concept, design and first implementation at 4.7 T and 7 T. *J. Magn. Reson.*, 273, 65–72.

Gabriel, C., Gabriel, S., Corthout, Y.E. (1996). The dielectric properties of biological tissues I: Literature survey. *Phys. Med. Biol.*, 41, 2231.

Griswold, M.A., Jakob, P.M., Heidemann, R.M., Nittka, M., Jellus, V., Wang, J., Kiefer, B., Haase, A. (2002). Generalized autocalibrating partially parallel acquisitions (GRAPPA). *Magn. Reson. Med.*, 47(6), 1202–1210.

Harrison, W.H., Arakawa, M., McCarten, B.M. (1987). RF coil coupling for MRI with tuned RF rejection circuit using coax shield choke. U.S. Patent, 4(682), 125.

Hosseinnezhadian, S., Frass-Kriegl, R., Goluch-Roat, S., Pichler, M., Sieg, J., Vít, M., Poirier-Quinot, M., Darrasse, L., Moser, E., Ginefri, J.C. et al. (2018). A flexible 12-channel transceiver array of transmission line resonators for 7 T MRI. *J. Magn. Reson.*, 296, 47–59.

Hoult, D.I. (2000). The principle of reciprocity in signal strength calculations – A mathematical guide. *Concepts Magn. Reson.*, 12(4), 173–187.

Hoult, D.I. and Lauterbur, P.C. (1979). The sensitivity of the zeugmatographic experiment involving human samples. *J. Magn. Reson.*, 34(2), 425–433.

Hurshkainen, A.A., Derzhavskaya, T.A., Glybovski, S.B., Voogt, I.J., Melchakova, I.V., van den Berg, C.A., Raaijmakers, A.J. (2016). Element decoupling of 7 T dipole body arrays by EBG metasurface structures: Experimental verification. *J. Magn. Reson.*, 269, 87–96.

Labbé, A., Authelet, G., Baudouy, B., Van Der Beek, C.J., Briatico, J., Darrasse, L., Poirier-Quinot, M. (2021). Recent advances and challenges in the development of radiofrequency HTS coil for MRI. *Front. Phys.*, 9, 386.

Ladd, M.E. and Quick, H.H. (2000). Reduction of resonant RF heating in intravascular catheters using coaxial chokes. *Magn. Reson. Med.*, 43(4), 615–619.

Macovski, A. (1996). Noise in MRI. *Magn. Reson. Med.*, 36(3), 494–497.

Matula, R.A. (1979). Electrical resistivity of copper, gold, palladium, and silver. *J. Phys. Chem. Ref. Data*, 8(4), 1147–1298.

Mispelter, J., Lupu, M., Briguet, A. (2015). *NMR Probeheads for Biophysical and Biomedical Experiments: Theoretical Principles and Practical Guidelines*. World Scientific Publishing Company, London.

Murphy-Boesch, J. and Koretsky, A.P. (1983). An in vivo NMR probe circuit for improved sensitivity. *J. Magn. Reson.*, 54(3), 526–532.

Nohava, L., Ginefri, J.C., Willoquet, G., Laistler, E., Frass-Kriegl, R. (2020). Perspectives in wireless radio frequency coil development for magnetic resonance imaging. *Front. Phys.*, 8, 11.

Peterson, D.M., Beck, B.L., Duensing, G.R., Fitzsimmons, J.R. (2003). Common mode signal rejection methods for MRI: Reduction of cable shield currents for high static magnetic field systems. *Concepts Magn. Reson. Part B*, 19(1), 1–8.

Pruessmann, K.P., Weiger, M., Scheidegger, M.B., Boesiger, P. (1999). SENSE: Sensitivity encoding for fast MRI. *Magn. Reson. Med.*, 42(5), 952–962.

Raki, H., Koon, K.T.V., Saniour, I., Souchay, H., Lambert, S.A., Robb, F., Beuf, O. (2020). Serial and parallel active decoupling characterization using RF MEMS switches for receiver endoluminal coils at 1.5 T. *IEEE Sensors Journal*, 20(18), 10511–10520.

Roemer, P.B., Edelstein, W.A., Hayes, C.E., Souza, S.P., Mueller, O.M. (1990). The NMR phased array. *Magn. Reson. Med.*, 16(2), 192–225.

Sarracanie, M. and Salameh, N. (2020). Low-field MRI: How low can we go? A fresh view on an old debate. *Front. Phys.*, 8, 172.

Schmitt, M., Potthast, A., Sosnovik, D.E., Polimeni, J.R., Wiggins, G.C., Triantafyllou, C., Wald, L.L. (2008). A 128-channel receive-only cardiac coil for highly accelerated cardiac MRI at 3 Tesla. *Magn. Reson. Med.*, 59(6), 1431–1439.

Sergeeva-Chollet, N., Dyvorne, H., Dabek, J., Herreros, Q., Polovy, H., Le Goff, G., Cannies, G., Pannetier-Lecoeur, M., Fermon, C. (2011). Low field MRI with magnetoresistive mixed sensors. *J. Phys. Conf. Ser.*, 303(1), 012055.

Sodickson, D.K. and Manning, W.J. (1997). Simultaneous acquisition of spatial harmonics (SMASH): Fast imaging with radiofrequency coil arrays. *Magn. Reson. Med.*, 38(4), 591–603.

Suits, B.H., Garroway, A.N., Miller, J.B. (1998). Surface and gradiometer coils near a conducting body: The lift-off effect. *J. Magn. Reson.*, 135(2), 373–379.

Webb, A.G. (2011). Dielectric materials in magnetic resonance. *Concepts Magn. Reson. Part A*, 38(4), 148–184.

Weiss, S., Vernickel, P., Schaeffter, T., Schulz, V., Gleich, B. (2005). Transmission line for improved RF safety of interventional devices. *Magn. Reson. Med.*, 54(1), 182–189.

Zhang, B., Sodickson, D.K., Cloos, M.A. (2018). A high-impedance detector-array glove for magnetic resonance imaging of the hand. *Nat. Biomed. Eng.*, 2(8), 570–577.

3

Fast Imaging and Acceleration Techniques

Nadège CORBIN, Sylvain MIRAUX, Valéry OZENNE, Émeline RIBOT and Aurélien TROTIER

CRMSB, CNRS, Université de Bordeaux, France

3.1. Introduction

MRI has become an indispensable clinical technology for patient diagnosis or therapy monitoring. It is also a powerful tool for studying and performing longitudinal follow-up of healthy and pathological models in small animals.

Given the large increase in the usage of this technology, the need for faster image acquisition has emerged. Other constraints, including physiological limitations and patient movement during the scan, as well as the need for dynamic image acquisitions and multi-contrast protocols, have spurred the development of acceleration methods. The numerous advances in the domain of acquisition sequences and image reconstruction have thus a goal of providing images with excellent quality while maintaining or reducing the acquisition time.

In this chapter, we will consider the notion of fast imaging by describing the most commonly used sequences and acceleration techniques. Finally, the last section will be dedicated to applications requiring rapid MRI acquisitions.

3.2. Definition of fast imaging

Fast imaging is associated with the notion of temporal resolution. In MRI, this concept concerns two aspects. The most intuitive one is the time required to acquire a full image. To visualize a dynamic phenomenon, such as a contrast agent entering inside a tissue, the image acquisition time has to be much shorter than the duration of the observed phenomenon. As an example, in functional brain imaging, current techniques acquire about 30 slices of the brain in less than 1 second (s). This temporal resolution permits, for example, following the activation states of cerebral structures during the execution of a task.

Advances in MRI have even provided this technology with "real-time" capabilities for some applications. However, the real-time notion is not only related to the acquisition time, but also to the time necessary for reconstructing and displaying an image. Nowadays, it is possible to perform surgical interventions with real-time MRI guidance (see Chapter 11).

Another way of considering the temporal resolution is related to the periodicity of an observed phenomenon and to the ways of decomposing such a behavior. For instance, let us take the example of cardiac imaging. Under normal physiological conditions, heart movement is regular and periodic. In humans, heartbeats occur approximately every second. Using MRI, it is possible to decompose this cardiac rhythm into several phases by acquiring images with a very high temporal resolution (of the order of 5 ms in mice). For this kind of acquisition, the sequence repetition time is going to define the temporal resolution. However, to acquire these images (i.e. to obtain full k-spaces), the acquisition will be repeated over several cardiac periods and will thus last several minutes.

3.3. Fast accelerated sequences

3.3.1. *Sequence optimization*

If MR image acquisitions have to be performed rapidly, the first step consists of exploiting the available time during an MR sequence in the most efficient way possible. Basic MRI sequences include many dead times useful for magnetization recovery that can be leveraged to "gain some time".

Hence, in a 2D gradient-echo MRI sequence with T_1 weighting (TE/TR = 5/400 ms), the dead time can be used to:

– acquire several slices;

– prepare the magnetization of an adjacent slice;

– introduce a useful contrast module, such as "fat suppression";

– acquire several k-space lines to accelerate the k-space filling.

3.3.2. *Turbo spin echo and echo-planar imaging*

Multi-echo sequences were already introduced in the early days of MRI with the idea of gathering several k-space lines during the sequence dead times. The two main types of such sequences are rapid imaging with refocused echoes (RARE) (Hennig et al. 1986) and *echo-planar imaging* (EPI) (Ordidge et al. 1988).

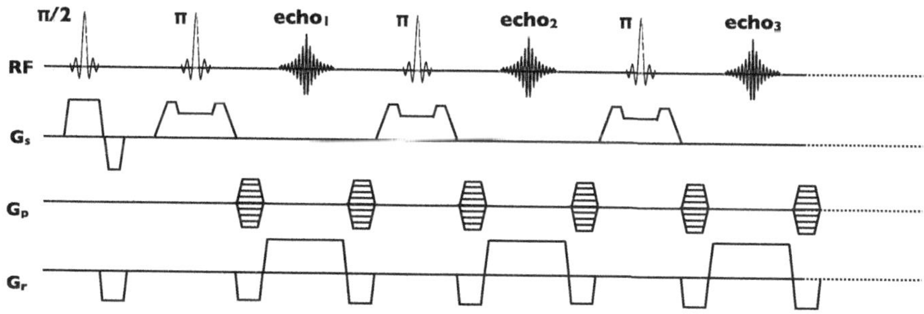

a)

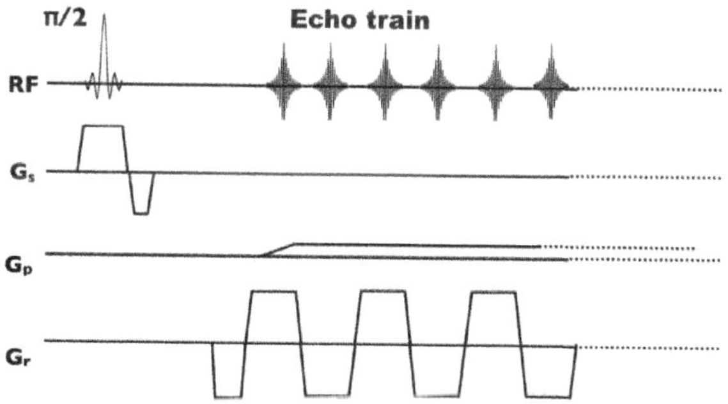

b)

Figure 3.1. *(a) Chronogram of a RARE sequence with the first three echoes of the echo train. (b) Chronogram of an EPI sequence with the first six echoes of the echo train*

A RARE sequence uses an RF excitation pulse followed by a train of refocusing pulses to produce multiple spin echoes. Each echo is spatially encoded such that several k-space lines can be sampled for each excitation pulse. As a result, acquisition times can be greatly reduced compared to a standard spin echo sequence.

RARE sequences are among the most used MRI sequences, especially for acquiring T_2-weighted scans. They are extremely versatile: their chronograms can be easily modified to acquire images in two or three dimensions, they can be adapted to non-Cartesian methods (PROPELLER, BLADE) and several modules (fat suppression, FLAIR) can be added. Moreover, image reconstruction is relatively simple as it requires very few corrections compared to EPI sequences.

The principle of an EPI sequence is comparable to that of a RARE sequence. However, the different echoes are generated from a gradient echo and not a spin echo. EPI sequences are therefore faster than RARE sequences. The former are usually used for functional brain imaging, for quickly encoding the signal after a diffusion module, or for first-pass imaging of a contrast agent during perfusion MRI. EPI sequences are T_2*-weighted.

3.3.2.1. *Echo train concept*

Echo train length (ETL) is an important parameter in RARE (and EPI) sequences. It defines the reduction of the acquisition time compared to a spin echo sequence. The longer the echo train is, the more the acquisition time is reduced. The maximum ETL is constrained by two factors: tissue relaxation time T_2 (i.e. the time during which the transverse magnetization decreases) and the elapsed time between the centers of two consecutive spin echoes. The latter is also called inter-echo time. In practice, for a T_2-weighted RARE sequence with TE = 80 ms, ETL is 32 with an inter-echo time of 5 ms.

3.3.2.2. *Notion of contrast manipulation in RARE*

Image contrast can be modified depending on the way in which the RARE sequence encodes the k-space. In simple terms, if the first echo of the echo train is used to encode the central line of the k-space, then the sequence's $TE_{effective}$ (time between the RF pulse and the echo of the k-space center) is short and the image will have a T_1 weighting. On the other hand, if the last echo is used to encode the center of the k-space, $TE_{effective}$ is long and the sequence becomes T_2-weighted.

3.3.3. *Non-Cartesian methods*

The most classical trajectory for sampling signals in the k-space is the Cartesian one. In this case, each signal is recorded along a horizontal line of the k-space. This approach is still the most used today as it provides high spatial resolutions in two and three dimensions. It is also very robust to hardware drifts, and in particular to errors in trajectories related to the execution of gradients. Nevertheless, other ways of sampling the k-space have been developed for accelerated acquisitions.

Today, the most common non-Cartesian imaging methods are the radial approaches (Lauterbur 1973). The signal is sampled along radial spokes or diameters of a disk, which provides ultra-short echo time sequences and projection-reconstruction (PR) sequences, respectively. In the case of a 2D sequence, these trajectories cover a disk, while in 3D sequences, they cover a sphere (Figure 3.2).

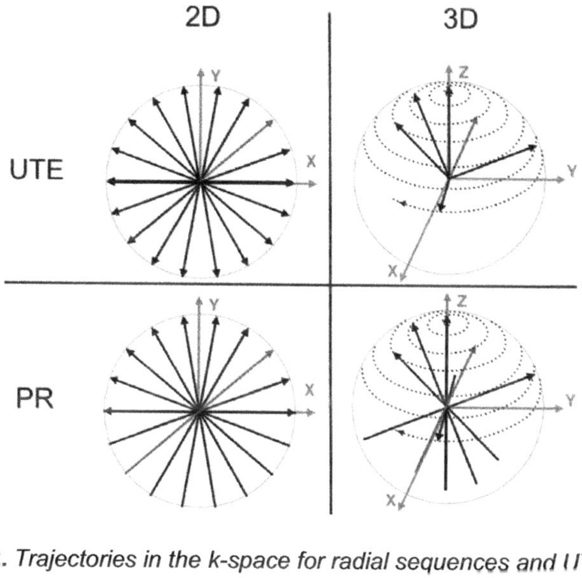

Figure 3.2. *Trajectories in the k-space for radial sequences and UTE, in 2D, and 3D. (UTE: ultra-short echo time; PR: projection-reconstruction). For a color version of this figure, see www.iste.co.uk/ratiney-beuf/challenges.zip*

Radial imaging techniques have several advantages such as the possibility of using high undersampling factors. In fact, since each radial spoke or diameter acquires the center of the k-space, it is possible to reconstruct an image even with a low number of projections. These sequences are also known to be less sensitive to flow or motion artifacts.

On the downside, compared to Cartesian methods, radial sequences often produce images with a lower spatial resolution because the edges of the k-space are undersampled (Figure 3.3).

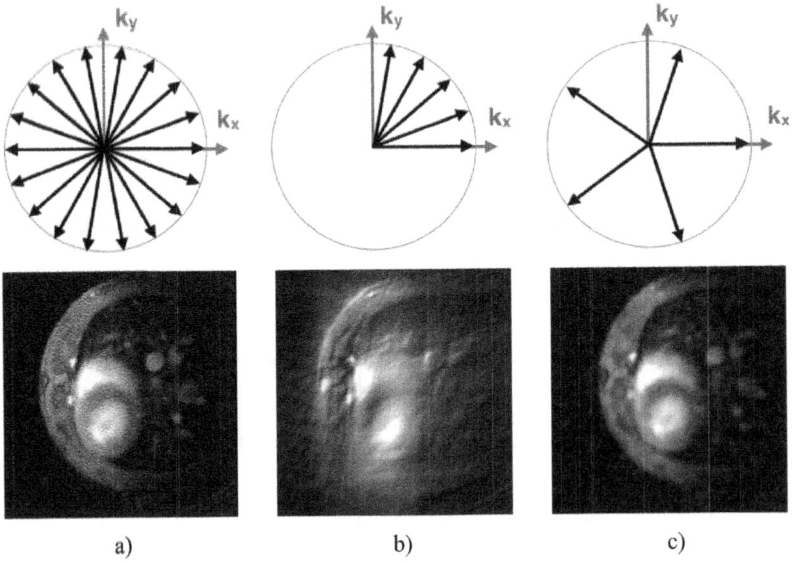

Figure 3.3. *k-Space trajectories and the corresponding images. (a) Radial sequences with number of projections corresponding to Nyquist criteria and a weak number of projections (b). The projections have to be uniformly distributed to obtain an image without artifacts (c)*

Among other non-Cartesian trajectories, the spiral acquisition developed by Ahn et al. (1986) consists of sampling the signal using sinusoidal gradients. Although seldom used in clinical and preclinical routines, this approach presents some advantages that make it robust and very versatile: (1) oversampling of the k-space center makes this method robust to flow and movement artifacts; (2) this type of trajectory acquires the full k-space in a single acquisition (single-shot approach), providing 2D or 3D images very quickly; (3) in the case of a so-called spiral-out trajectory, that is, a spiral trajectory starting from the center of the k-space and ending at the edges, very short or even ultra-short echo times (UTE) can be achieved. Variations of this encoding exist, for example, using Cartesian encoding in the slice-selection direction that permits acquiring spiral planes (Stacks-of-Spirals method) with a cylindric-shaped k-space. Hybrid radial/spiral encoding has also proven useful for abdominal imaging in mice (Castets et al. 2017).

This method also presents several disadvantages, such as sensitivity to chemical shifts, to variations of the magnetic field, and to gradients imperfections altering the trajectories (in particular, eddy currents or fluctuations in communication delays). However, these technical obstacles can be overcome owing to recent advances in terms of hardware and MRI methods. For example, spiral acquisitions can be easily combined with different fat-signal saturation modules. Trajectory monitoring methods can compensate for the gradients' imperfections. Multi-shot encoding can also represent a solution, at the cost of longer acquisition time however. Nevertheless, it has recently been shown that spiral encoding can be combined with parallel imaging (Chen et al. 2016) or compressed sensing methods (Zhao et al. 2015) to accelerate acquisitions.

Other methods based on spiral encoding have been developed, such as the twisted projection imaging (TPI) method (Boada et al. 1997b). Due to its very short TE, TPI has been used for the quantification and imaging of sodium in different organs. Similarly, the Cones method (Boada et al. 1997a) samples the signal very quickly and preserves excellent image quality in studies of short-T_2* tissues. Finally, the spiral projection imaging technique (Boada et al. 1997a) consists of rotating the spirals by a certain angle around the rotation axis. This method keeps the scan time very short, albeit with lower image quality in terms of spatial resolution and signal intensity in tissues with short T_2*.

Today, the main method employing spiral single-shot encoding is fingerprinting (Bipin Mehta et al. 2019), which acquires several signals with different acquisition parameters and thus enables the reconstruction of multiparametric maps (see Chapter 10).

Wave-Caipirinha (Wave-Caipi) trajectory (Bilgic et al. 2015) is another recent and particularly useful method for accelerating image acquisitions. In this encoding scheme, sinusoidal gradients Gy and Gz (with a phase shift of pi/2 between the two) are simultaneously applied during the readout of each k-space line, thereby creating offsets between the slices by modifying k-space phase and partition encodings. The result is a very efficient sampling model of the k-space that is uniformly filled in all the spatial directions (x, y and z). Given that this approach takes advantage of the spatial variation of the coils' 3D sensitivity profiles, it enables highly accelerated volumetric imaging with negligible disadvantages in terms of signal-to-noise ratio (SNR).

All of these encoding approaches provide images from undersampled k-spaces. In fact, according to Nyquist's criterion, the sampling frequency has to be twice the highest frequency of the measured signal. In the cases when this criterion is not complied with, artifacts can appear in the final image. Several methods can improve the robustness of random undersampling schemes. Among these, using the golden angle leads to a random k-space filling while significantly reducing artifacts from the magnetic field heterogeneity. Some literature examples have demonstrated the possibility of combining spiral acquisitions with 2D or 3D golden angles thanks to hybrid radial/spiral encoding. Indeed, radial encoding (Lauterbur 1973) is particularly robust to undersampling. The principle of this technique consists of sampling the signal along diameters symmetrically centered at the origin of the k-space. This method oversamples the k-space center. Moreover, it is also very robust to physiological fluid motion, such as blood flow. This encoding enables the use of a sliding window to reconstruct images with a variable amount of raw data (GRASP) (Feng et al. 2014), and thus to reconstruct dynamic (cine) images, that is, resolving the movement of an organ (heart or lungs, for example). In practice, signal acquisition is either synchronized with the movement (prospective synchronization) or performed continuously until all of the k-spaces have been filled (retrospective synchronization). In both cases, the TR of the employed sequence has to be much shorter than the duration of a physiological movement cycle (cardiac or respiratory). The distribution of information is performed after the acquisition by sorting the k-space echoes according to each phase of the physiological cycle. Thus, the number of undersampled images per cycle can be chosen a posteriori. Radial encoding is quite suitable for obtaining dynamic images as it can avoid acquiring signals via external sensors (ECG or respiratory bellows) by recording the signal caused by the movement at each TR (self-gating or auto-synchronization method). This approach is particularly useful in the case of physiological cycle disruptions, such as arrhythmias. Many applications use this versatile acquisition method such as free-breathing acquisitions or first-pass transits of contrast agents, for example.

3.4. Acceleration methods

In addition to modifying the main sequence parameters, there are other ways for accelerating scans, such as changing the undersampling of the k-space.

Sections 3.4.1–3.4.4 present three types of commonly used undersampling strategies and the corresponding reconstruction approaches (Figure 3.4).

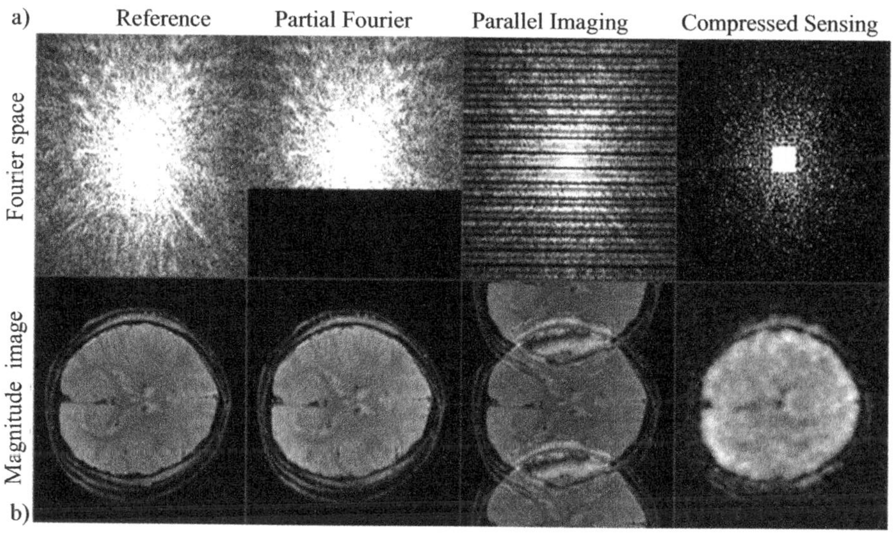

Figure 3.4. *(a) Typical k-space acquisition strategies with different sampling approaches. (b) k-Transform of the corresponding k-spaces showing the typical artifacts caused by these techniques*

3.4.1. *Partial Fourier*

The *partial Fourier* (PF) acceleration approach makes use of the k-space's Hermitian symmetry property:

$$S(-k_x, -k_y) = S(k_x, k_y)^* \qquad [3.1]$$

where S is a point of the k-space at k_x, k_y coordinates and * corresponds to the complex conjugate operation.

This relation is valid only when the image has a purely real component, which implies the absence of B_0 field inhomogeneities, magnetic susceptibility differences between tissues, etc., which would produce phase variations in the image. In the ideal case, half of the k-space can be acquired and the second half can be retrieved because of equation [3.1], in order to reconstruct an image with good quality.

In order to compensate for the phase variations appearing during an MRI scan, a minimum of 60–90% of the k-space has to be acquired (Figure 3.1). This enables the reconstruction of a low-resolution phase image using the central symmetric region of the sampled k-space. This phase estimation is then used to obtain an image where the phase is equal to 0 and is thus purely real, such that Hermitian symmetry can be applied.

Several PF reconstruction approaches have been developed: Margosian (Margosian et al. 1986), Homodyne (Noll et al. 1991), as well as the iterative *projection onto convex sets* (POCS) method (Haacke et al. 1991). A Matlab implementation of these algorithms has been made available by Mark Chiew[1]. Many variations of these methods exist, concentrating mainly on the combination of PF with parallel-imaging reconstructions (Bydder and Robson 2005; Uecker and Lustig 2017; Kettinger et al. 2019) or on the estimation of a higher resolution phase image (Koopmans and Pfaffenrot 2021) which reduces the artifacts in the regions with large phase variations.

This acceleration method is used very often as it can be applied in 2D or 3D and it reduces the acquisition time by 20–40%. Another possibility consists of applying partial Fourier along the readout direction (rather than along the phase direction) to reduce the sequence's echo time.

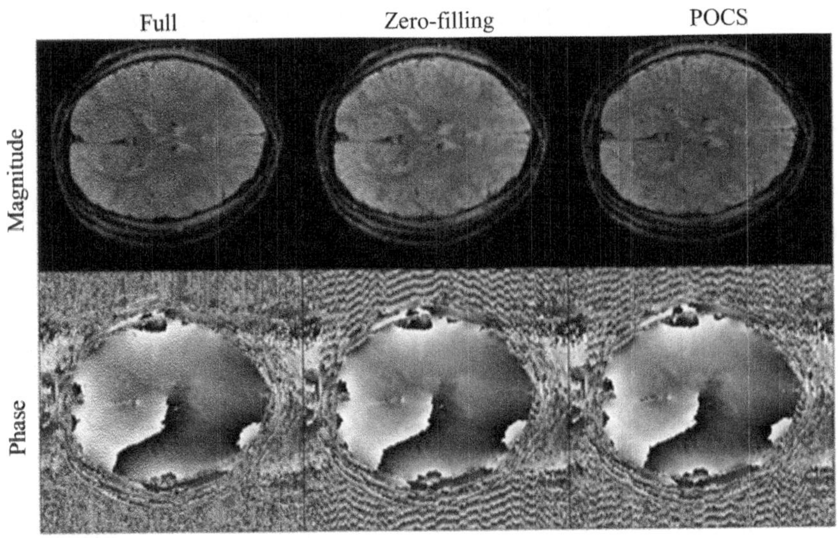

Figure 3.5. *Image reconstruction using the POCS algorithm. Improvements in spatial resolution of the magnitude image are visible but the phase image has a resolution equivalent to a zero-filled image*

1 See: https://users.fmrib.ox.ac.uk/~mchiew/docs/PartialFourier.html [Accessed May 6, 2021].

The main PF's limitations are the low SNR, due to the reduction of the number of acquired lines, and the appearance of artifacts in the images whenever rapid phase variations are present (e.g. at tissue/air or tissue/biomedical material interfaces, etc.). Furthermore, this approach is not recommended for applications that require phase information such as susceptibility or temperature mapping (Figure 3.5).

3.4.2. *Parallel imaging*

The improvement of MRI hardware and, in particular, the use of phased arrays with coils spatially distributed on the sample have enabled higher SNRs by reducing the field of view of each coil element. This led to the idea that fully encoding the phase direction via magnetic field gradients is not strictly necessary, giving birth to the so-called parallel imaging method.

Parallel imaging consists of accelerating MRI scans by skipping some lines of the k-space (Figure 3.4). When images are reconstructed from such an incomplete k-space, filling artifacts appear. These artifacts can be explained by the following property of the k-space:

$$\mathrm{FOV} = \frac{1}{\Delta(k)} \qquad [3.2]$$

For example, according to this equation, if a line is acquired every three lines along k_y, the field of view will be divided by three and the signals coming from three different spatial locations will be superposed in the same pixel:

$$\mathrm{im}_{R_y=3}(x, y) = \mathrm{im}(x, y) + \mathrm{im}(x, y + N/3) + \mathrm{im}(x, y + 2 \times N/3)$$

where im is the image without artifacts, $\mathrm{im}_{R_y=3}$ corresponds to the image reconstructed from an undersampled k-space and N is the number of lines along the y-axis.

In order to obtain unwrapped images, two main types of parallel imaging reconstruction algorithms can be used: those operating in the image domain (SENSE) (Pruessmann et al. 1999) and those acting on the k-space (GRAPPA) (Griswold et al. 2002). Although they are different from a mathematical point of view, the two methods are similar:

– They require multi-channel receive coils. Since the coils are positioned at different locations around the object to be scanned, they will have different sensitivities that depend on their location. This situation can be mathematically described as:

$$\mathrm{im}_l(x, y) = C_l(x, y) \times \mathrm{im}(x, y)$$

where im_l is the image obtained after Fourier transformation of the k-space acquired by coil L, C_l corresponds to the sensitivity map and im is the object. In the case of the GRAPPA algorithm, using one receive coil leads to a convolution of the object's k-space with the Fourier transform of this coil.

– They require reference data: a sensitivity map for the SENSE method or a fully sampled portion of the k-space for the GRAPPA method.

The acquisition of the sensitivity map is performed at the beginning of a scan or is integrated into the sequences by, for instance, using a fast gradient echo sequence with a large field of view and low spatial resolution (few seconds of acquisition time). The knowledge of such a sensitivity map and the acceleration factor (and thus of the superposed voxels) enables writing for each image voxel the following matrix system:

$$\begin{bmatrix} im_1(x,y) \\ im_2(x,y) \\ \vdots \\ im_L(x,y) \end{bmatrix} = \begin{bmatrix} C_1(x,y) & C_1(x+N_x/2,y) \\ C_2(x,y) & C_2(x+N_x/2,y) \\ \vdots & \\ C_L(x,y) & C_L(x+N_x/2,y) \end{bmatrix} \begin{bmatrix} im(x,y) \\ im(x+N_x/2,y) \end{bmatrix}$$

This problem can be solved using the Moore–Penrose pseudoinverse.

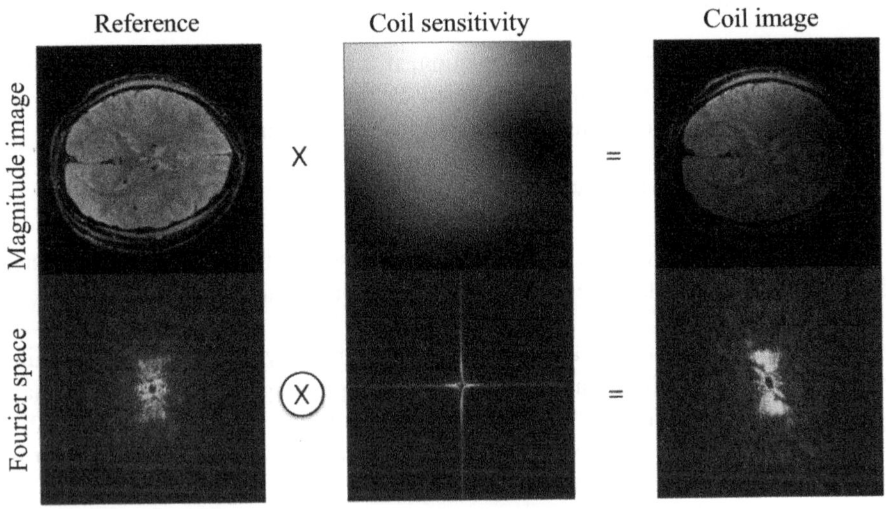

Figure 3.6. *The image acquired by a coil array element is the product of the coil's sensitivity profile and the object. In the k-space domain, this corresponds to a convolution of the object's and coil profile's k-spaces. For a color version of this figure, see www.iste.co.uk/ratiney-beuf/challenges.zip*

In the case of a GRAPPA reconstruction, data that are missing in the k-space are recovered as a weighted average of the adjacent sampled data points coming from the k-spaces of all of the coils. In fact, the information at a point of the k-space is convoluted with the coil and thus it is also contained in the adjacent point of the k-space (Figure 3.6). To measure the weights, all of the lines of a portion of k-space have to be acquired. Usually, for SNR reasons, the fully sampled portion is the central one.

Various Python implementations of these two algorithms have been made available by Nicholas McKibben (see: https://github.com/mckib2/pygrappa) for comparing the results of the reconstructions and their implementations.

In both reconstruction methods, the maximum theoretical acceleration factor is equal to the number of coils. However, in practice, it is equal to two or three for reconstructions with sufficient image quality. In fact, the SNR obtained with parallel imaging methods follows the equation:

$$\mathrm{RSB}(x, y) \propto \frac{1}{g(x, y)\sqrt{R}}$$

where R corresponds to the acquisition's acceleration factor, g is the geometrical factor and x,y are the coordinates of the reconstructed image.

The origin of the square root of the acceleration factor corresponds to the fact that fewer lines are acquired in the k-space. The geometrical factor (also called the g-factor) represents the increase of the image noise caused by solving ill-conditioned matrix problems of the two reconstruction methods. It varies with the position in the image and depends on the location of the coils with respect to the object and to each other, as well as on the number of voxels wrapping one upon another at a given position.

Although differences in the acquisition of calibration data or sensitivity maps exist, they do not imply significant differences in terms of image quality after reconstruction and thus do not favor using the SENSE method rather than the GRAPPA method. The different availability of these methods on the scanners can usually be explained by historical or patent reasons.

Parallel imaging is compatible with the acceleration of 3D acquisitions along the second phase encoding direction, which increases the applied acceleration factor. Moreover, the SENSE and GRAPPA algorithms are the foundation of simultaneous multislice acquisition reconstructions.

3.4.3. *Simultaneous multislice imaging*

Simultaneous multislice imaging consists of exciting several slices at the same time. Therefore, multislice acceleration increases the number of slices acquired within a fixed TR and provides better volumetric coverage of the object of interest. The corresponding images, reconstructed via Fourier transform, contain the sum of the signals from all of the slices and are called "wrapped" images. The reconstruction process thus consists of "unwrapping" the image by isolating the signal of each slice.

This concept was initially proposed by Larkman in 2001 (Larkman et al. 2001). The reconstruction method was analogous to the SENSE reconstruction and employed the sensitivity of the receive channels to unwrap the image. If the k-space is not fully sampled, multislice imaging does not cause SNR loss, contrary to what was described for parallel imaging in section 3.4.2. However, signal leakage can occur from slice A to slice B and vice versa, described by a slice leakage factor, which corresponds to an unwrapping error that can be quantified during the reconstruction. Although promising, this method remained marginal until the beginning of the 2010s when several major publications enhanced the technique by combining it with novel acquisition and reconstruction methods.

In 2010, Moeller et al. (2010) applied this method to an EPI sequence dedicated to functional imaging at 7T. The authors demonstrated the use of multislice EPI in combination with undersampling in the phase direction, which allowed for reaching an acceleration factor of 16. On the downside, an SNR penalty due to the geometrical factor is introduced into the reconstruction process. To tackle this problem, Setsompop et al. (2012) proposed a new implementation with a phase shift in the slice direction in order to increase the signal separation in the wrapped slice.

The multislice imaging reconstruction method is based on SENSE or GRAPPA concepts (Barth et al. 2016). They are compatible with an undersampling of the k-space in the phase direction. Here, we present briefly the slice-GRAPPA method.

The slice-GRAPPA reconstruction consists of (1) acquiring separate calibration images (called single-band) of each slice (without multislice acceleration); (2) synthetically calculating the multislice images (called multi-band) by summing up the k-spaces; and finally, (3) estimating the operator for unwrapping the multislice image. Acquiring calibration data increases the acquisition time, but for a given spatial coverage, the acquisition time of the next repetitions is divided by the number of slices acquired simultaneously.

3.4.4. *Iterative reconstruction*

Increasing the acceleration factor can be done by sampling the k-space in a more random way (Figure 3.1). Such methods exploit the sparsity and redundancy of information contained in the k-space. In these conditions, the conventional methods based on the Fourier transform become suboptimal. Therefore, the encoding approaches require iterative reconstruction methods.

In MRI, the reconstruction process can be described by distinguishing the object signal v (image) that has to be reconstructed, the measurement m (k-space) and the encoding operator E (often written in a matrix form) that symbolizes the acquisition process. Applying the encoding operator to the object yields the signal ρ of the k-space measured during the acquisition.

Consequently, a so-called direct transformation $Ev = m$ can be written. As an example, in the case of several receive channels and undersampling, the encoding operator can be written as:

$$E = T.F.C$$

where C is the coil's sensitivity map, F is the Fourier transform, T is the mask that represents the undersampling or the non-Cartesian trajectory used during the acquisition.

The reconstruction consists of estimating v by knowing E and m. The most direct mathematical method requires inverting E to perform the so-called inverse transformation: $v = E^{-1}m$.

This equation can be solved directly if, for example, the E matrix is invertible, which is not usually the case (e.g. in an undersampled acquisition). In the opposite case, iterative methods have to be employed to indirectly estimate v. We have to find the best v that satisfies $Ev = m$.

However, the equation is incomplete as it is missing the acquired noise.

One approach for solving this system is to estimate the solution iteratively. The process can be described in the following way:

1) instead of directly inverting the encoding operator E, the iterative method calculates an approximate temporary solution;

2) a direct transformation of this temporary solution is performed to calculate estimated data;

3) a comparison between the acquired and estimated data is performed;

4) if the comparison is correct (according to a user-defined criterion), the solution has been found.

Alternatively, the difference between the two types of data can be used to modify the estimated image. Mathematically, the problem can be written in the following way:

$$\hat{v} = \underset{v}{\operatorname{argmin}} \|m - Ev\|^2$$

The goal is to find $\hat{v}$, and this minimizes the error between acquired and estimated data. This problem can be reformulated by differentiating this equation. In fact, the local minimum of the derivative represents, in the case of a convex problem, the solution to the problem.

A classical method for this purpose is the gradient descent method, in which the error evolution (the descent direction toward the minimum and the optimal step to minimize this error) is estimated at each iteration. To improve the conditioning of the system, some a priori knowledge about the solution can be introduced via regularization terms. The a priori data can be a low-resolution image or criteria on the spatial or temporal variation of the signal in the reconstructed images.

The equation becomes as follows:

$$\hat{v} = \underset{v}{\operatorname{argmin}} \|m - Ev\|^2 + \lambda \|R\|$$

with λ the regularization parameter and R the regularization term.

Some methods employ the l2 norm (Tikhonov method), while others use the l1 norm (total variation, wavelet methods) and are more commonly called compressed sensing (CS) methods (Lustig et al. 2008). The latter require a modification of the solving method as the l1 norm is not differentiable and has to be approximated.

Starting from the 2010s, several algorithms dedicated to iterative solving of l1 methods have been developed and applied in MRI (Ye 2019).

3.5. Applications

MRI acceleration methods are as numerous as the motivations for using them, even if the benefits of these speed-ups always carry some disadvantages.

Clearly, accelerating MRI acquisitions reduces the total duration of the clinical examinations with maximized patient comfort and a decreased waiting time. In 2017, the average waiting time before getting an MRI scan in the context of suspected metastasis or cancer relapse was of 31.4 days, whereas the Cancer 2014–2019 program recommends a maximum waiting time of 20 days (Detournay and Courouve 2017). Reducing the scan durations also enables more acquisitions with different contrasts to provide as much information on the patient as possible and thus allow radiologists to refine their diagnosis.

Typically, MRI acquisition durations increase with spatial resolution. Reducing the voxel size means acquiring extra points of the k-space, further away from its center. The acceleration techniques make it possible to cover the k-space more quickly (at the expense of sampling density) and thus improve the spatial resolution without increasing the acquisition time. A Poisson-density undersampling combined with a CS (iterative method) reconstruction has led, for example, to increased spatial resolutions of T_1 maps (MP2RAGE) while maintaining the same scan duration, thereby improving the detection of small-sized metastases in mice (Trotier et al. 2019).

Depending on the application, the acceleration time gain can be used more wisely to increase the temporal resolution rather than the spatial resolution. In fact, temporal resolution is critical whenever a sequence of images is acquired, such as in the case of dynamic MRI.

MRI studies of capillary microcirculation in tissues can be performed by acquiring a sequence of temporal T_1-weighted images after intravenous injection of contrast agent (DCE-MRI method). The propagation of the contrast agent via blood vessels can be observed in time to detect lesions. By analyzing the blood flow, it is possible to distinguish malignant tumors from benign ones. However, this requires a temporal resolution of at least one image every 45 s (El Khouli et al. 2009), hence the need for acceleration methods.

Interventional MRI consists of a real-time evaluation of a lesion's thermal ablation treatment. Images are acquired during the entire procedure to provide real-time observation of any change in the lesion and the surrounding tissue. Having access to markers, such as needle position, temperature and mechanical or magnetic tissue properties, allows interventional radiologists to confirm lesion destruction as well as the preservation of surrounding healthy tissue. A very frequent update of these markers and, therefore, a high temporal resolution is critical for proper monitoring of the procedure. For example, the CS method has led to a 55% increase in temporal resolution for interventional MRI-dedicated sequences such as SEMAC (Sonnow et al. 2018). These acquisitions have a low sensitivity to artifacts created by the needles that are typically used in MRI, but they are quite time consuming. The acceleration techniques were able to tackle this limitation.

Temporal resolution is equally crucial in functional MRI. In this technique, the hemodynamic response to neural stimulation is observed. Such a response lasts between 10 and 20 s and reaches a peak after 4–5 s. Therefore, a temporal resolution of at least an image every 4 s is required to observe the response. Thanks to acceleration methods, we can obtain one image of the entire human brain per second with sufficient spatial resolution. This enables an increased statistical accuracy if the total scan duration is unchanged, a filtering of the physiological noise (cardiac and respiratory), and observations of more rapid events (Feinberg and Setsompop 2013). For example, it has been demonstrated that epileptic phenomena can only be observed with a temporal resolution of at least one image per second (Sahib et al. 2018), which can be only reached via acceleration methods. However, a too-quick acceleration can become counterproductive in functional MRI as temporal correlations can skew the statistical tests (Olszowy et al. 2017; Corbin et al. 2018) and leakage phenomena can occur (Todd et al. 2016), which may lead to an incorrect localization of active regions.

More generally, accelerated MRI scans offer the opportunity to acquire more data in a given time. These data can be used to increase the spatial or temporal resolutions or the field of view, but they can also provide a greater number of contrasts for quantitatively estimating parameters that are characteristic of the tissue microstructure via biophysical models. For example, in diffusion MRI, it can be useful to acquire several images with diffusion gradients applied along multiple directions in order to characterize the fibers of interest more accurately. However, the scan time is proportional to the number of directions. Thanks to the CS method, it was possible, for example, to take images of the density and orientation of mice neurites with a resolution of 50 μm by acquiring 234 diffusion directions in 66 hours (h) with an acceleration factor of 4 (Wang et al. 2019a). Similar achievements are possible for most quantitative MRI applications. Relaxometry, which consists of the quantitative estimation of the relaxation times T_2, T_2*, or T_1, benefits from an increased number of acquisitions with varying critical parameters, such as echo time or inversion time. By accelerating the acquisitions, more contrasts, and therefore more information, are achievable within a reasonable scan duration. In this way, the biophysical models that have to be inverted to estimate the quantitative parameters benefit from a greater amount of input data. For example, thanks to an optimized k-space sampling, the echo planar time resolved imaging (EPTI) method (Wang et al. 2019b) can provide 8 × 48 images with different contrasts with a resolution of 1.5 mm^3 at 3 T in only 5 min (Dong et al. 2021). With these multiple contrasts, a myelination map of the entire brain can be produced once the relaxation parameters have been estimated.

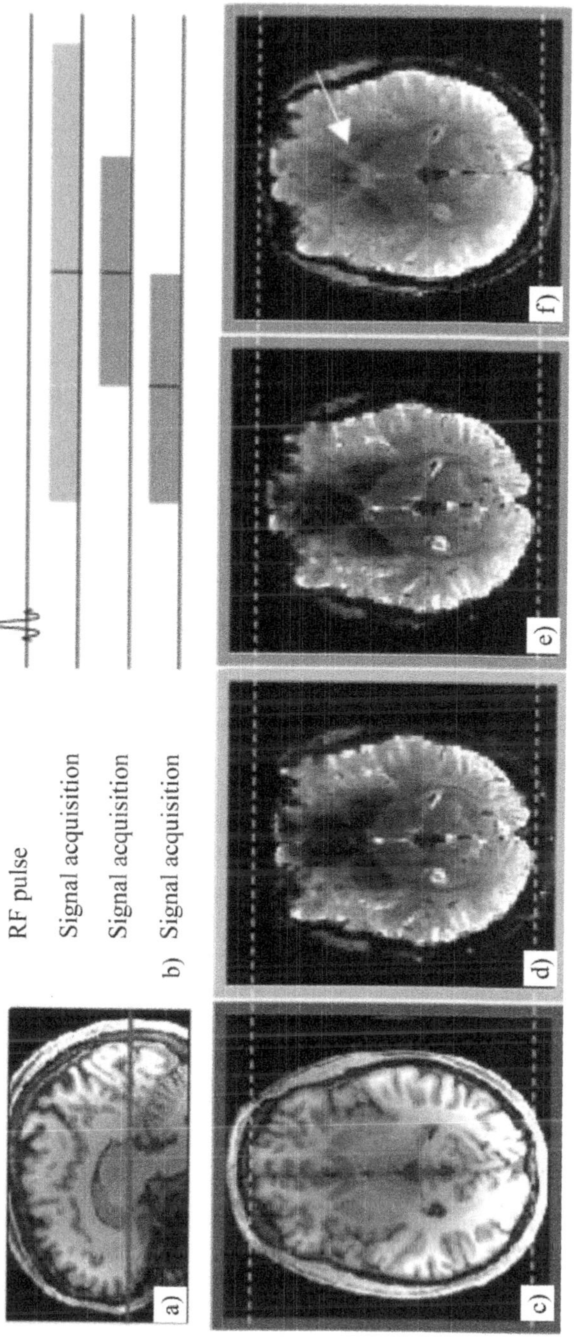

Figure 3.7. *Reducing EPI scan artifacts thanks to an acceleration factor. For a color version of this figure, see www.iste.co.uk/ratiney-beuf/challenges.zip*

COMMENT ON FIGURE 3.7.– *Sagittal (a) and axial (c) slices of an MPRAGE acquisition. Same axial slice for three EPI scans (d, e, f) and their simplified chronograms (b). With an EPI echo train of 128 echoes and a TE of 60 ms (yellow [b-d]), the distortions and signal loss in the medial frontal brain region are significant. An acceleration factor of 2 (green [b–e]) shortens the echo train and thus reduces the distortions (the brain has a normal shape, dashed line). Thanks to the shorter echo train, TE can be reduced to 30 ms (blue [b–f]) that allows for recovering the signal in the medial frontal regions (white arrow).*

Although acceleration techniques often cause image artifacts, using them to get rid of some artifacts is not so uncommon. EPI, which is often used in diffusion and functional MRI, is very sensitive to magnetic field inhomogeneities that introduce distortion artifacts and regions without any signal (dropouts). In EPI, several lines of the k-space, called echo train, are acquired after a single radiofrequency pulse. The inhomogeneities of the B_0 magnetic field, caused by the variations in magnetic susceptibility among tissues, can be modeled as an intrinsic magnetic field gradient that is superposed to the imaging gradients employed to encode the k-space. The presence of these intrinsic gradients hinders a correct sampling of the k-space, which induces distortion artifacts that change the shape of the scanned object. The higher the strength of the imaging gradients with respect to the intrinsic gradients, the less the signal is displaced in mm (Jezzard and Balaban 1995). In such cases, resorting to parallel imaging along the encoding direction of the EPI trains increases the moment of the phase encoding gradients (blips) that is proportional to the distance between the lines of the k-space, thus enabling a reduction of distortion artifacts (Figures 3.7(d) and 3.7(e)). In EPI, regions of absent signal are often observed as a consequence of the long TE, typical of EPI and short T_2* of these regions. In order to reduce TE, especially at ultra-high fields (Aitken et al. 2020), where T_2* is shorter, the scans often employ parallel imaging to shorten the echo train and/or the partial Fourier technique to acquire the center of the k-space as early as possible (Figures 3.7(e) and 3.7(f)). Shortening the echo train also reduces the variation of the signal amplitude over the k-space lines that are acquired during the signal decay. Limiting the variation of intensity along the echo train can therefore reduce the blurring effect in the images. The acceleration methods have also enabled the development of 3D acquisitions, which have the advantage of increasing the SNR compared to 2D scans, as both phase encoding directions can be accelerated in a similar way to drastically reduce the acquisition time.

Physiological patient motion (breathing, cardiac beating, peristalsis) is another source of critical artifacts. By shortening the acquisition time, the sensitivity to motion is reduced. This is particularly the case for 3D scans, which are very sensitive to motion since each volume is reconstructed from all of the data of the k-space, which could have been acquired over a non-negligible time. By employing acceleration techniques, the duration for acquiring a volume is shortened, thus minimizing the sensitivity to motion. However, using parallel imaging can have the opposite effect. In fact, often, a reference volume is acquired at the beginning of the scans to estimate the sensitivity maps of the coil elements, a crucial step for reconstructing images. If the patient is not stable during this reference scan or if they change, even just a little, their position between the reference and the actual images, reconstruction may be heavily impaired (Yanasak and Kelly 2014).

3.6. References

Ahn, C.B., Kim, J.H., Cho, Z.H. (1986). High-speed spiral-scan echo planar NMR imaging I. *IEEE Transactions on Medical Imaging*, 5(1), 2–7.

Aitken, F., Menelaou, G., Warrington, O., Koolschijn, R.S., Corbin, N., Callaghan, M.F., Kok, P. (2020). Prior expectations evoke stimulus-specific activity in the deep layers of the primary visual cortex. *PLoS Biology*, 18(12), e3001023.

Barth, M., Breuer, F., Koopmans, P.J., Norris, D.G., Poser, B.A. (2016). Simultaneous multislice (SMS) imaging techniques. *Magnetic Resonance in Medicine*, 75(1), 63–81.

Bilgic, B., Gagoski, B.A., Cauley, S.F., Fan, A.P., Polimeni, J.R., Grant, P.E., Wald, L.L., Setsompop, K. (2015). Wave-CAIPI for highly accelerated 3D imaging. *Magnetic Resonance in Medicine*, 73(6), 2152–2162.

Bipin Mehta, B., Coppo, S., Frances McGivney, D., Ian Hamilton, J., Chen, Y., Jiang, Y., Ma, D., Seiberlich, N., Gulani, V., Alan Griswold, M. (2019). Magnetic resonance fingerprinting: A technical review. *Magnetic Resonance in Medicine*, 81(1), 25–46.

Boada, F.E., Gillen, J.S., Shen, G.X., Chang, S.Y., Thulborn, K.R. (1997a). Fast three dimensional sodium imaging. *Magnetic Resonance in Medicine*, 37(5), 706–715.

Boada, F.E., Shen, G.X., Chang, S.Y., Thulborn, K.R. (1997b). Spectrally weighted twisted projection imaging: Reducing T_2 signal attenuation effects in fast three-dimensional sodium imaging. *Magnetic Resonance in Medicine*, 38(6), 1022–1028.

Bydder, M. and Robson, M.D. (2005). Partial Fourier partially parallel imaging. *Magnetic Resonance in Medicine*, 53(6), 1393–1401.

Castets, C.R., Lefrançois, W., Wecker, D., Ribot, E.J., Trotier, A.J., Thiaudière, E., Franconi, J.M., Miraux, S. (2017). Fast 3D ultrashort echo-time spiral projection imaging using golden-angle: A flexible protocol for in vivo mouse imaging at high magnetic field. *Magnetic Resonance in Medicine*, 77(5), 1831–1840.

Chen, Y., Lee, G.R., Aandal, G., Badve, C., Wright, K.L., Griswold, M.A., Seiberlich, N., Gulani, V. (2016). Rapid volumetric T_1 mapping of the abdomen using three-dimensional through-time spiral GRAPPA. *Magnetic Resonance in Medicine*, 75(4), 1457–1465.

Corbin, N., Todd, N., Friston, K.J., Callaghan, M.F. (2018). Accurate modeling of temporal correlations in rapidly sampled fMRI time series. *Human Brain Mapping*, 39(10), 3884–3897.

Curtis, A.D. and Cheng, H.L.M. (2020). Primer and historical review on rapid cardiac CINE MRI. *Journal of Magnetic Resonance Imaging*, 2022(55), 373–388.

Detournay, B. and Courouve, L. (2017). Les insuffisances en matière d'équipements d'imagerie médicale en France : étude sur les délais d'attente pour un rendez-vous IRM en 2017. Report, SNITEM, 3, 2017–099 [Online]. Available at: https://fnmr.fr/wp-content/uploads/2022/12/Les-insuffisances-en-matiere-dequipements-dimagerie-medicale-en-France-Etude-SNITEM-2017.pdf [Accessed May 3 2021].

Dong, Z., Wang, F., Chan, K.S., Reese, T.G., Bilgic, B., Marques, J.P., Setsompop, K. (2021). Variable flip angle echo planar time-resolved imaging (vFA-EPTI) for fast high-resolution gradient echo myelin water imaging. *NeuroImage*, 232, 117897.

El Khouli, R.H., Macura, K.J., Barker, P.B., Phil, D., Habba, M.R., Jacobs, M.A., Bluemke, D.A. (2009). The relationship of temporal resolution to diagnostic performance for dynamic contrast enhanced (DCE) MRI of the breast. *Journal of Magnetic Resonance Imaging: JMRI*, 30(5), 999–1004.

Feinberg, D.A. and Setsompop, K. (2013). Ultra-fast MRI of the human brain with simultaneous multi-slice imaging. *Journal of Magnetic Resonance*, 229, 90–100.

Feng, L., Grimm, R., Block, K.T., Chandarana, H., Kim, S., Xu, J., Axel, L., Sodickson, D.K., Otazo, R. (2014). Golden-angle radial sparse parallel MRI: Combination of compressed sensing, parallel imaging, and golden-angle radial sampling for fast and flexible dynamic volumetric MRI. *Magnetic Resonance in Medicine*, 72(3), 707–717.

Griswold, M.A., Jakob, P.M., Heidemann, R.M., Nittka, M., Jellus, V., Wang, J., Kiefer, B., Haase, A. (2002). Generalized autocalibrating partially parallel acquisitions (GRAPPA). *Magnetic Resonance in Medicine*, 47(6), 1202–1210.

Haacke, E.M., Lindskogj, E.D., Lin, W. (1991). A fast, iterative, partial-Fourier technique capable of local phase recovery. *Journal of Magnetic Resonance*, 92(1), 126–145.

Hennig, J., Nauerth, A., Friedburg, H. (1986). RARE imaging: A fast imaging method for clinical MR. *Magnetic Resonance in Medicine*, 3(6), 823–833.

Jezzard, P. and Balaban, R.S. (1995). Correction for geometric distortion in echo planar images from B_0 field variations. *Magnetic Resonance in Medicine*, 34(1), 65–73.

Kettinger, A.O., Setsompop, K., Kannengiesser, S.A.R., Breuer, F.A., Vidnyanszky, Z., Blaimer, M. (2019). Full utilization of conjugate symmetry: Combining virtual conjugate coil reconstruction with partial Fourier imaging for g-factor reduction in accelerated MRI. *Magnetic Resonance in Medicine*, 82(3), 1073–1090.

Koopmans, P.J. and Pfaffenrot, V. (2021). Enhanced POCS reconstruction for partial Fourier imaging in multi-echo and time-series acquisitions. *Magnetic Resonance in Medicine*, 85(1), 140–151.

Larkman, D.J., Hajnal, J.V., Herlihy, A.H., Coutts, G.A., Young, I.R., Ehnholm, G. (2001). Use of multicoil arrays for separation of signal from multiple slices simultaneously excited. *Journal of Magnetic Resonance Imaging: JMRI*, 13(2), 313–317.

Lauterbur, P.C. (1973). Image formation by induced local interactions: Examples employing nuclear magnetic resonance. *Nature*, 242(5394), 190–191.

Lustig, M., Donoho, D.L., Santos, J.M., Pauly, J.M. (2008). Compressed sensing MRI. *IEEE Signal Processing Magazine*, 25(2), 72–82.

Margosian, P., Schmitt, F., Purdy, D. (1986). Faster MR imaging: Imaging with half the data. Proceedings paper, 0593. doi: 10.1117/12.952139.

Moeller, S., Yacoub, E., Olman, C.A., Auerbach, E., Strupp, J., Harel, N., Uğurbil, K. (2010). Multiband multislice GE-EPI at 7 tesla, with 16-fold acceleration using partial parallel imaging with application to high spatial and temporal whole-brain fMRI. *Magnetic Resonance in Medicine*, 63(5), 1144–1153.

Noll, D.C., Nishimura, D.G., Macovski, A. (1991). Homodyne detection in magnetic resonance imaging. *IEEE Transactions on Medical Imaging*, 10(2), 154–163.

Olszowy, W., Williams, G.B., Rua, C., Aston, J. (2017). Autocorrelation bias still exists in fMRI results. *arXiv:1711.09877* [Online]. Available at: http://arxiv.org/abs/1711.09877 [Accessed November 28, 2017].

Ordidge, R.J., Coxon, R., Howseman, A., Chapman, B., Turner, R., Stehling, M., Mansfield, P. (1988). Snapshot head imaging at 0.5 T using the echo planar technique. *Magnetic Resonance in Medicine*, 8(1), 110–115.

Pruessmann, K.P., Weiger, M., Scheidegger, M.B., Boesiger, P. (1999). SENSE: Sensitivity encoding for fast MRI. *Magnetic Resonance in Medicine*, 42(5), 952–962.

Sahib, A.K., Erb, M., Marquetand, J., Martin, P., Elshahabi, A., Klamer, S., Vulliemoz, S., Scheffler, K., Ethofer, T., Focke, N.K. (2018). Evaluating the impact of fast-fMRI on dynamic functional connectivity in an event-based paradigm. *PLoS One*, 13(1), e0190480.

Setsompop, K., Gagoski, B.A., Polimeni, J.R., Witzel, T., Wedeen, V.J., Wald, L.L. (2012). Blipped-controlled aliasing in parallel imaging for simultaneous multislice echo planar imaging with reduced g-factor penalty. *Magnetic Resonance in Medicine*, 67(5), 1210–1224.

Sonnow, L., Gilson, W.D., Raithel, E., Nittka, M., Wacker, F., Fritz, J. (2018). Instrument visualization using conventional and compressed sensing SEMAC for interventional MRI at 3T. *Journal of Magnetic Resonance Imaging*, 47(5), 1306–1315.

Todd, N., Moeller, S., Auerbach, E.J., Yacoub, E., Flandin, G., Weiskopf, N. (2016). Evaluation of 2D multiband EPI imaging for high-resolution, whole-brain, task-based fMRI studies at 3T: Sensitivity and slice leakage artifacts. *NeuroImage*, 124, 32–42.

Trotier, A.J., Rapacchi, S., Faller, T.L., Miraux, S., Ribot, E.J. (2019). Compressed-sensing MP2RAGE sequence: Application to the detection of brain metastases in mice at 7T. *Magnetic Resonance in Medicine*, 81(1), 551–559.

Uecker, M. and Lustig, M. (2017). Estimating absolute-phase maps using ESPIRiT and virtual conjugate coils. *Magnetic Resonance in Medicine*, 77(3), 1201–1207.

Wang, F., Dong, Z., Reese, T.G., Bilgic, B., Manhard, M.K., Chen, J., Polimeni, J.R., Wald, L.L., Setsompop, K. (2019a). Echo planar time-resolved imaging (EPTI). *Magnetic Resonance in Medicine*, 81(6), 3599–3615.

Wang, F., Zhang, J., Cofer, G., Qi, Y., Anderson, R.J., White, L.E., Allan Johnson, G. (2019b). Neurite orientation dispersion and density imaging of mouse brain microstructure. *Brain Structure and Function*, 224(5), 1797–1813.

Yanasak, N.E. and Kelly, M.J. (2014). MR imaging artifacts and parallel imaging techniques with calibration scanning: A new twist on old problems. *Radiographics: A Review Publication of the Radiological Society of North America, Inc*, 34(2), 532–548.

Ye, J.C. (2019). Compressed sensing MRI: A review from signal processing perspective. *BMC Biomedical Engineering*, 1, 8.

Zhao, L., Fielden, S.W., Feng, X., Wintermark, M., Mugler, J.P., Meyer, C.H. (2015). Rapid 3D dynamic arterial spin labeling with a sparse model-based image reconstruction. *NeuroImage*, 121, 205–216.

4

The Basics of Diffusion and Intravoxel Incoherent Motion MRI

Giulio GAMBAROTA

Laboratoire de biophysique, Université de Rennes, France

4.1. Introduction

This chapter is dedicated to the measurements of water diffusion in vivo using magnetic resonance imaging (MRI). Since performing in the early days mostly for clinical application in brain, nowadays diffusion-weighted imaging (DWI) is a well-established technique for clinical MRI examinations of different tissues/organs. It has a major role in many therapeutic domains, including oncology and neurology, for both diagnosis and assessment of treatment efficacy.

We will first introduce the basic physics of diffusion; then, the measurements of water diffusion using nuclear magnetic resonance (NMR) will be described. Finally, we will illustrate clinical applications of DWI.

4.2. The history and physics of diffusion

Here, we present a brief account of the history and physics of diffusion. A simple way to visualize the phenomenon of diffusion is to put a drop of ink into a Petri dish

---

For a color version of all the figures in this chapter, see www.iste.co.uk/ratiney-beuf/challenges.zip.

The Challenges of MRI,
coordinated by Hélène RATINEY and Olivier BEUF.

filled with water. Afterward, we observe that the ink particles will spread in time in all directions around their initial position, which can be chosen for simplicity as the origin of a coordinate system (Figure 4.1). The size of the spot will increase with time, as ink particles will diffuse. In general, the phenomenon of diffusion of particles in solution – in the presence of a concentration gradient – was known to scientists of the 19th century. In 1855, the physiologist Adolf Fick described the diffusion of salt in water by the following equation, named Fick's second law:

$$\frac{\partial C}{\partial t} = D\frac{\partial^2 C}{\partial x^2} \qquad [4.1]$$

where C, the concentration expressed as the number of particles of solute per unit volume of solution, is a function of time and space, that is, $C(x,t)$, and D is the diffusion coefficient. The dimensional analysis of equation [4.1] shows that the diffusion coefficient has dimensions $[D] = L^2T^{-1}$, that is, $length^2 \cdot time^{-1}$.

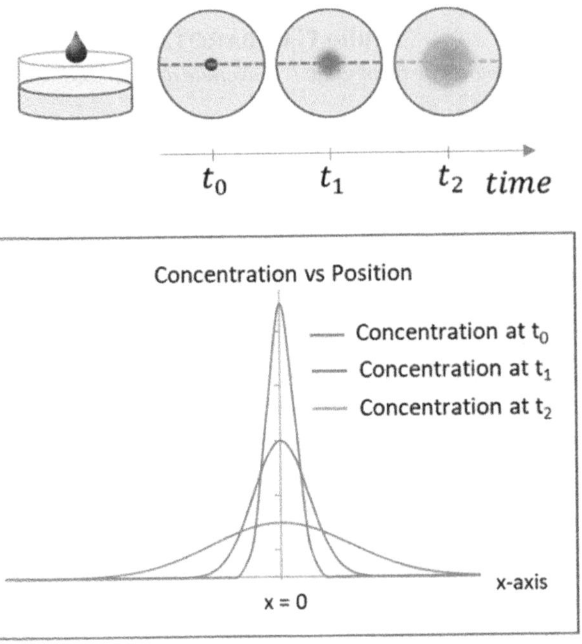

Figure 4.1. *A drop of ink into a Petri dish filled with water. Upper panel: the ink particles will diffuse in time in all directions. Lower panel: the concentration of ink particles is plotted as a function of time along the radial direction at three time points*

For simplicity, we consider the diffusion motion just along the x-axis. Under the condition that at time $t = 0$, the ink drop is concentrated at the origin, that is, in mathematical terms the initial condition is a Dirac delta function, the solution of equation [4.1] is the Gaussian function:

$$C(x,t) = \frac{1}{\sqrt{4\pi Dt}} e^{-\frac{x^2}{4Dt}} \qquad [4.2]$$

where $C(x,t)$ is the concentration and D is the diffusion coefficient. In Figure 4.1 (lower panel), the concentration is represented at three different time points. Three observations are of interest: (1) this physical system consists of two chemical species (salt and water or ink and water, for instance); (2) strictly speaking, D is the so-called *mutual diffusion coefficient*, as we are in a two-component, solvent–solution system; (3) the molecules of solvent diffuse under a macroscopic concentration gradient.

We consider now the spot size, which is a metric characterizing how particles diffuse in the solution. The displacement of ink particles could be taken as a measure of this diffusion process. However, when averaged over all particles, the mean displacement will be zero since particles equally spread in all directions. To overcome this problem, the mean *square* displacement is considered; thus, by taking the displacement of each particle, calculating the square of this value and then averaging over all particles, we obtain a metric that defines and characterizes the phenomenon of diffusion.

We can calculate the mean displacement – this is simple, since it is the integral of an odd-function (x) multiplied by an even function (C). Thus, by symmetry arguments the integral is zero, as expected:

$$\langle x \rangle = \int_{-\infty}^{\infty} xC(x,t)dx = 0 \qquad [4.3]$$

The calculation of the mean square displacement is more complicated and here we provide just the solution:

$$\langle x^2 \rangle = \int_{-\infty}^{\infty} x^2\, C(x,t)dx = 2Dt \qquad [4.4]$$

From this formula, we see that (1) the mean square displacement grows proportionally with time and (2) for a given time, the higher the diffusion coefficient, the bigger the spot size.

In 1905, Albert Einstein developed the theoretical framework of the diffusion phenomenon. For the interested reader, the collection of Einstein's papers related to diffusion are available and translated into English in Einstein and Fürth (1956). Einstein derived the following equation, for particles in a solution:

$$D = \frac{R}{N_a}\frac{T}{6\pi r\eta} \quad [4.5]$$

where R is the ideal gas constant, N_a is the Avogadro constant, T is the temperature, η is the viscosity of solvent and r is the effective radius of the diffusing particles; it should be noted that the Boltzmann constant k is equal to R/N_a.

From equation [4.5], we learn that (1) the diffusion coefficient depends on the temperature: the higher the temperature, the higher the diffusion coefficient; (2) the bigger the particle, the lower the diffusion coefficient; and (3) in contrast to Fick's law, which requires a concentration gradient for the diffusion to take place, equation [4.5] indicates that particles would undergo a diffusion motion even in the absence of a concentration gradient (!), as long as the temperature is different to 0 K. Thus, the thermal energy of the system drives a constant, random motion of particles in solution. In the same year, equation [4.5] was independently obtained by the physicist William Sutherland (1905). As part of Einstein's theory, which was based on the viscosity studies by the physicist George Stokes (1819–1903), equation [4.5] is called the Stokes–Einstein–Sutherland equation.

Now let us go back to the ink-water experiment and repeat the same experiment, but instead of using a drop of ink we use a drop of water. What happens to the water molecules contained in the water drop? If we could label these water molecules, we would observe a phenomenon similar to that observed with the ink, that is, the water molecules of the drop would diffuse and mix with the other water molecules in the Petri dish, driven by the thermal energy. All of this occurs in the *absence of a concentration gradient* as there is one chemical species only, that is, a one-component system. Here, strictly speaking, D is the so-called *self-diffusion coefficient*, since the molecules diffuse in an environment of identical molecules. Now, what would be the formula that governs the diffusion behavior of water molecules in water? Einstein found that the mean square displacement was given by the formula:

$$\langle x^2 \rangle = 2Dt \quad [4.6]$$

This formula is referred to as the Einstein diffusion equation, and it is valid in the case of diffusion along one dimension. For the case of two-dimensional and three-dimensional diffusion, the formula of the mean square displacement is $\langle x^2 \rangle = 4Dt$ and $\langle x^2 \rangle = 6Dt$, respectively.

The combination of the Einstein diffusion equation [4.6] with the Stokes–Einstein–Sutherland equation [4.5] would provide a new way, as Einstein suggested, to determine the Avogadro constant (by eliminating D from the two equations and measuring all of the remaining physical variables: the viscosity, the temperature and so on). This is exactly what Perrin (1910) did a few years later and his successful experiments were rewarded with the Nobel Prize in Physics in 1926.

One year after Einstein's work, the physicist Marian Smoluchowski (1906) derived the Einstein diffusion equation using a completely different approach: the concept of random walk, which is nowadays often employed to describe self-diffusion processes.

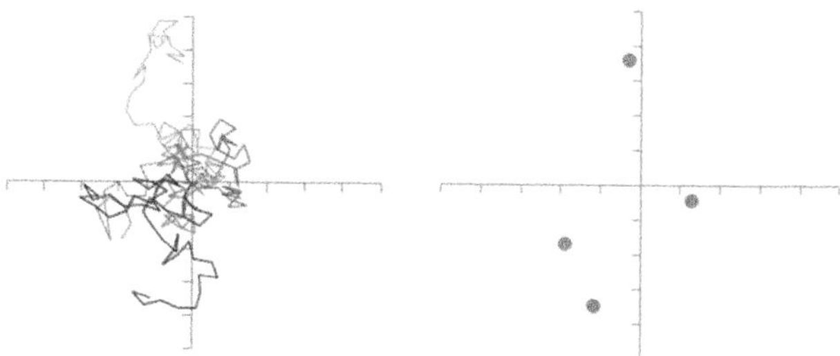

Figure 4.2. *Example of 2D random walk of four particles. Left panel: four particles start at the origin of the coordinate system and undergo 50 steps in random directions. Each path is shown in a different color. Right panel: the final position of each particle after 50 steps is illustrated by the gray markers*

In Figure 4.2, the random walk of four particles is illustrated. In this simple case, the mean square displacement can be determined by taking the average over the four particles of their square displacement (square displacement = the distance squared from the origin). In a real scenario for water molecules: each step corresponds to a collision with neighboring molecules and the number of collisions for a single molecule of water in a second is about 10^{14} (Feynman 1964). It should be also noted that, keeping in mind that $\langle x^2 \rangle$ is proportional to Dt, the displacement of a particle in random motion increases with the square-root of the time $\sqrt{t}$. This is in contrast to the displacement of a particle moving with a constant velocity along a straight line, where the displacement increases with the time t.

Before going to the next section, we take a step back to 1827, when the botanist Robert Brown (1828) observed under the microscope grains of pollen suspended in water that were constantly moving in a random fashion. Where was the energy animating these microscopic particles coming from? Were these particles a living organism? Intrigued by his first observations, Brown conducted a series of experiment to further investigate this phenomenon. He concluded that no biological factor was associated to this constant, random motion, since he observed that microscopic particles obtained from stones and suspended in a fluid would display a similar motion. Simply put, Brown took the life out of this random motion, which was later called "the Brownian motion". Almost a century later, Einstein demonstrated that the random motion of these particles (whether grains of pollen or stone powder) was due to the collision with water molecules and the thermal energy of the system was responsible for this random motion. At last, the scientific saga of Brownian motion that started in 1828 found its end with Einstein's work in 1905. Further details, information and anecdotes illustrating the impact of Brown's observations on the scientific community (over a century worth!) can be found in enlightened review articles (Brush 1968; Maiocchi 1990; Haw 2002; Duplantier 2006; Bigg 2008).

4.3. Diffusion and NMR

4.3.1. *First NMR measurements of diffusion*

Already in the very early NMR studies, such as the *Spin echoes* article by Erwin Hahn in 1950, the effect of the diffusion on the MR signal was detected and investigated (Hahn 1950). Simply put, the random motion of water molecules, in the presence of magnetic field inhomogeneity, resulted in a loss of signal. Hahn indeed observed that the diffusion of water molecules generated a signal attenuation, which could be written as:

$$\frac{S}{S_0} = e^{-\frac{1}{12}\gamma^2 G^2 TE^3 D} \qquad [4.7]$$

where S_0 is the signal in the absence of the magnetic field gradient G, TE is the echo time, D is the diffusion coefficient and γ is the gyromagnetic ratio. It is important to notice that in the experimental apparatus employed by Hahn, the magnetic field gradient G originated from the intrinsic inhomogeneity of the static magnetic field B_0.

In 1954, Carr and Purcell (1954) conducted more detailed investigations with the dual aim of (1) reducing the confounding factor introduced by the diffusion in the measurement of T_2 relaxation time and (2) measuring the diffusion coefficient of water. For the first aim, they introduced the idea of using a train of 180° pulses. For achieving the second aim, they applied a magnetic field gradient of 0.28 gauss/cm, generated with two circular turns of current-carrying wire. The gradient was always on throughout the measurement. The measured value of the diffusion coefficient of water at 25°C was equal to $2.5 \times 10^{-5}\ \mathrm{cm^2/s}$. They concluded that: *all methods for measurement of diffusion depend on somehow "labeling" molecules. To the extent that the 'label' has a negligible effect on the diffusion process itself, a method may be said to measure truly the "self-diffusion" constant. In the method here described a molecule is in effect labelled by the direction of the nuclear magnetic moment it carries; a more innocuous label would be difficult to imagine.*

4.3.2. Measurements of diffusion with pulsed gradients: the Stejskal and Tanner method

The major methodological improvement in the measurement of diffusion coefficients was proposed by Stejskal and Tanner in 1965. This approach, designed to eliminate certain experimental limitations of the method used by Carr and Purcell, represents the basis of diffusion MRI measurements nowadays. Stejskal and Tanner proposed the use of *magnetic field gradient pulses*, in contrast to the previous method where the magnetic field gradient was continuously on throughout the measurement. The gradient pulses are illustrated in Figure 4.3.

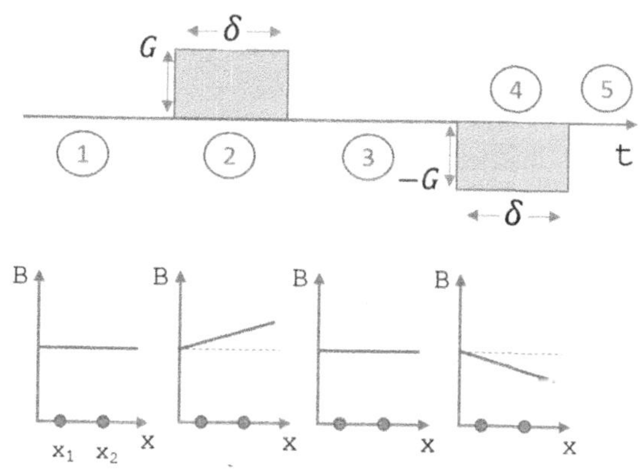

Figure 4.3. *The magnetic field gradient pulses employed in the Stejskal and Tanner method. Upper panel: G is the strength of the gradient pulse and δ the duration. Five time intervals are identified. Lower panel: the total magnetic field (B) as a function of the position along the x-axis. Two stationary water molecules, depicted on the x-axis, are located in position x_1 and x_2. In the absence of gradient pulses (time interval 1, 3 and 5), the total magnetic field is equal to the applied static magnetic field B_0*

We will analyze in detail the effect of gradient pulses, taken for simplicity along the x-direction, on the spin precession and therefore on the NMR signal. It should be pointed out that the direction of the magnetic field generated by a gradient pulse is always along the z-direction. For a G_x (G_y or G_z) gradient, it is just the magnetic field strength that changes linearly along the x-direction (y-direction or z-direction).

We consider five time intervals, as indicated in Figure 4.3. One water molecule is located in x_1 and another in x_2, along the x-axis. For the sake of clarity, we focus on one hydrogen nucleus only on each water molecule. We denote with s_1 (s_2) the spin of one hydrogen nucleus belonging to the water molecule located in x_1 (x_2). In the first time interval, in the absence of a gradient, the magnetic field along the x-axis will be uniform and equal to the static applied magnetic field B_0 (Figure 4.3, lower panel). During the second interval, a gradient pulse of strength G and duration δ is applied; the total magnetic field B varies linearly along the x-axis. Thus, the two water molecules will experience a different magnetic field and their spins will precess at different angular frequency, as dictated by the Larmor equation, $\omega = \gamma B$, where ω is the angular frequency, γ the gyromagnetic ratio and B the total magnetic field. The spin s_2 will precess faster than the spin s_1, since it experiences a stronger magnetic field. As a result of their different resonance frequency, at the end of the second interval there will be a dephasing between s_1 and s_2, which can be calculated as follows. The relation between the phase φ and angular frequency is $\omega = \varphi/t$, where t is the time. Thus, $\varphi = \omega t = \gamma B t$. Neglecting the contribution of B_0, since this contribution is similar for s_1 and s_2, the magnetic field in x_1 is Gx_1 and in x_2 is Gx_2. At the end of the gradient pulse ($t = \delta$), the phase acquired by the spin s_1 is $\varphi_1 = \gamma G x_1 \delta$ and for the spin s_2 is $\varphi_2 = \gamma G x_2 \delta$.

In the third interval, the dephasing is not changing, as s_1 and s_2 precess at the same angular frequency. During the fourth interval, the spin s_1 will precess faster than the spin s_2. At the end of the second gradient pulse, this gradient has induced a phase equal to $\varphi_1 = -\gamma G x_1 \delta$ for s_1 and $\varphi_2 = -\gamma G x_2 \delta$ for s_2; in other words, a phase equal and opposite to the one induced by the first gradient. Thus, for stationary spins, this second gradient has compensated the dephasing induced by the first gradient. During the fifth interval, as s_1 and s_2 are precessing at the same angular frequency and, more importantly, have the same phase. This is the case for stationary, nondiffusing water molecules.

What happens in the presence of diffusion? The water molecules will change position (during the third interval, for example, and the new position is x_1' and x_2'); the dephasing induced by the second gradient $\varphi_1 = -\gamma G x_1' \delta$ and $\varphi_2 = -\gamma G x_2' \delta$ will not compensate the one induced by the first gradient and we will observe a signal loss.

For a general formulation of the problem in three dimensions, we consider a magnetic field gradient $\boldsymbol{G}$ applied along an arbitrary direction. The resonance angular frequency is given by:

$$\omega(\boldsymbol{r}) = \gamma(B_0 + \boldsymbol{G} \cdot \boldsymbol{r}) \qquad [4.8]$$

where $\boldsymbol{r}$ is the position of the molecule. Given that in general $\omega = d\varphi/dt$, by integrating this equation we obtain the general formula of the gradient-induced phase for any type of gradient shape (trapezoidal or sinusoidal shape, for example) and timings:

$$\varphi(\boldsymbol{r}) = \gamma \int_0^t \boldsymbol{G}(\tau) \cdot \boldsymbol{r}(\tau) d\tau \qquad [4.9]$$

In the case of a rectangular gradient along the x-axis, the integral can be easily solved and we find back the formulae of φ previously developed for s_1 and s_2.

We are now ready to set up an experiment for measuring the diffusion coefficient of water using NMR. Following Stejskal and Tanner, we include two gradient pulses into a spin-echo sequence to obtain the pulsed gradient spin echo (PGSE) scheme, as shown in Figure 4.4. It should be noted here that the polarity of the second gradient is the same as that of the first gradient – in contrast to the scheme of Figure 4.3 – since the refocusing RF pulse has the effect of reversing the phase induced by the first gradient.

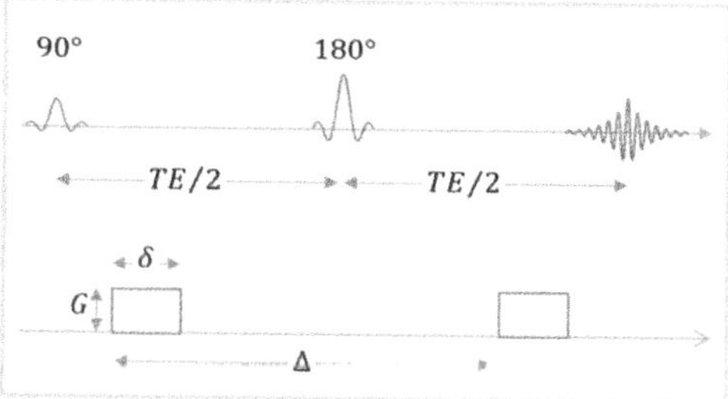

Figure 4.4. *The pulsed gradient spin echo (PGSE) sequence proposed by Stejskal and Tanner in 1965. TE is the echo time; G and δ are the strength and duration of the diffusion sensitizing gradient, respectively. Increasing the diffusion time Δ comes at the expense of an increased TE*

The PGSE scheme is the most commonly used approach nowadays. Other ways to generate a diffusion-weighted (DW) signal include: (1) the stimulated echo

(PGSTE) scheme (Tanner 1970), shown in Figure 4.5, where the gradients are positioned during the TE/2 time intervals; (2) the double echo; and (3) the steady-state free precession (SSFP) (Buxton 1993). When comparing the PGSTE to PGSE: the disadvantage of the PGSTE is the well-known 50% signal loss compared to the PGSE (Tanner 1970). On the other hand, the advantage of the PGSTE is that the time interval Δ, also called diffusion (or observation) time, can be extended without increasing the echo time. In other words, longer diffusion times will not yield a signal loss from T_2 relaxation decay when using the PGSTE. We will see later that varying the diffusion time could be useful for investigations of tissue microstructure. It should be noted that magnetic field gradient pulses are ubiquitous in the MRI sequences, in particular for the spatial encoding of the MR signal. When gradient pulses are employed to generate dephasing of diffusing spins, they are typically called "diffusion-sensitizing gradients".

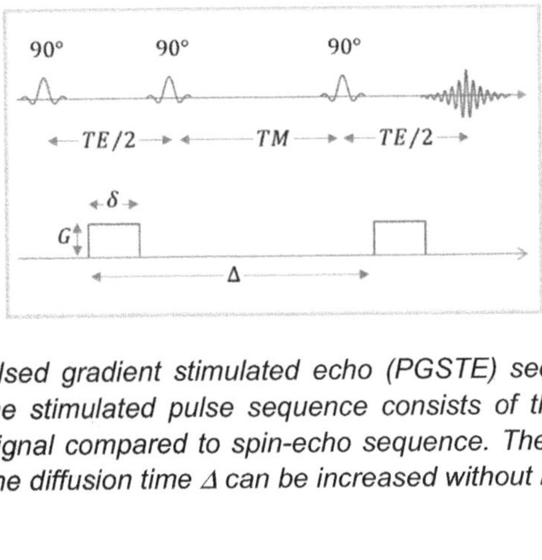

Figure 4.5. *The pulsed gradient stimulated echo (PGSTE) sequence proposed by Tanner in 1970. The stimulated pulse sequence consists of three 90° pulses and yields 50% of the signal compared to spin-echo sequence. The TM is the so-called mixing time. Here, the diffusion time Δ can be increased without increasing the TE*

In general, the signal intensity for an MR diffusion experiment can be written as:

$$\frac{S}{S_0} = e^{-bD} \qquad [4.10]$$

where S_0 is the signal intensity without the diffusion-sensitizing gradients; it depends on experimental settings and in particular on the echo time TE; thus, S_0 includes the decay due T_2 relaxation. D is the diffusion coefficient, measured along the direction of the diffusion-sensitizing gradients. The parameter b, called b-value, is given by the following formula:

$$b = \gamma^2 G^2 \delta^2 (\Delta - \delta/3) \qquad [4.11]$$

The b-value includes all of the factors that determine the diffusion weighting, that is, G, δ and Δ. It should be noted that the b-value in DW MRI has the same role as the echo time TE in T_2-weighted MR imaging. The greater the b-value, the stronger the diffusion weighting. With respect to the units of D and b: the most intuitive unit of the diffusion coefficient, when dealing with diffusion phenomena of water in tissues, would be $\mu m^2/ms$ since over a time scale of milliseconds the displacement of water molecules is micrometers. A number of MR scientists have used this unit over the years. However, nowadays the most established unit of the diffusion coefficient in the MR community is mm^2/s. As a result, from equation [4.10], it can noted that the unit of b is s/mm^2.

CALCULATION OF B-VALUES.–

Example 1. The reader can verify by a simple calculation that a b-value close to $1{,}000\ s/mm^2$ ($b = 993\ s/mm^2$) can be obtained with the following parameters: $G = 20$ mT/m, $\delta = 35$ ms and $\Delta = 40$ ms. The value of the gyromagnetic ratio is $\gamma = 2.675 \times 10^8 s^{-1}T^{-1}$. With this choice of parameters, the minimum echo time would not be less than 75 ms (i.e. $\Delta + \delta$) in the PGSE scheme.

Example 2. A b-value ($b = 1{,}016\ s/mm^2$) similar to the one of Example 1 could be obtained by increasing the gradient strength to $G = 39$ mT/m and with $\delta = 20$ ms and $\Delta = 30$ ms. This experimental set-up allows for a shorter TE, thus minimizing the signal loss due to T_2 relaxation.

The gradient strength of typical MRI clinical systems nowadays is around 40 mT/m, with high-performance systems achieving 80 mT/m and even 300 mT/m (McNab et al. 2013). Equation [4.11] of the b-value is valid for the scheme shown in Figures 4.4 and 4.5. In general, the b-value for gradients of any given shape (trapezoidal or sinusoidal shape, for example) and timings, applied between $t = 0$ and $t = TE$, can be obtained by calculating the following integral:

$$b = \gamma^2 \int_0^{TE} \left(\int_0^t G(t')dt' \right)^2 dt \qquad [4.12]$$

From equation [4.10], it can be observed that to measure the diffusion coefficient D it is sufficient to acquire two data sets: one data set with a b-value $b = 0\ s/mm^2$, which will provide S_0, and a second data set (S_1) with a nonzero b-value. This value can be chosen to be equal to the reciprocal of the expected value of diffusion coefficient, that is, $b = 1/D$. The value of D will be easily calculated as:

$$D = \frac{1}{b} ln\left(\frac{S_0}{S_1}\right) \qquad [4.13]$$

In practice, for improved accuracy and better characterization of the diffusion signal decay, multiple measurements are performed with different b-values, obtained by increasing the gradient strength G. The diffusion coefficient D is then determined by an exponential fitting of the data, as of equation [4.10].

The most common approach of increasing the b-value is to change the gradient strength G. Another strategy is to increase the diffusion (or observation) time Δ. The diffusion time is the time interval during which the diffusion process is being observed. It provides a means to gain insight into tissue microstructure; in particular, by changing the value of Δ, we can gain information on restricted diffusion and on the compartment size of the biological structures that contribute to impede the free motion of water. Specifically, as shown in Figure 4.6, by using a "long" diffusion time Δ, we have the opportunity to distinguish tissues where water molecules remain confined from tissues where there is no restriction to water diffusion. With this MR diffusion-based approach, in 1968, Tanner and Stejskal investigated a number of systems displaying restricted diffusion and determined, for instance, the size of yeast cells (Tanner and Stejskal 1968).

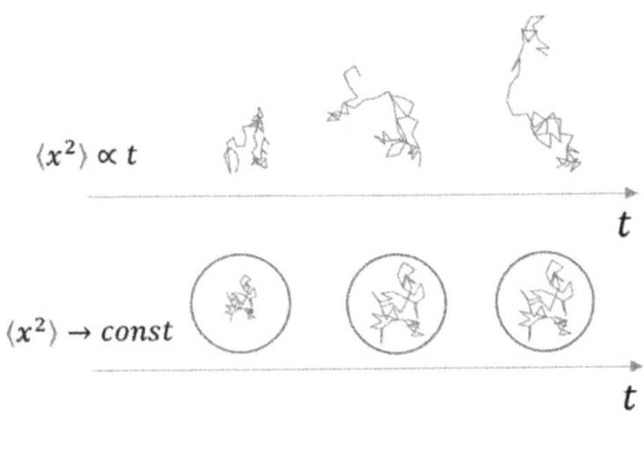

Figure 4.6. *The random walk of a particle for free, unrestricted diffusion (top) and restricted diffusion – in a spherical confinement, for instance – (bottom), at three time points. The mean square displacement increases linearly with time in unrestricted diffusion, whereas in a restricted environment it tends to a constant value*

Before going on to the section dedicated to diffusion MRI, we will make two observations. Firstly, in 1965, Stejskal (1965) referred to the diffusion coefficient as *apparent diffusion coefficient*, in reference to a previous work by Woessner (1963), where the diffusion coefficient of water molecules confined in porous rocks was measured. This was an example of restricted diffusion. Stejskal used the term *apparent* diffusion coefficient to indicate that the measured value of the diffusion coefficient was dependent on the experimental parameters (namely, the diffusion time, as seen Figure 4.6). Secondly, in the same study, Stejskal considered the case of anisotropic diffusion and introduced the concept of diffusion tensor into the Bloch-Torrey equations. In 1956, years before the work by Stejskal and Tanner, Torrey (1956) included the effect of diffusion into the Bloch equations, by introducing the diffusion coefficient D, as a scalar. It is only afterwards that Stejskal replaced the scalar D in the Bloch–Torrey equations with the diffusion tensor to account for the situation where particles undergo an anisotropic diffusion (Stejskal 1965). We will provide more details regarding the diffusion tensor in the next sections.

4.4. Water diffusion in biological tissues

Over the timescale of milliseconds, the displacements of water molecules in biological tissues are of the order of micrometers (see equation [4.6]), which correspond to the dimension of cells, organelles, etc. Thus, water molecules can be viewed as molecular probes to investigate tissue microstructure. In general, the diffusion coefficient of water in tissues is smaller than in pure water; this is because the water displacements in tissues are impeded by tissue components (cell membranes, macromolecules and so on), which may act as permeable, semi-permeable or impermeable barriers to the diffusion motion. The different scenarios of water diffusion in biological tissues can be generally classified in four broad categories and two examples are depicted in Figure 4.7.

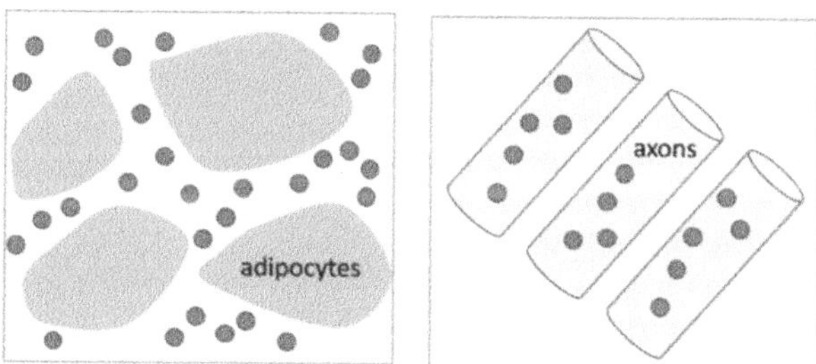

Figure 4.7. Hindered versus restricted diffusion. The blue circles represent water molecules. Left panel: an example of hindered diffusion; water diffusion is strongly impeded by the adipocytes (fat-containing cell) in bone marrow. Right panel: an example of restricted diffusion; water molecules diffuse inside the myelinated axons in white matter

(1) Free, unrestricted diffusion: the water molecules diffuse as in a liquid, without obstacles that impede the random motion. This is the case for water in the CSF, for instance. (2) Hindered diffusion: water diffusion is impeded by

impermeable barriers, as it occurs in bone marrow for instance, where the adipocytes (fat-storing cells) represent impermeable barriers to the water motion as shown in Figure 4.7 (left panel). (3) Restricted diffusion: the water molecules are confined within a tissue structure by impermeable barriers, as it occurs in white matter axons (Figure 4.7, right panel). Furthermore, the water diffusion is also anisotropic given the axon cylindrical geometry. It should be noted that the water molecules are also present outside the axons (extra-axonal water molecules). For clarity, these molecules have not been illustrated in Figure 4.7. The extra-axonal water molecules do undergo hindered diffusion, since their motion is impeded by impermeable barriers (Assaf et al. 2004). (4) The fourth scenario includes the behavior of water diffusion in many tissues/organs, such as muscle, liver and prostate. This is the case where the water diffusion motion is generally impeded by tissue structures that behave as semi-permeable barriers (such as cell membranes) and by interaction with organelles and macromolecules, for instance: yet, in this case, the diffusion is neither purely hindered nor purely restricted.

Previously in this chapter we observed that the diffusion of water molecules in pure water is characterized by a Gaussian behavior that results in the mono-exponential signal decay, as given in equation [4.10]. On the other hand, biological tissues are a complex environment that affect water diffusion and, as a result, the diffusion signal as a function of the b-value may deviate from a mono-exponential decay. This deviation becomes more evident when acquiring data at higher b-values (Figure 4.8). A number of models have been proposed to account for this non-mono-exponential diffusion behavior (Yablonskiy and Sukstanskii 2010).

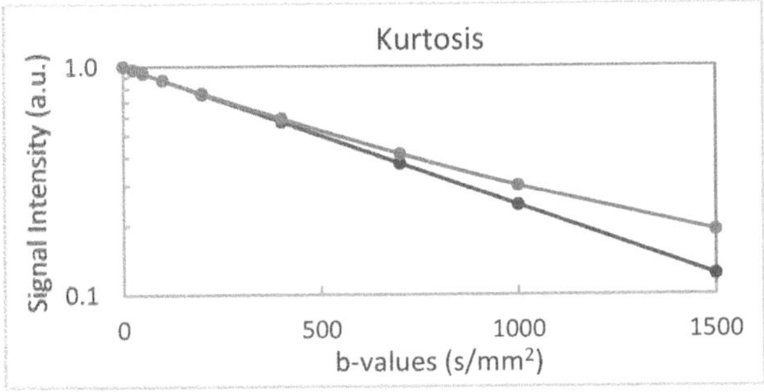

Figure 4.8. *The diffusion decay of the signal intensity for the kurtosis model (line in orange color) with* $D = 1.4 \times 10^{-3}\, mm^2/s$ *and* $K = 0.6$. *For reference, a mono-exponential signal decay is also illustrated (line in blue color). Data are plotted on a logarithmic scale for the vertical axis to highlight the deviation of the kurtosis model from the mono-exponential behavior*

The kurtosis model is one of these models (Jensen and Helpern 2010) and is represented in Figure 4.8, where we employ a plot with a logarithmic scale on the vertical axis (semi-log plot). The advantage of using this semi-log plot is that mono-exponential decays appear as a straight line, so any deviation from the mono-exponential behavior results in a deviation from a straight line, which is then easily observable by simple visual inspection. The formula of the kurtosis signal is provided in equation [4.14], where S_0, D and b have the same meaning as in equation [4.10] and K is the kurtosis coefficient. The origin of the non-Gaussian diffusion behavior can be ascribed to the presence of diffusion barriers and compartments in tissues; thus, K is strongly dependent on the tissue microstructure, and it can be viewed as *a measure of the heterogeneity of the diffusion environment* (Jensen and Helpern 2010).

$$\frac{S}{S_0} = e^{-bD+(bD)^2K/6} \qquad [4.14]$$

Overall, in biological tissues, the order of magnitude of the diffusion coefficient D is $10^{-3}\ \mathrm{mm^2/s}$. The reader should be aware that the measured value of D depends on the MRI pulse sequence parameters, such as the choice and the number of b-values, and in the literature we may find different values of D for the same given tissue (Taouli and Koh 2010). For pure water, the diffusion coefficient value is $D \sim 3 \times 10^{-3}\ \mathrm{mm^2/s}$ at body temperature (37°C) and $D \sim 1 \times 10^{-3}\ \mathrm{mm^2/s}$ at 0°C (Holz et al. 2000), with the temperature dependence being highlighted in equation [4.5]. As a matter of fact, a water phantom surrounded by an ice bath that keeps the temperature stable at 0°C can be used as a test phantom for quality control measurements of MRI pulse sequences and clinical scanners (Chenevert et al. 2011).

4.5. Diffusion magnetic resonance imaging

4.5.1. *Diffusion MRI pulse sequences*

Nowadays, diffusion MRI is a well-established technique, routinely employed in diagnostic MRI protocols, for different organs and therapeutic domains. It is also a technique in continuous development for both novel data-acquisition and data-modeling methods. To generate DW MR images, that is, images with a signal intensity sensitive to the diffusion characteristics of water molecules, it is necessary to combine a diffusion preparation module with an imaging module. In Figure 4.8, a scheme of a diffusion MRI sequence is illustrated: the PGSE proposed by Stejskal and Tanner, which was shown in Figure 4.4, is followed by a single-shot echo planar imaging (SS-EPI) module. SS-EPI is the most commonly used imaging module for DW MRI. The advantages of SS-EPI include speed, which also makes this sequence robust to motion; disadvantages include image artifacts such as spatial and intensity distortions. These image artifacts may arise from (1) magnetic field inhomogeneity, as it occurs around tissue/air interfaces due to susceptibility differences, for instance, and (2) eddy currents, which can be particularly intense as they originate from the strong diffusion-sensitizing gradients.

Many methods to mitigate these image artifacts have been developed in recent years. As an example, one method for correcting distortions originating from magnetic field inhomogeneity is the reversed gradient polarity method (Andersson et al. 2003), which requires the acquisition of an additional image with the phase encoding gradient of opposite polarity compared to the first acquisition. With respect to the eddy currents, the dual spin echo approach, for instance, helps for reducing the eddy-current-induced distortions (Reese et al. 2003). This method consists of combining diffusion-sensitizing gradients into a double spin echo, rather than into a single spin echo module, at the expenses of a longer echo time.

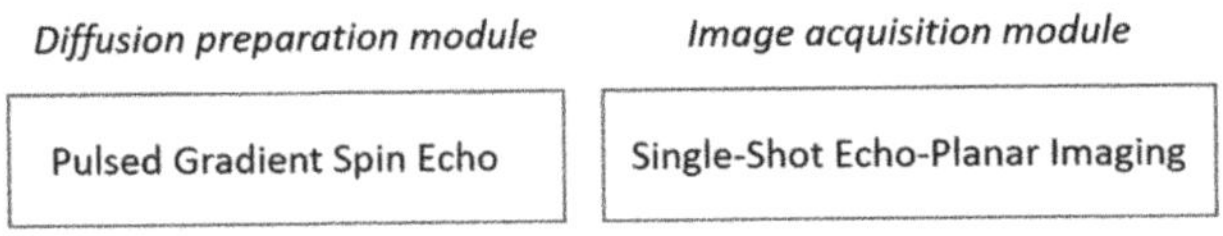

Figure 4.9. *A simplified scheme of a typical diffusion-weighted MR imaging sequence. A diffusion preparation module, usually the pulsed gradient spin echo (PGSE) is followed by the spatial encoding of the signal, often done with single-shot echo planar imaging (SS-EPI)*

To overcome some of the limitations of the single-shot EPI, multi-shot EPI approaches have been proposed. A notable example is the read-out segmentation of long variable echo train (RESOLVE) sequence, which employs 2D navigator correction with readout-segmented EPI acquisitions of the k-space (Porter and Heidemann 2009). The advantages of the RESOLVE sequence over SS-EPI include (1) the acquisition of images at higher spatial resolution and (2) the shortening of the EPI echo train, which helps to mitigate image distortions and blurring artifacts. The disadvantage of the RESOLVE sequence, in comparison to the single-shot approach, is the longer acquisition time.

4.5.2. *Applications of DW-MRI*

DW MR images are routinely acquired in many clinical MRI protocols. This is particularly true in patients with suspected cancer. As an example, we consider firstly the case of prostate cancer. DW-MRI is one of the three modalities of the multiparametric MRI (mpMRI) protocol for prostate cancer, with the other two modalities being T_2-weighted (T_2w) imaging and dynamic contrast-enhanced MRI (DCE-MRI). The MR images obtained with the mpMRI protocol are evaluated within the framework of the Prostate Imaging Reporting and Data System (PI-RADS) (Weinreb et al. 2016). The PI-RADS was developed to standardize image acquisition, interpretation and reporting of mpMRI, with the aim of improving detection, localization and characterization of prostate cancer. Figure 4.10 shows an example of parametric map of the apparent diffusion coefficient, obtained by exponential fitting of the signal from images acquired at multiple b-values in the range $0 - 1{,}000\ \mathrm{s/mm^2}$. It should be noted that in the MRI literature the term *apparent diffusion coefficient* and *diffusion coefficient* are often used interchangeably.

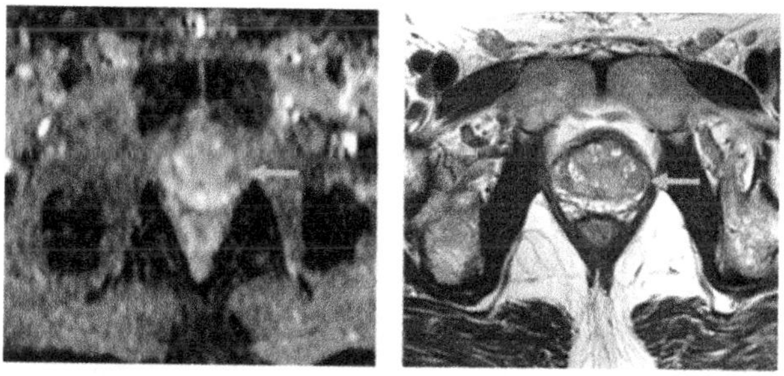

Figure 4.10. *Axial MR images of the pelvis of a prostate cancer patient. Left panel: the parametric apparent diffusion coefficient (ADC) map, with the arrow indicating the location of the cancer. The ADC in prostate cancer is lower than that in healthy prostate tissue, due to the higher cell density that impedes the diffusion of water molecules. Right panel: T_2-weighted (T_2w) MR image*

Another example of DW-MRI with application in the field of oncology is shown in Figure 4.11, with MR images of brain in a patient with meningioma.

An axial DW MR image and the ADC parametric map are illustrated in Figure 4.11, central and right panel, respectively. Here, the ADC map is obtained from data acquired at two b-values only. In this example, it is of interest to note that the MR image at $b = 0\ \mathrm{s/mm^2}$ (Figure 4.11, left panel) displays a T_2-weighting. As a matter of fact, in order to accommodate the diffusion gradients in the spin-echo diffusion preparation module, a relatively long TE (typically ~100 ms) is necessary. Thus, the ensuing T_2-weighting yields a high signal intensity for tissues with a long T_2 relaxation time, like the peritumoral edema in this case. In the diffusion parametric map (Figure 4.11, right panel), the edema region displays a diffusion coefficient value higher than the one of the surrounding brain tissue, as the water molecules can move more freely in the edematous tissue environment.

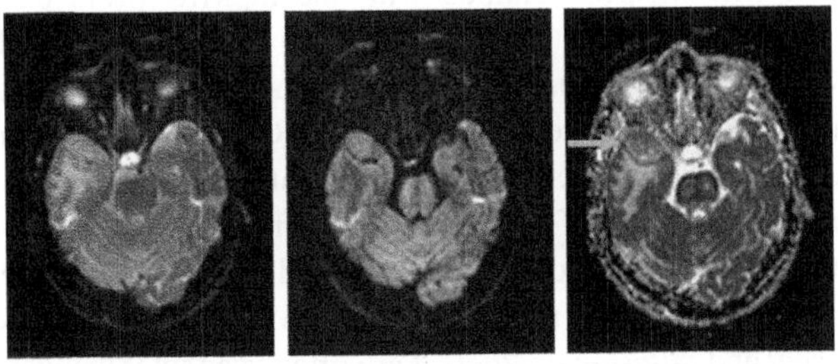

$b = 0\ (s/mm^2)$ $b = 1000\ (s/mm^2)$ $ADC\ map$

Figure 4.11. *Axial diffusion MR images and diffusion parametric map of brain in a patient with meningioma. The meningioma is indicated by the arrow on the ADC map and can also be easily identified as the round shaped structure on the image at* $b = 1{,}000\ s/mm^2$. *The vasogenic peritumoral edema, characterized by a long* T_2 *relaxation time, displays a high signal intensity on the image at* $b = 0\ s/mm^2$

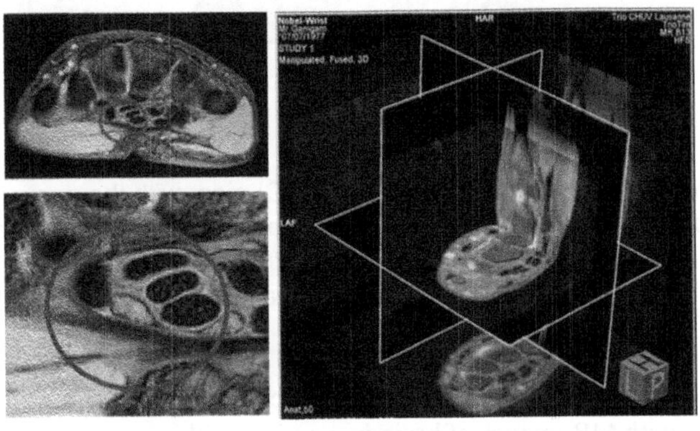

Figure 4.12. *MRI of median nerve in a healthy volunteer. Left panel, top: axial MR image of the wrist. Left panel, bottom: zoom-in of the carpal tunnel, with the median nerve at the center of the red circle. Left panel: nerve tractography, with the nerve depicted in blue colors*

Another important application of DW-MRI is the diffusion tensor imaging (DTI), which allows for *tracking* tissue structures characterized by anisotropic diffusion (Basser et al. 1994). This modality has been extensively applied to brain imaging and is useful both in clinical settings – for neurosurgical planning, for instance – and in a research setting, for investigating brain structure and function (Assaf and Pasternak 2008; Alexander et al. 2007; McNab et al. 2013). DTI applications also include investigations of other tissues that are characterized by anisotropic diffusion of water, such as peripheral nerve and muscle, etc. An example of DTI applied to peripheral nerve tracking is shown in Figure 4.12: in this case, the DTI approach is of interest to assess peripheral nerve axonal degeneration and regeneration, for instance (Howe et al. 1992; Takagi et al. 2009).

We provide here some details about the DTI formalism (Basser et al. 1994; Alexander et al. 2007). It was previously mentioned that when dealing with anisotropic diffusion, the diffusion coefficient being a scalar (i.e. is a single numeric value) cannot adequately describe the diffusion characteristics of the tissue. A more sophisticated mathematical approach is necessary, where diffusion is characterized by the diffusion tensor, represented by a 3 × 3 matrix as follows:

$$\begin{pmatrix} D_{xx} & D_{xy} & D_{xz} \\ D_{yx} & D_{yy} & D_{yz} \\ D_{zx} & D_{zy} & D_{zz} \end{pmatrix} \qquad [4.15]$$

This matrix is symmetric (i.e. $D_{ij} = D_{ji}$), thus is characterized by six distinct elements. As a result, six measurements with diffusion gradients applied in six noncollinear directions, plus one measurement with $b = 0\ \text{s/mm}^2$, are necessary to identify the elements of the matrix. In practice, many gradient directions (for instance, 30 or more) are acquired, as proposed in methods such as the high angular resolution diffusion imaging (HARDI) (Tuch 2004). Once the matrix is diagonalized, we obtain the following matrix:

$$\begin{pmatrix} \lambda_1 & 0 & 0 \\ 0 & \lambda_2 & 0 \\ 0 & 0 & \lambda_3 \end{pmatrix} \qquad [4.16]$$

where λ_1, λ_2 and λ_3 are the diffusion tensor eigenvalues, ranged in descending order with respect to their magnitude. For each eigenvalue λ_i, we have an associated eigenvector $\boldsymbol{\epsilon}_i$. The eigenvalue λ_1 represents the diffusion along the direction of maximal diffusivity $\boldsymbol{\epsilon}_1$. For example, in the case of white matter axons, λ_1 is the diffusion coefficient along the direction of the axon and the eigenvector $\boldsymbol{\epsilon}_1$ provides the direction of the axon; the eigenvalues λ_2 and λ_3 represents the diffusion coefficient along the directions $\boldsymbol{\epsilon}_2$ and $\boldsymbol{\epsilon}_3$ perpendicular to the axon. A number of useful metrics can be derived from the DTI formalism; among these metrics, we point out the mean diffusivity (MD), defined as the average value of the three eigenvalues:

$$MD = \frac{1}{3}(\lambda_1 + \lambda_2 + \lambda_3) \quad [4.17]$$

The MD provides a global measure of tissue diffusion. It is the equivalent to the diffusion coefficient D for tissues with isotropic diffusion. Another important metric is the fractional anisotropy (FA) defined as:

$$FA = \sqrt{\frac{3}{2}}\sqrt{\frac{(\lambda_1 - MD)^2 + (\lambda_2 - MD)^2 + (\lambda_3 - MD)^2}{\lambda_1^2 + \lambda_2^2 + \lambda_3^2}} \quad [4.18]$$

The FA provides the degree of anisotropy, that is, a measure of the departure from the isotropic diffusion behavior. The values of FA are between 0 and 1. When $\lambda_1 = \lambda_2 = \lambda_3$ (isotropic diffusion), FA is zero. When $\lambda_1 \gg \lambda_2, \lambda_3$, as it occurs in tissues with a highly anisotropic water diffusion, like white matter, for instance, the FA approaches the value of 1.

In Figure 4.12, we have shown an example of fiber tracking (i.e. tractography) applied to peripheral nerve. For brain imaging, we invite the reader to explore the spectacular 3D images visualizing the white matter fiber architecture, with association pathways connecting cortical areas, on websites such as the Human Connectome Project (see: http://www.humanconnectomeproject.org).

To conclude this section, we will point to another important application of diffusion MRI: the radiological examination of patients who have suffered a stroke. In particular, on DW MR images the signal of the infarct area is hyperintense compared to the healthy tissue, that is, the diffusion motion of water molecules is slower in the infarct area. From a historical point of view, this was the first striking application of diffusion MRI: in preclinical model of acute cerebral ischemia it was observed by Moseley et al. (1990) that (1) the DW MR images allowed for an early detection of the infarct area and (2) the change in the signal intensity of diffusion MR images would precede any change in signal intensity of T_2-weighted images. As such, the diffusion coefficient of water could be considered to be a biomarker of early detection of tissue damage following cerebral ischemia.

4.6. IntraVoxel Incoherent Motion MRI

Biological tissues are heterogeneous and complex; furthermore, they are characterized by multiple compartments. One compartment virtually ubiquitous in all tissues is the capillary network. Thus, for a given tissue we can consider a two-compartment model that consists of the capillary component (the intravascular compartment) and the remaining tissue component (the extravascular compartment, which will be simply denoted here as tissue compartment). This is the IntraVoxel Incoherent Motion (IVIM) model (Le Bihan et al. 1986). The tissue compartment is characterized by the diffusion coefficient D. But how about the intravascular compartment? Given the intricate and random layout of the capillary network, when blood is flowing in the capillaries, the flow of water molecules mimics a random motion similar to the water diffusion in tissues (Figure 4.13). To quantify this diffusion-like motion of water in capillaries, a pseudo-diffusion coefficient, called D^*, is introduced. The pseudo-diffusion coefficient turns out to be higher than the tissue diffusion coefficient D, since the velocity of water in capillaries is faster than in tissues.

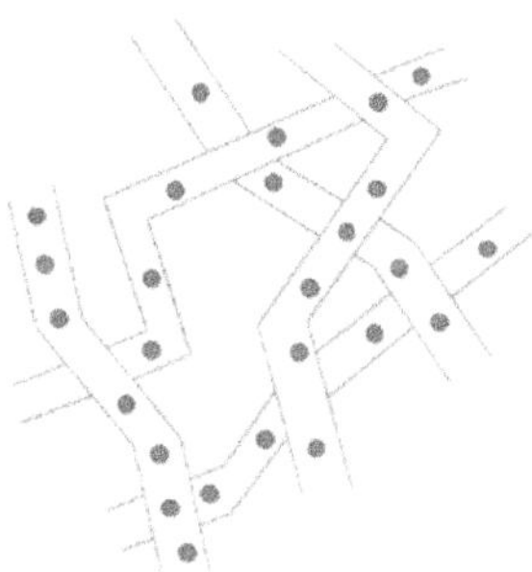

Figure 4.13. *The IntraVoxel Incoherent Motion (IVIM). The capillary component is illustrated here, with the blue circles representing the water molecules. Given the random and intricate configuration of the capillary network, the flow of water molecules in capillaries resembles to a random, diffusion motion, characterized by a pseudo-diffusion coefficient* D^*

The two-compartment IVIM model can be represented using the following formalism:

$$\frac{S(b)}{S_0} = f \cdot e^{-bD^*} + (1-f) \cdot e^{-bD} \qquad [4.19]$$

where S_0 is the signal intensity without the diffusion-sensitizing gradients, f is denoted as the *perfusion fraction*, D is the tissue diffusion coefficient and D^* is the pseudo-diffusion coefficient ($D^* \gg D$). In other words, the MRI signal as a function of the b-values displays two components, with the fast diffusion component being associated to the tissue perfusion and the slower component representing the tissue diffusion. It should be noted that in the IVIM model the perfusion fraction f is equivalent to capillary blood volume fraction in a voxel (Bihan and Turner 1992).

From an experimental point of view, to quantify the IVIM parameters D, D^* and f, DW-MR images are acquired with different diffusion-sensitizing gradients, from small ($0 - 100\ \mathrm{s/mm^2}$) to greater ($100 - 1{,}000\ \mathrm{s/mm^2}$) b-values. A schematic representation of the IVIM MRI data acquisition, data analysis and output is provided in Figure 4.14.

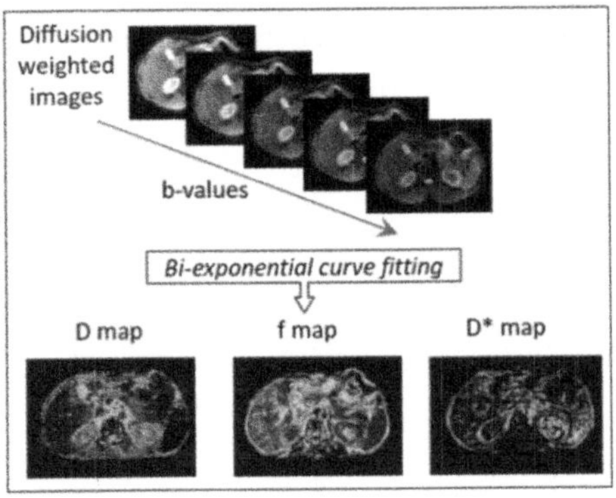

Figure 4.14. *The IntraVoxel Incoherent Motion (IVIM) MRI. MR images are acquired at different b-values; fitting the data to a bi-exponential function yields parametric maps of D (the tissue diffusion coefficient), f (the perfusion fraction) and D* (the pseudo-diffusion coefficient). In this example, axial MR images of the liver are shown*

The MR signal corresponding to the IVIM bi-exponential model is shown in Figure 4.15. The tissue parameters used in this plot are the following: $D = 1.4 \times 10^{-3}\ \mathrm{mm^2/s}$, $D^* = 40 \times 10^{-3}\ \mathrm{mm^2/s}$ and $f = 0.20$. For reference, the mono-exponential signal decay corresponding to single compartment with $D = 1.4 \times 10^{-3}\ \mathrm{mm^2/s}$ is plotted. It can be noted that in the IVIM bi-exponential model, the fast decaying signal at small b-values corresponds to the tissue perfusion component. Tissue perfusion and diffusion measurements, using the IVIM-MRI have been performed nowadays on all main organs/tissues, such as brain, breast, liver, muscle, bone marrow and prostate (Bihan et al. 2018).

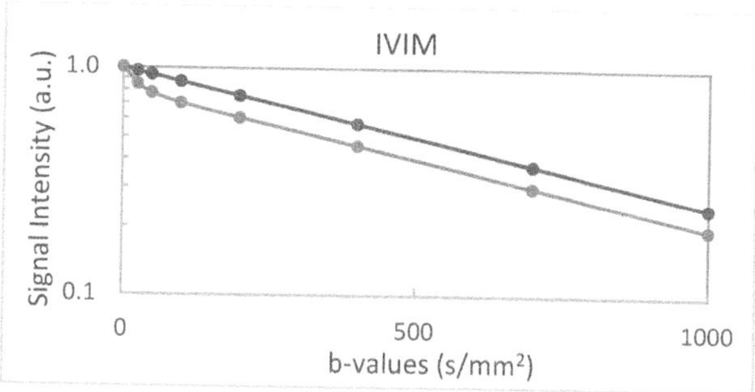

Figure 4.15. *The bi-exponential diffusion decay of the signal intensity for the IVIM model (line in orange color). For reference, a mono-exponential signal decay is also illustrated (line in blue color). Data are plotted on a logarithmic scale for the vertical axis to highlight the two components of the IVIM model*

4.7. Conclusion

In this chapter, we have provided a brief overview of the phenomenon of diffusion: from the observations of Brown in 1827 to the physical model of Einstein – in his 1905 *annus mirabilis* – and then to the breakthrough 1965 MR experiments of Stejskal and Tanner, to finally arrive to the clinical MRI applications. MRI is a unique imaging modality that allows for noninvasive measurement of the diffusion properties of water molecules in tissues. In diffusion MRI, water molecules can be viewed as microscopic probes to investigate tissue microstructure. Nowadays, diffusion MRI is an essential diagnostic tool with applications to different organs and therapeutic domains. It is a very active domain of research that continues to inspire ruminations (Mulkern et al. 2009), novel biophysical models and experimental approaches (Jelescu and Budde 2017), to improve our knowledge of the human body.

4.8. References

Alexander, A.L., Lee, J.E., Lazar, M., Field, A.S. (2007). Diffusion tensor imaging of the brain. *Neurotherapeutics*, 4(3), 316–329.

Andersson, J.L.R., Skare, S., Ashburner, J. (2003). How to correct susceptibility distortions in spin-echo echo-planar images: Application to diffusion tensor imaging. *NeuroImage*, 20(2), 870–888.

Assaf, Y. and Pasternak, O. (2008). Diffusion tensor imaging (DTI)-based white matter mapping in brain research: A review. *Journal of Molecular Neuroscience*, 34(1), 51–61.

Assaf, Y., Freidlin, R.Z., Rohde, G.K., Basser, P.J. (2004). New modeling and experimental framework to characterize hindered and restricted water diffusion in brain white matter. *Magnetic Resonance in Medicine*, 52(5), 965–978.

Basser, P.J., Mattiello, J., LeBihan, D. (1994). MR diffusion tensor spectroscopy and imaging. *Biophysical Journal*, 66(1), 259–267.

Bigg, C. (2008). Evident atoms: Visuality in Jean Perrin's Brownian motion research. *Studies in History and Philosophy of Science Part A*, 39(3), 312–322.

Bihan, D.L. and Turner, R. (1992). The capillary network: A link between ivim and classical perfusion. *Magnetic Resonance in Medicine*, 27(1), 171–178.

Bihan, D.L., Iima, M., Federau, C., Sigmund, E.E. (2018). *Intravoxel Incoherent Motion (IVIM). MRI: Principles and Applications.* Jenny Stanford Publishing, Boca Raton.

Brown, R. (1828). XXVII. A brief account of microscopical observations made in the months of June, July and August 1827. *The Philosophical Magazine*, 4(21), 161–173.

Brush, S.G. (1968). A history of random processes. *Archive for History of Exact Sciences*, 5(1), 1–36.

Buxton, R.B. (1993). The diffusion sensitivity of fast steady-state free precession imaging. *Magnetic Resonance in Medicine*, 29(2), 235–243.

Carr, H.Y. and Purcell, E.M. (1954). Effects of diffusion on free precession in nuclear magnetic resonance experiments. *Physical Review*, 94(3), 630–638.

Chenevert, T.L., Galbán, C.J., Ivancevic, M.K., Rohrer, S.E., Londy, F.J., Kwee, T.C., Meyer, C.R., Johnson, T.D., Rehemtulla, A., Ross, B.D. (2011). Diffusion coefficient measurement using a temperature-controlled fluid for quality control in multicenter studies. *Journal of Magnetic Resonance Imaging*, 34(4), 983–987.

Duplantier, B. (2006). Brownian motion, "diverse and undulating". In *Einstein, 1905–2005. Progress in Mathematical Physics*, Damour, T., Darrigol, O., Duplantier, B., Rivasseau, V. (eds). Birkhäuser, Basel. doi: 10.1007/3-7643-7436-5_8.

Einstein, A. and Fürth, R. (1956). *Investigations on the Theory of Brownian Movement.* Dover Publications, New York.

Feynman, R. (ed.) (1964). The Brownian movement. In *The Feynman Lectures on Physics.* Addison-Wesley, Reading.

Hahn, E.L. (1950). Spin echoes. *Physical Review*, 80(4), 580–594.

Haw, M.D. (2002). Colloidal suspensions, Brownian motion, molecular reality: A short history. *Journal of Physics: Condensed Matter*, 14(33), 7769–7779.

Holz, M., Heil, S.R., Sacco, A. (2000). Temperature-dependent self-diffusion coefficients of water and six selected molecular liquids for calibration in accurate 1H NMR PFG measurements. *Physical Chemistry Chemical Physics*, 2(20), 4740–4742.

Howe, F.A., Filler, A.G., Bell, B.A., Griffiths, J.R. (1992). Magnetic resonance neurography. *Magnetic Resonance in Medicine*, 28(2), 328–338.

Jelescu, I.O. and Budde, M.D. (2017). Design and validation of diffusion MRI models of white matter. *Frontiers in Physics*, 5, 61.

Jensen, J.H. and Helpern, J.A. (2010). MRI quantification of non-Gaussian water diffusion by kurtosis analysis. *NMR in Biomedicine*, 23(7), 698–710.

Le Bihan, D., Breton, E., Lallemand, D., Grenier, P., Cabanis, E., Laval-Jeantet, M. (1986). MR imaging of intravoxel incoherent motions: Application to diffusion and perfusion in neurologic disorders. *Radiology*, 161(2), 401–407.

Maiocchi, R. (1990). The case of Brownian motion. *The British Journal for the History of Science*, 23(3), 257–283.

McNab, J.A., Edlow, B.L., Witzel, T., Huang, S.Y., Bhat, H., Heberlein, K., Feiweier, T., Liu, K., Keil, B., Cohen-Adad, J. et al. (2013). The Human Connectome Project and beyond: Initial applications of 300mT/m gradients. *NeuroImage*, 80, 234–245.

Moseley, M.E., Cohen, Y., Mintorovitch, J., Chileuitt, L., Shimizu, H., Kucharczyk, J., Wendland, M.F., Weinstein, P.R. (1990). Early detection of regional cerebral ischemia in cats: Comparison of diffusion- and T_2-weighted MRI and spectroscopy. *Magnetic Resonance in Medicine*, 14(2), 330–346.

Mulkern, R.V., Haker, S.J., Maier, S.E. (2009). On high b diffusion imaging in the human brain: Ruminations and experimental insights. *Magnetic Resonance Imaging*, 27(8), 1151–1162.

Perrin, J. (1910). Mouvement brownien et molécules. *Journal de physique théorique et appliquée*, 9(1), 5–39.

Porter, D.A. and Heidemann, R.M. (2009). High resolution diffusion-weighted imaging using readout-segmented echo-planar imaging, parallel imaging and a two-dimensional navigator-based reacquisition. *Magnetic Resonance in Medicine*, 62(2), 468–475.

Reese, T.G., Heid, O., Weisskoff, R.M., Wedeen, V.J. (2003). Reduction of eddy-current-induced distortion in diffusion MRI using a twice-refocused spin echo. *Magnetic Resonance in Medicine*, 49(1), 177–182.

von Smoluchowski, M. (1906). Zur kinetischen Theorie der Brownschen Molekularbewegung und der Suspensionen. *Annalen der Physik*, 326(14), 756–780.

Stejskal, E.O. (1965). Use of spin echoes in a pulsed magnetic-field gradient to study anisotropic, restricted diffusion and flow. *The Journal of Chemical Physics*, 43(10), 3597–3603.

Stejskal, E.O. and Tanner, J.E. (1965). Spin diffusion measurements: Spin echoes in the presence of a time-dependent field gradient. *The Journal of Chemical Physics*, 42(1), 288–292.

Sutherland, W. (1905). LXXV. A dynamical theory of diffusion for non-electrolytes and the molecular mass of albumin. *The London, Edinburgh, and Dublin Philosophical Magazine and Journal of Science*, 9(54), 781–785.

Takagi, T., Nakamura, M., Yamada, M., Hikishima, K., Momoshima, S., Fujiyoshi, K., Shibata, S., Okano, H.J., Toyama, Y., Okano, H. (2009). Visualization of peripheral nerve degeneration and regeneration: Monitoring with diffusion tensor tractography. *NeuroImage*, 44(3), 884–892.

Tanner, J.E. (1970). Use of the stimulated echo in NMR diffusion studies. *The Journal of Chemical Physics*, 52(5), 2523–2526.

Tanner, J.E. and Stejskal, E.O. (1968). Restricted self-diffusion of protons in colloidal systems by the pulsed-gradient, spin-echo method. *The Journal of Chemical Physics*, 49(4), 1768–1777.

Taouli, B. and Koh, D.-M. (2010). Diffusion-weighted MR imaging of the liver. *Radiology*, 254(1), 47–66.

Torrey, H.C. (1956). Bloch equations with diffusion terms. *Physical Review*, 104(3), 563–565.

Tuch, D.S. (2004). Q-ball imaging. *Magnetic Resonance in Medicine*, 52(6), 1358–1372.

Weinreb, J.C., Barentsz, J.O., Choyke, P.L., Cornud, F., Haider, M.A., Macura, K.J., Margolis, D., Schnall, M.D., Shtern, F., Tempany, C.M. et al. (2016). PI-RADS prostate imaging – Reporting and data system: 2015, Version 2. *European Urology*, 69(1), 16–40.

Woessner, D.E. (1963). NMR spin-echo self-diffusion measurements on fluids undergoing restricted diffusion. *The Journal of Physical Chemistry*, 67(6), 1365–1367.

Yablonskiy, D.A. and Sukstanskii, A.L. (2010). Theoretical models of the diffusion weighted MR signal. *NMR in Biomedicine*, 23(7), 661–681.

5

Functional MRI

Laura Adela HARSAN[1], Laetitia DEGIORGIS[1], Marion SOURTY[1], Éléna CHABRAN[1] and Denis LE BIHAN[2]

[1] *ICUBE, CNRS, Université de Strasbourg, France*

[2] *NeuroSpin, CEA, Gif-sur-Yvette, France*

5.1. BOLD-contrast functional imaging and brain connectivity

5.1.1. *Introduction*

A century before the first functional MRI scans, Roy and Sherrington (1890) wrote:

> We conclude then, that the chemical products of cerebral metabolism contained in the lymph which bathes the walls of the arterioles of the brain can cause variations of the caliber of the cerebral vessels: that in this re-action the brain possesses an intrinsic mechanism by which its vascular supply can be varied locally in correspondence with local variations of functional activity.

The authors were thus already describing a mechanism that would later be called neurovascular coupling (NVC). This phenomenon is the foundation of hemodynamic imaging techniques, such as blood oxygenation level dependent (BOLD) functional magnetic resonance imaging, or BOLD-contrast fMRI, which detects the cerebral activity related to a task or, more recently, the synchronous activity of neural networks at rest.

For a color version of all the figures in this chapter, see www.iste.co.uk/ratiney-beuf/challenges.zip.

The Challenges of MRI,
coordinated by Hélène RATINEY and Olivier BEUF. © ISTE Ltd 2024.

The first part of this chapter presents the basics of the BOLD signal's origin and describes how the variations of this signal are related to transient changes in neuronal activity. Subsequently, we present the principles of functional connectivity mapping based on resting state fMRI data modeling and examples of clinical applications and translational animal studies. Functional MRI data pre-processing and subsequent statistical analysis is very complex and will not be described in this chapter.

5.1.2. *BOLD-contrast functional MRI principles*

BOLD-contrast functional MRI is an indirect method to produce images of cerebral activity based on the detection of local variations in blood flow and oxygenation induced by neuronal activity (Ogawa et al. 1990). This technique links (1) the paramagnetic nature of deoxyhemoglobin (DHb), modifying the magnetic susceptibility of blood and causing a change in T_2*, with (2) the NVC based on the dynamic relationship between cerebral metabolism, cerebral blood flow (CBF), cerebral blood volume (CBV) and neuronal activity. NVC depends on the vasoreactivity of the cerebrovascular system.

5.1.2.1. *Cerebral circulation*

Red blood cells transport oxygen via hemoglobin, gathering oxygen in the pulmonary circulation system and offloading it in the capillaries to meet the tissue needs (Figure 5.1(a)). Therefore, hemoglobin circulates in the blood in two states: an oxygenated state (OHb) and a deoxygenated one (DHb).

a)

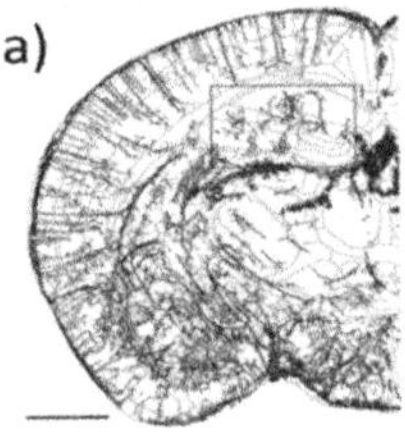

b)

Blood hemoglobin	Arteries arterioles	Capillaries	Veins venules
Oxygenated hemoglobin OHb	100%	100% – 60%	60%
Deoxygenated hemoglobin DHb	0%	0% - 60%	40%

Figure 5.1. *Cerebral blood circulation. (a) Coronal slice of a mouse brain acquired with a multiphotonic microscope, showing the arteries in red and the veins in blue (modified with permission from Kirst et al. 2020). (b) Percentage of OHb and DHb in cerebral blood vessels*

These changes lead to a modification of the oxygen saturation (SO_2) in the blood, which is a measure of the OHb percentage. Arterial blood is oxygenated at 100%, but exchanges in the capillary network reduce the oxygen saturation level in the venous blood to levels that vary overall between 70% and 60% (Figure 5.1(b)) depending on the region.

5.1.2.2. *Paramagnetic properties of DHb*

In 1936, Linus Pauling (Nobel prize in Chemistry in 1954) and Charles Coryell demonstrated that the hemoglobin molecule has different magnetic properties depending on its state of association with oxygen (Pauling and Coryell 1936; Figure 5.2). On the one hand, OHb is diamagnetic, showing no unpaired electrons and a magnetic moment equal to zero. On the other hand, DHb is paramagnetic with two unpaired electrons and a non-zero magnetic moment. When located within a static magnetic field, DHb causes a local perturbation of the magnetic field. This induces changes in magnetic susceptibility, leading to the production of magnetic field gradients in intravascular and perivascular spaces. The non-uniform field around vessels leads to a decrease in the relaxation time T_2* and therefore reduces the MRI signal intensity. Thus, DHb is an authentic endogenous contrast agent. Later, Ogawa et al. performed an in vivo study at 7 T in anesthetized rats, hypothesizing that modifications of the blood oxygen proportion would affect the detectability of cerebral blood vessels on T_2*-weighted images. The authors showed that the cortical surface had a uniform texture when the rats were breathing pure oxygen (Figure 5.2(a), right), while a 21% decrease in oxygen – that is, while rats were breathing normal air – led to regions with a signal loss in areas matching blood vessel locations (Figure 5.2(b), right).

Since cerebral metabolic processes require oxygen provided through blood circulation, Ogawa suggested using this contrast, called blood oxygenation level dependent (BOLD), as an indirect measure of changes in cerebral activity (see Kim and Ogawa 2012; Huettel et al. 2014).

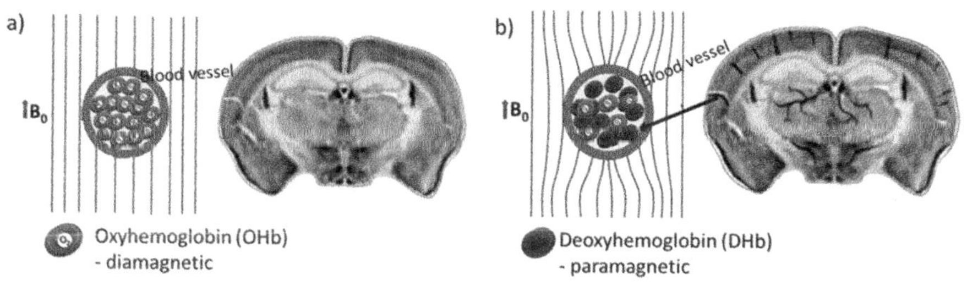

Figure 5.2. *Magnetic properties of oxyhemoglobin (OHb-A) and deoxyhemoglobin (DHb-B)*

COMMENT ON FIGURE 5.2.– *(a) Diamagnetic properties of OHb. On the right, a schematic illustration of a coronal slice in the brain of a rat breathing pure oxygen, with a uniform cortical surface. (b) Paramagnetic properties of DHb. Deoxygenated blood locally perturbs the magnetic field B_0. The coronal slice shows the blood vessels (loss of signal in black – in T_2* weighting) after inhaling air, correlated to an increased DHb concentration. Figure adapted from Ogawa et al. (1990).*

5.1.2.3. *Physiology of neurovascular response*

The physiological foundations behind BOLD fMRI are complex. Here, we present a summary of this topic and highlight excellent literature reviews (Kim and Ogawa 2012; Huettel et al. 2014; Howarth et al. 2021).

5.1.2.3.1. Resting brain metabolism

At rest, the cerebral metabolic rates of O_2 ($CMRO_{2:}$ ~5 mL/min/100 g) and glucose ($CMR_{glu:}$ ~ 31 µmol/min/100 g) represent 20% and 25%, respectively, of the total consumption of our bodies (Ter-Minassian 2006). The blood flow is also very high in the entire brain, with some variations depending on cerebral areas, and constitutes 20% of the cardiac flow at rest. This resting energy metabolism is mainly related to synaptic activity (Shulman et al. 2004), and thus to intercellular communication.

To satisfy these high metabolic needs, the brain has access to only one source of energy – the glucose delivered through blood circulation. Astrocytes (glial cells in brain tissue) have been reported to play a major role in cerebral metabolism by regulating the microcirculation and the distribution of energetic substrates according to neuronal activity (Magistretti 2011).

However, 80% of the glucose consumption is related to synaptic activity at rest. Therefore, the resting state, conceptualized by the American neurologist Marcus Raichle as a "default mode" (Raichle et al. 2001), is a particularly energy-consuming activity.

5.1.2.3.2. Neurovascular coupling

The neuronal activity increase following a stimulation (Figure 5.3), a cognitive task or activity, leads to local synaptic and electrical responses, increasing the tissue's energy needs. In that case, a fast metabolic response occurs, increasing the glucose (CMRglu between 20 and 40%) and oxygen consumption ($CMRO_2$ between ~5% and 20%) (Figure 5.3c(1)).

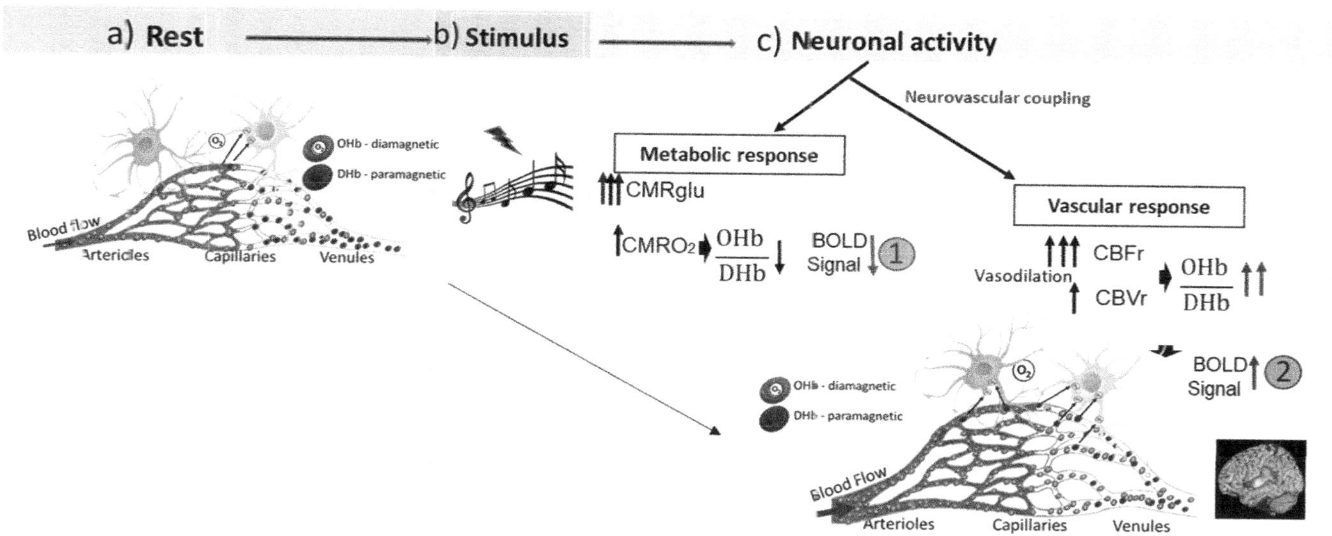

Figure 5.3. *Physiological principle of BOLD fMRI*

COMMENT ON FIGURE 5.3.– *(a) In basal conditions (before stimulation), the arteries are 100% oxygen-saturated, compared to about 60% saturation in the veins.* O_2 *is exchanged at the capillaries. (b) Cerebral activation due to a stimulus produces (c) a rapid local metabolic and vascular response with increased consumption of glucose* (CMR_{glu}) *and oxygen* ($CMRO_2$)*, as well as an increased cerebral blood flow (CBF) and cerebral blood volume (CBV). The local* O_2 *supply exceeds the exchanges in capillaries, leading to an excess of OHb in the venules and an increased OHb/DHb ratio. This translates into decreased magnetic susceptibility effects and a small increase in BOLD fMRI signal.*

Vasoactive signals are sent to surroundings of arterioles and capillaries, thereby dilatating the upstream arterial vessels. A hemodynamic response occurs 1–2 s after a stimulation, inducing an increase in the regional cerebral blood flow (rCBF) by 30–70% of the CBF by 5–30%. According to the so-called Balloon model (Buxton et al. 1998), an arteriole vasodilation and an increased CBF lead to a passive vasodilation of venules and veins thanks to their elasticity. While the increased rCBF addresses the higher needs in glucose in the active region, the local oxygen supply exceeds the more moderate increase in its extraction at the capillaries. Therefore, the oxygenation rate in veinous blood changes, showing higher oxyhemoglobin (diamagnetic) in venous capillaries of the activated area relatively to the DHb (paramagnetic) concentration (Figure 5.3c(2)).

The signal increase reaches a peak 5–7 s after the beginning of a stimulation, a cognitive task or activity. The maximum amplitude is maintained for the duration of the activation time. Once the activation phase ends, blood flow and volume decrease, which translates into a gradual return of the signal intensity to the basal level. Since the intensity of the BOLD effect depends on the static magnetic field B_0, the observed signal variations are between 1 and 5% for a 1.5 T magnetic field, while they are greater than 20% at a 4 T field (Turner et al. 1993).

5.1.2.3.3. Hemodynamic response function

The dynamic of the neurovascular system making the link between stimuli and measured BOLD signals is characterized by the hemodynamic response function (HRF, Figure 5.4). The hemodynamic response induced by a short stimulation (Figure 5.4(a)) can be decomposed into several phases related to NVC: (1) an initial decrease in the signal at least 2 s after the stimulation (known as "initial dip") related to an immediate oxygen extraction that precedes the blood flow increase; (2) a much greater increase in the amplitude of the signal from 5 to 7 s after the stimulation; (3) a signal undershoot below its basal level before stabilizing within about 20 s. Therefore, there is a time delay between the cerebral activation and the detection of the peak signal in BOLD fMRI. The maximum amplitude of the hemodynamic response will be maintained depending on the duration of the stimulation (Figure 5.4(b)).

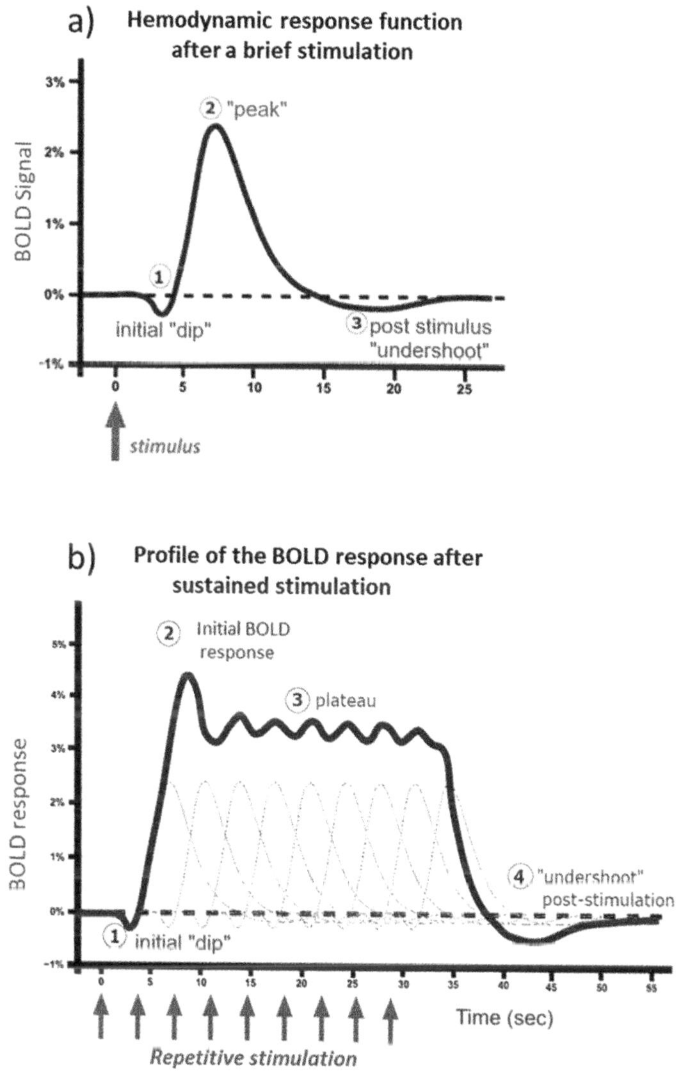

Figure 5.4. *Theoretical representation of the hemodynamic response following a short stimulus (a) and sustained stimulation (b)*

5.1.2.3.4. What kind of neuronal activity for BOLD fMRI signal?

Several electrophysiological methods have been combined with BOLD fMRI to test the relationship between neuronal activity and BOLD signal in a more direct way (Logothetis and Wandell 2004). Using electrical recordings of the visual cortex of anesthetized monkeys, Logothetis and Wandell showed that the BOLD signal would be much more correlated with the local field potentials (LFPs) than with multi-unit activity (MUA) of the axons.

The authors concluded that the BOLD signal mainly reflects electrical inputs and their intracortical processing rather than output discharges. However, in some regions, multi-unit neuronal discharges are only temporary, while the LFP is sustained, suggesting a more linear relationship between the BOLD signal and the local potential.

In rodents, neuronal activity can be controlled using optogenetic approaches (Deisseroth 2011) while recording the BOLD signal via MRI (Kahn et al. 2011). Kahn et al. used an optogenetic stimulation to induce a BOLD MRI signal that accurately reflected the imposed neuronal discharges and showed an excellent linearity (Kahn et al. 2011). Despite these breakthroughs, understanding the cerebral activity mechanisms underlying the BOLD signal remains a very active research topic (Schwalm et al. 2017). The recent combination of calcium imaging (measuring the variations in intraneuronal and/or intra-astrocyte calcium concentration as a marker of cellular activity) with BOLD fMRI in preclinical studies (Pradier et al. 2021) offers new ways of studying the direct relationship between brain cell activity, the physiological response following the activity of these cells and the detected fMRI signal.

Thus, the association between neuronal activity and BOLD signal is indirect. Moreover, it is modulated by a great number of parameters such as the quality and intensity of neuronal response to a stimulus, the NVC, the intrinsic features of the hemodynamic response in the different brain regions, as well as the hardware parameters of fMRI acquisitions.

5.1.2.4. *BOLD signal detection*

Several methodological aspects must be considered to detect the BOLD effect in MRI with good *sensitivity* and *specificity* associated with neuronal activity. *Sensitivity* is described as the capability of BOLD fMRI to reveal brain activity with an increase in neuronal activity. It is defined by hardware characteristics, such as magnetic field intensity, voxel size, bandwidth, sequences, echo time (TE) or spatial encoding. *Specificity* describes the ability to properly localize signals related to neuronal activity changes. This specificity is disturbed by the higher sensitivity of the BOLD signal to the venous drainage network compared to the neurons. In fact, the BOLD signal is divided into two components: an intravascular component related to T_2* variations in the vessels and an extravascular component originating from perivascular tissue in contact with the activated neurons. Thus, increasing the fMRI specificity means being able to better discriminate between the intravascular and extravascular components of the BOLD signal, and therefore detection of activations closer to the recruited neurons (Uludağ et al. 2009).

5.1.2.5. *BOLD fMRI acquisition methods and sequences*

The BOLD effect causes variations of T_2* (ΔR_2*, R_2* = 1/T_2*). This requires the use of ΔR_2* sensitive sequences, that is, T_2* weighted, the premium choice being gradient echo (GE) sequences. Using such sequences, the first fMRI studies in humans (Menon et al. 1993) found a link between the echo time (TE) and the sensitivity to detect BOLD signal variations following a stimulation (here, a photic stimulation). If *S* is the signal intensity in a voxel of an image obtained at an echo time *TE*, then the percentage of BOLD signal change (ΔS/S) after stimulation can be calculated using the following approximation (Menon et al. 1993; Uludağ and Blinder 2018):

$$\boldsymbol{S \sim S_0 . e^{-TE \times R_2^*}} \qquad [5.1]$$

In this formula, S_0 represents the intrinsic MRI signal at TE = 0. By deriving the expression, the BOLD signal can be estimated as:

$$\boldsymbol{\Delta S} = \left|\frac{\partial S}{\partial R_2^*}\right| . \boldsymbol{\Delta R_2}^* = \boldsymbol{TE.S.\Delta R_2}^* \qquad [5.2]$$

The BOLD signal change (ΔS/S) in percent can thus be estimated as:

$$\frac{\Delta S}{S} \sim \boldsymbol{TE.\Delta R_2}^* \qquad [5.3]$$

showing a direct dependency with *TE* value.

To model this relationship in a more accurate way, the effects of different tissue behaviors (extravascular, intravascular) must be considered (Havlicek et al. 2017). Gradient-echo echo-planar imaging (GE-EPI) is the standard approach for BOLD fMRI scans. In conventional GE-EPI protocols, the signal is measured for a single *TE*, specifically chosen to match the mean T_2* of the tissue and maximize the sensitivity. However, T_2* values vary a lot across brain areas and tissues and depend on the intensity of the magnetic field (Cheng et al. 2015). Using multi-echo (ME) scan protocols, BOLD-contrast sensitivity can be optimized through weighting schemes that combine fMRI signals of different TEs (Posse 2012). The optimization of TE can also improve spatial specificity: since the T_2* of the venous system is quite shorter than the T_2* in tissues, the extravascular BOLD signal component can be emphasized using a higher *TE*. The combination of ME sequences with multiband (MB) techniques provides a way of obtaining high temporal and/or spatial resolution images (Cohen et al. 2021).

5.1.2.5.1. Spatial and temporal resolution in fMRI

Spatial resolution refers to the ability to distinguish changes in images across different spatial locations, while temporal resolution refers to the ability to distinguish activity changes at a given location over time. Spatial resolution is closely related to spatial activation specificity. In conventional GE-EPI protocols, spatial resolution is about a few millimeters (2–3 mm). High magnetic fields (3T and above) are without a doubt of great benefit for fMRI as they provide better spatial imaging resolution, higher BOLD contrast sensitivity and better microvascular specificity. High-field applications demonstrate the feasibility of very accurate functional mapping (Figure 5.5; Yang et al. 2021) when BOLD fMRI is compared to alternative fMRI techniques, such as those based on CBV mapping (Huber et al. 2021).

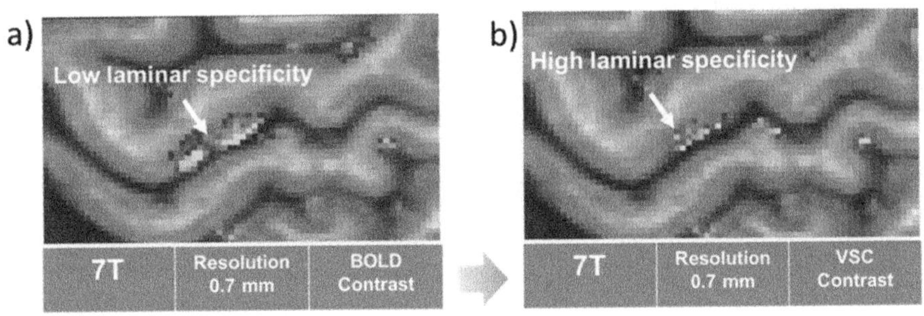

Figure 5.5. *Mapping of cerebral activity within various neuronal layers of the motor cortex following activation of alternated movements of the right thumb and index. (a) Activation detected via BOLD fMRI (GE-EPI) at 7 T. (b) Mapping of cerebral blood volume via a VASO (vascular space occupancy) sequence. Figure modified with permission from Yang et al. (2021)*

Temporal resolution in fMRI relies on the acquisition of repeated measures over time for each voxel to explore the brain function. In such contexts, echo-planar acquisitions are fast and cover the entire brain (a volume of images) in only 2–3 s. Each image is acquired in 20–150 ms depending on the sequence parameters and the employed hardware. fMRI signals are thus usually described as "time-courses".

Decreasing the repetition time (TR) for a better sampling of the hemodynamic fMRI response is beneficial as it improves the estimation of the response. Thanks to important technical advancements, higher temporal resolutions have been recently achieved. For example, the MB (Demetriou et al. 2018) and simultaneous multislice (SMS) (Bhandari et al. 2020) acquisitions decrease TR (from 2 s to 300 ms).

5.1.3. *fMRI activation paradigms*

Experimental design is a key point in activation fMRI studies and the timeline of the stimulation paradigm is fundamental as it has to be synchronized with the image acquisition. A paradigm design consists of a temporal sequence of stimuli received and/or tasks performed by the subject, whose goal is to trigger the cerebral activity of interest. fMRI does not allow for quantification of the level of cerebral activity in absolute terms; it detects the difference in cerebral activity during the execution of the chosen task with respect to a reference state (at rest or while performing another task). The alternation of the different conditions defines the type of paradigm design. *"Block" paradigms* consist of a successive stimulus train (or block) of a few tens of seconds during which stimuli occur repeatedly at regular intervals. In *event-related paradigms*, short-duration stimuli are induced individually in a pseudo-random time sequence to prevent anticipation effects from the participant.

Whatever the paradigm design implemented, the delay between the neuronal activation and the measured hemodynamic response is taken into account. Theoretical curves of the hemodynamic response can be established and then modeled to perform statistical analyses to identify voxels whose signal variation is related to the paradigm.

5.1.3.1. fMRI with stimulation paradigms in preclinical studies

Animal imaging studies (Gil et al. 2021) have demonstrated their importance for the better understanding of the physiological (NVC) or pathological aspects of the cerebral response following a stimulation or regarding questions about the specificity of the BOLD signal at very high fields (Jung et al. 2021). The use of magnetic fields higher than 7 T is now common in preclinical imaging studies in rodents. Using a sequence with high spatial and temporal resolutions at 15.2 T in anesthetized mice, Jung et al. (2021) have recently shown that the detection timeline of the first BOLD responses (from one active cerebral area to another) reflects the direction of neuronal information flow (Figure 5.6). In fact, sensory stimulation in mice (electrical stimulus of the left paw) using a block paradigm produces a sequence of fast activations of thalamic nuclei, sensorial cortex and motor cortex. This coincides with the known sequence of neural activation.

fMRI studies involve several image pre-processing steps that are fundamental for further statistical group analyses. Data processing fMRI pipelines can vary depending on the type of acquisition and target analysis. These analyses are not within the scope of this chapter, but they are nevertheless important for interpreting the results.

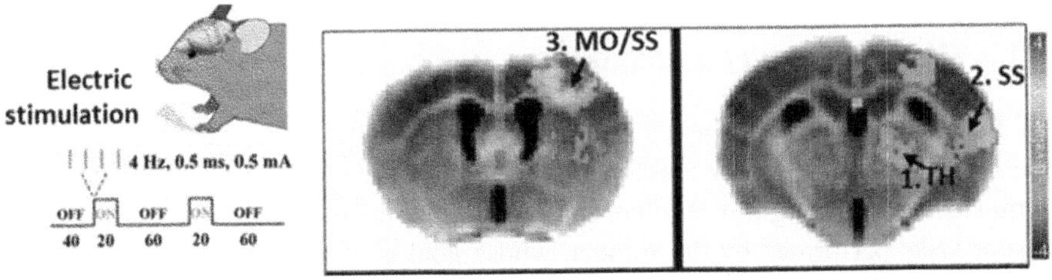

Figure 5.6. *Block paradigms for fMRI stimulation in mice, using an electrical stimulus of the left paw and corresponding functional maps of the BOLD response. The timeline of the first detected BOLD responses is the following: (1) thalamus (TH), (2) somatosensory cortex (SS) and (3) motor cortex (MO). Figure modified with permission from Jung et al. (2020)*

5.1.4. *Resting fMRI and functional cerebral connectivity mapping*

5.1.4.1. *Observing and modeling the brain as a large-scale network*

The large-scale organization of cerebral functioning is based on two fundamental principles: segregation and integration of information (Park and Friston 2013). Functional segregation refers to the existence of brain regions specialized in a given function. However, these brain areas do not work in an isolated way among each other: they are defined as nodes that interact in a coherent and dynamic way to process information, giving rise to the concept of functional integration (Varela et al. 2001). Due to the interaction between cerebral regions, the brain can be studied as a network, leading to the notion of connectivity. A brain structure supporting a given function can thus be considered as a set of specialized cortical areas linked by functional integration (Friston 2005). Therefore, functional specialization and integration are not mutually exclusive but rather complementary and are mediated via cerebral "connectivity", a fundamental notion in neuroscience (Park and Friston 2013).

In this context, three types of cerebral connectivities are considered: (i) *structural connectivity (SC)*, mapped using diffusion tensor MRI (DTI) and tractography and allowing anatomical connectivity to be studied through the analysis of white matter fibers; (ii) *functional connectivity (FC)*, studied via resting-state fMRI based on the analysis of the statistical correlations between time courses of the BOLD signal in different brain regions; (iii) *effective connectivity (EC)*, for investigating the direct influence of one brain region to another. Here, causal interactions related to a task or information flows are studied and described by dynamic causal models.

5.1.4.2. *Resting fMRI and functional cerebral connectivity mapping*

Resting-state fMRI (rs-fMRI) maps the intrinsic cerebral activity to identify its functional networks. In such acquisitions in humans, subjects are scanned "at rest" and asked to relax, not think about anything in particular, close their eyes or focus on a specific point in their field of view for the entire scan.

In animals, rs-fMRI scans can be performed under anesthesia/sedation or awake (e.g. in rat studies). This represents one of the biggest challenges of fMRI in rodents: anesthesia can prevent animal stress and potential movement artifacts, but it can also affect the cerebral functional response. Currently, studies converge toward a consensus on the utilization of a combination of low doses of isoflurane (vasodilator gas) and medetomidine (α-adrenergic receptors agonist, vasoconstrictor) administrated subcutaneously to sedate mice. This anesthetizing combination should sufficiently preserve the basal cerebral activity and the brain's ability to respond to external stimuli. Recent exploratory studies (Chen et al. 2020; Tsurugizawa et al. 2021) have proposed experimental configurations with awake mice, which were trained and accustomed to the MRI environment to reduce animal stress (Chen et al. 2020).

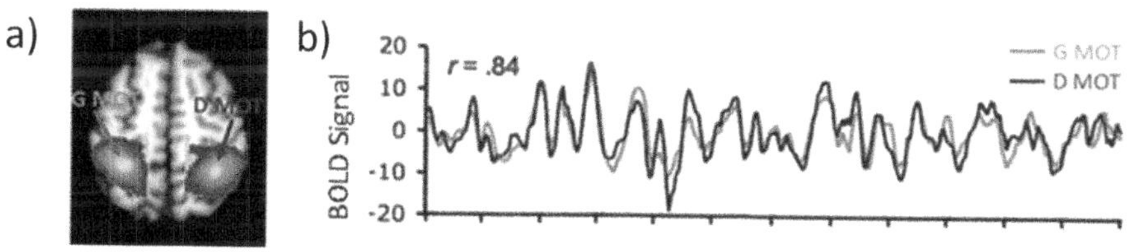

Figure 5.7. *BOLD signal fluctuations are correlated in time for regions that belong to the same functional system. (a) Motor network connectivity map, identifying the left motor cortex (L MOT) and the right motor cortex (R MOT). (b) Example of the average time course of the BOLD signal in a healthy subject at rest, highlighting a correlation between the BOLD signals of the left and right motor cortexes, with r being the correlation coefficient. Modified from Van Dijk et al. (2010)*

5.1.4.2.1. Functional connectivity mapping methods

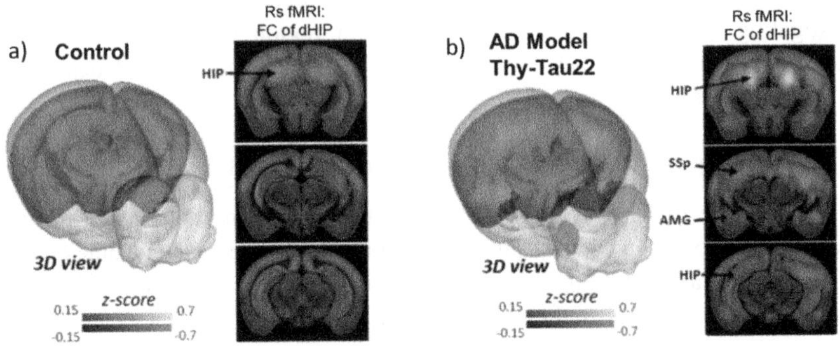

Figure 5.8. *Functional connectivity maps of the dorsal hippocampus (dHIP) in healthy mice (controls, a) and in mice at the so-called prodromal stage for a genetic model (Thy-Tau22) of Alzheimer's disease (AD). rs-fMRI was performed at 7 T in anesthetized mice. The maps obtained via the seed (HIP)-to-voxel approach show a more extended functional network in dHIP of AD model (b) toward the regions of the sensory cortex (SS) and amygdala (AMG). Figure adapted from Degiorgis et al. (2020)*

To map brain functional connectivity, resting-state fMRI studies consider the spontaneous fluctuations of the BOLD signal at low frequencies (typically lower than 0.1 Hz). Statistical data analysis aims to identify the cerebral regions where the BOLD signal spontaneously fluctuates in a synchronized way and which will be then defined as connected regions from the functional point of view (Figure 5.7). Using resting-state fMRI, Biswal et al. (1995) were the first to show that spontaneous fluctuations exhibited coherence within specific neuroanatomical systems such as the somatomotor system. Their results have been confirmed and extended to several other systems, including the visual and auditory systems, as well as the language processing networks, thus showing that a resting brain is far from being inactive (Fox and Raichle 2007; Raichle 2015). To extract functional cerebral networks, different methods can be utilized:

i) *Seed-based approaches* consider the connectivity of one region (e.g. the hippocampus in Figure 5.8, a key memory region). This method consists of measuring the correlation between the average time course in a source region and the average time course measured in one or many other regions of interest (ROI-to-ROI analysis), or else, measured voxel by voxel in the entire brain to obtain a functional connectivity map (seed-to-voxel analysis; see Figure 5.8).

ii) *Independent components analysis* (ICA, Figure 5.9) – most often a spatial analysis in fMRI – is a method in which the observations are the image volumes acquired during a scan session and the sought sources correspond to clusters of voxels showing correlated time courses. The so-identified clusters (components) are spatially independent and allow for a mapping of functional co-activations (Figures 5.10(a) and (b)).

iii) *Mathematical graph-theory approaches* model brain networks as nodes and edges. Nodes represent the brain regions and each edge corresponds to a connection between two nodes. Functional networks can thus be distinguished and their topology and efficiency can be studied by quantifying different metrics (Cao et al. 2016), such as the degree of a node, which corresponds to the number of significant connections that it forms with other nodes or the property of being a central node (hub) in a network.

5.1.4.2.2. Functional architecture of the brain at rest

Since the discovery of an existing synchronous activity between several brain regions in the absence of tasks, rich and complex functional networks have been defined with a common spatial configuration among individuals (Figure 5.9). The most studied rest network – and also one of the first to be identified – is the "default mode network" (DMN). It is characterized by a higher activity at resting state than during the execution of cognitive tasks and is activated when the subject's thoughts flow freely, thus underpinning a cerebral state of wandering thoughts. According to the DMN description in humans, this network includes the dorsal and ventral prefrontal cortexes, the posterior cingulate cortex, the precuneus and the lateral parietal cortex (Raichle et al. 2001). Several studies have linked DMN alteration with pathological states such as depression (Guo et al. 2014), schizophrenia (Mingoia et al. 2012) and Alzheimer's disease (Greicius et al. 2004), making DMN the focus of many functional connectivity studies. Besides DMN, other cerebral networks have been identified and are widely studied today (Figure 5.10(a)) such as the salience network, the executive control network, the sensorimotor network, the auditory network and the attention network (Raichle 2011). Through the exploration of these functional networks, rs-fMRI has been established as a key tool to non-invasively identify potential diagnostic biomarkers and the evolution of neuropathologies (Fornito et al. 2015) Finally, several preclinical explorations have used similar methodological approaches as in humans studies to explore animal models (Degiorgis et al. 2020; Mandino et al. 2021) and identified comparable network confirgurations (Figure 5.10(b)).

5.1.4.2.3. Observations of dynamic functional connectivity (DFC)

Recent studies have shown the existence of connectivity variations over time between networks and between brain areas within these networks (Calhoun et al. 2014; Iraji et al. 2019). These variations are detected by comparing the time course of the BOLD of various brain regions between several very short temporal windows (tens of seconds), suggesting a change in the functional configuration over time. These time courses can be correlated or anti-correlated, and their connectivity strength can vary also. Because of this behavior, a region can be included or not with a given network following a gain or loss of relationship strength. The functional connectivity variations constitute several "functional connectivity states". A state is usually represented by a spatial map of cerebral areas that are functionally connected at a time *t* or over a very short and reproducible period of time. Currently, the *sliding window* approach is the most common investigation technique for extracting the dynamic features of functional connectivity. This method evaluates the connectivity between brain regions from the correlation between pairs of the signal's time courses over a temporal interval called a temporal window (Calhoun et al. 2014). This computation is then repeated by shifting the window by a specific step every time to cover the whole acquisition time and create a connectivity time course corresponding to functional connectivity dynamics between regions (Figure 5.11). Using this approach, neurological pathology studies have been able to distinguish between schizophrenic and healthy subjects based on the connectivity patterns and strength of dynamic states (Du et al. 2016). Regarding neurodegenerative diseases, differences in state durations between Alzheimer's patients and healthy subjects have been described (Jones et al. 2012).

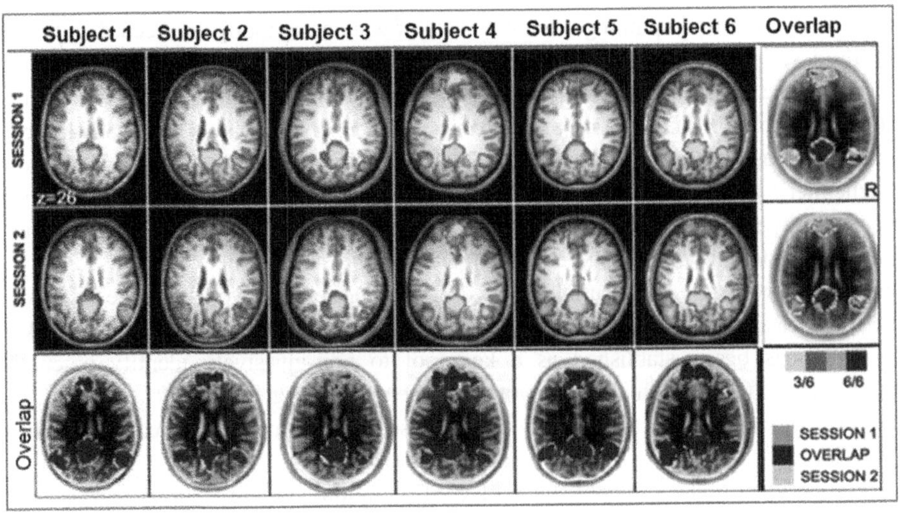

Figure 5.9. *Visualization of the default mode network using independent components analysis that shows reproducibility between subjects (healthy volunteers) and between scan sessions. Modified from Van Dijk et al. (2010)*

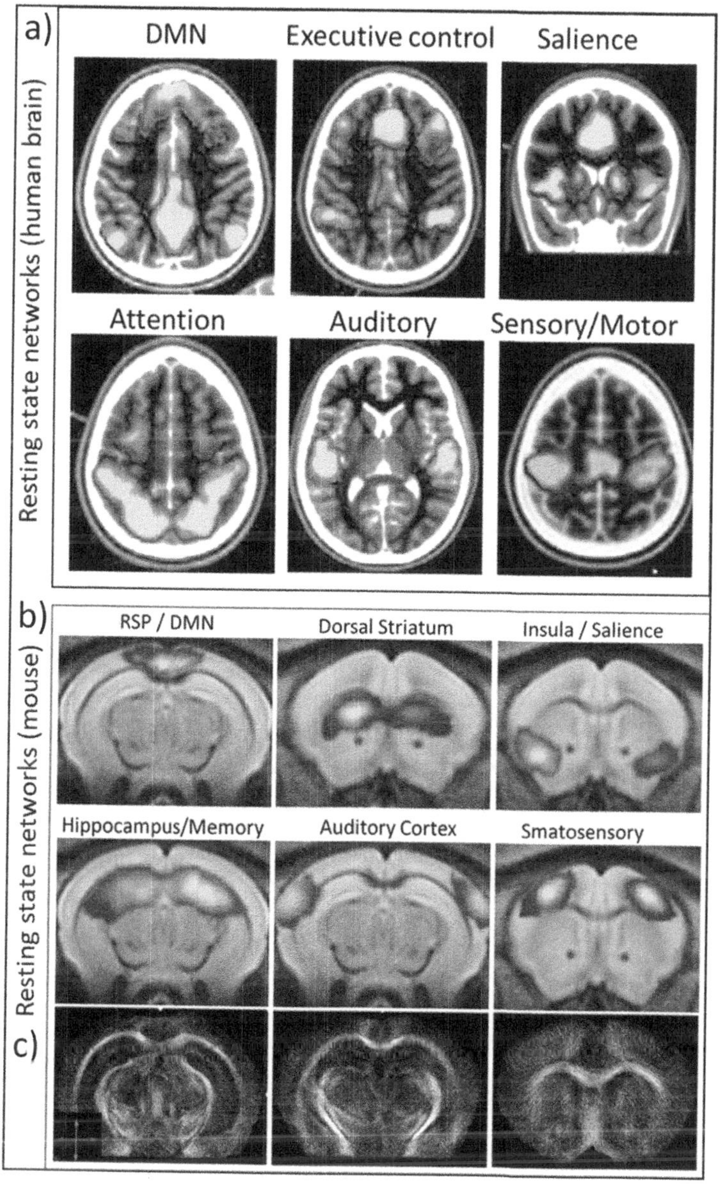

Figure 5.10. *Comparable functional networks identified in humans (a) and mice (b) using independent components analysis. (c) Example of mapping of the structural brain connectivity in a mouse. Fiber tractography maps (color-coded orientation) are obtained from diffusion tensor MRI acquired at 7 T. Panel A: images modified from Raichle et al. (2011)*

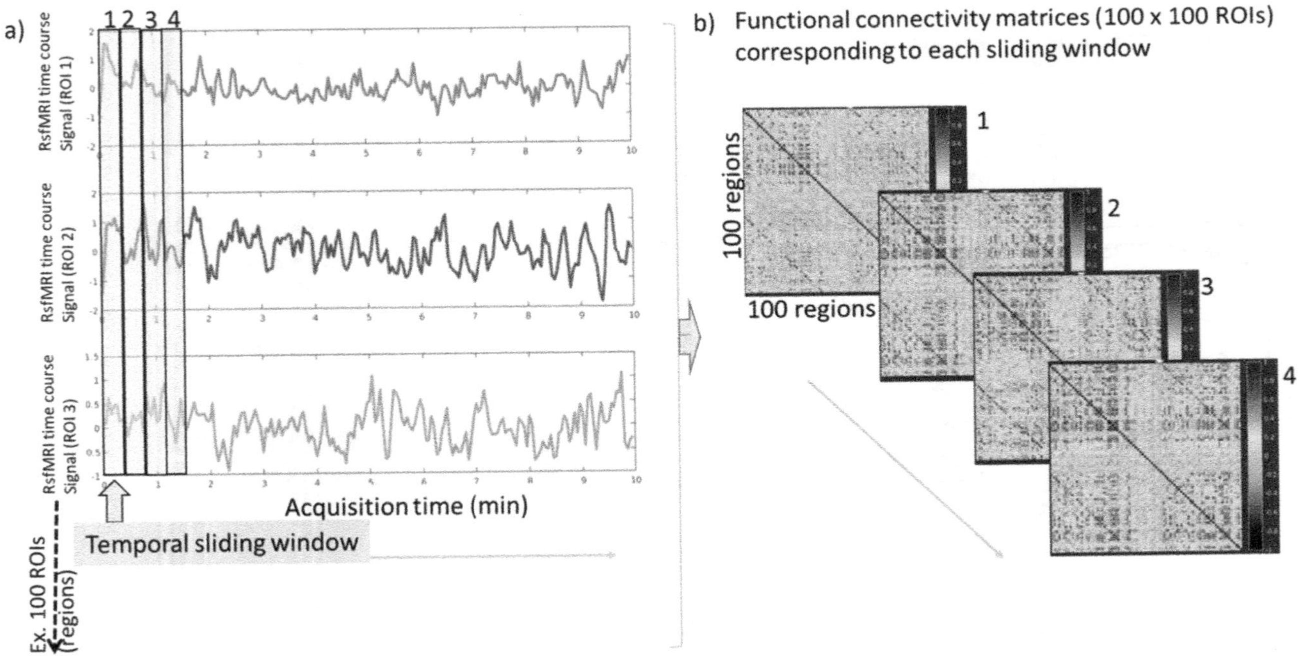

Figure 5.11. *Schematic representation of the dynamic functional connectivity characterization approach based on sliding windows. (a) Time course of the rs-fMRI signal in the studied regions (ROI). (b) Examples of functional connectivity matrices corresponding to the sliding windows, which show the networks' dynamics over time*

Similarly, dynamic functional connectivity has been studied in mouse models using the sliding window approach (Grandjean et al. 2017). Several dynamic connectivity states, which fluctuated depending on the anesthesia and stress levels in the mice, have been described. Dynamic connectivity state alterations have been observed in Alzheimer's disease (Belloy et al. 2018) and autism (Gutierrez-Barragan et al. 2019) models.

These recent fMRI results open a large number of opportunities for non-invasive biomarkers. By mapping the activities' fluctuations at rest, we have the following questions: Would it be possible to (i) uncover new and relevant mechanisms of brain functioning? (ii) Would it be possible to characterize and trace drug kinetics inside cerebral circuits? (iii) Would it be possible to identify specific connectivity states that are specific to different pathology stages and/or related to characteristic symptoms? (iv) Would it be possible to predict the evolution of a pathology for a specific individual and the response to treatments depending on the network dynamics and configuration? Moreover, exploring the dynamic functional cerebral networks in murine models (the most used model organism in fundamental neuroscience) represents a fundamental step in translational research that bridges the gap between preclinical and clinical investigations.

In this first section of this chapter, we only presented principles and applications of BOLD-contrast fMRI, which depends on the NVC for indirect measurement of neuronal activity. However, this method can fail in some physiological or pathological conditions that hinder this coupling. In such cases, alternative methods can be explored, one of them being diffusion fMRI (DfMRI), whose principles are described in the following section.

5.2. Diffusion MRI and brain function

5.2.1. *Introduction*

In his doctoral thesis (as well as in an article published in 1905 in the famous issue of *Annals of Physics* together with the articles on the photoelectric effect and the theory of relativity), Einstein (1905) linked diffusion (a visible phenomenon) to the Brownian motion (a microscopic phenomenon) in the context of heat theory to prove the existence of invisible atoms and molecules. Einstein supposed that Brownian motion resulted from particles being displaced by individual molecules and showed how their movement was related to the diffusion coefficient of Fick laws (see Chapter 4). Unexpectedly, several decades later, it became possible to obtain images representing the diffusion of water molecules in biological tissue in a completely non-invasive way thanks to MRI (Le Bihan and Breton 1985; Le Bihan et al. 1986).

The key concept underlying diffusion MRI that can explain the enormous success of the technique is that during their diffusion motion, the water molecules probe the tissue structure at a micrometric scale, much finer than the usual millimetric resolution, as a sort of virtual and functional biopsy (Le Bihan 2014). Diffusion MRI provides magnificent maps of brain connections, in color and in three dimensions. In this chapter, we shall see how water diffusion is intimately linked to cerebral function, and thus not only does it provide a way to study the brain, maybe this is also one of the mechanisms of neuronal activation. Since its inception, diffusion MRI has been generalized to all the translational movements that present a distribution of velocities, orientations or amplitudes within a given voxel and an interval of time via the concept of intravoxel incoherent motion (IVIM), because it has been realized that blood flow in capillary networks (perfusion) resembles the diffusion process and affects diffusion MRI measurements. Perfusion and diffusion effects were shown to be separable, such that independent images and measurements of molecular diffusion and perfusion can be obtained (Le Bihan et al. 1986, 1988) (see Chapter 4).

DfMRI (Le Bihan et al. 2006) has been proposed as an imaging method for non-invasively studying brain function, as an alternative to BOLD-contrast fMRI (Ogawa et al. 1992), which is widely used for cerebral activity studies. The latter method relies on the NVC hypothesis and does not directly measure neural activity (Logothetis et al. 2001; O'Herron et al. 2016) and it can thus fail in some conditions that affect the NVC. BOLD fMRI is also sensitive to global or local variations of CBF and diffusion that are not necessarily temporally and spatially related to the underlying neural activity (Abe et al. 2017b).

In addition, the spatial resolution of the functional neuroimaging based on the NVC is intrinsically limited because the vessels responsible for the increase in blood flow and volume feed or drain relatively large areas and are not necessarily co-localized with the neural networks that potentially perform different functions (Logothetis et al. 2001; O'Herron et al. 2016). Furthermore, the temporal resolution of BOLD fMRI is intrinsically limited by the physiological delay in triggering the vascular response after the activation. DfMRI is by definition more directly related to neuronal activation and represents the changes induced by neuronal activation at the very level of neuropil, such as the swelling of neurons or neuronal structures (dendritic spines) (Le Bihan 2014).

5.2.2. *IVIM fMRI*

In the mid-1980s, one of the major goals of IVM imaging was to obtain cerebral perfusion maps for studying brain function due to the known coupling between neuronal activation, metabolism and blood flow (called NVC) (Roy and Sherrington 1890). The first results were encouraging, yet insufficient to be published. IVIM-based fMRI has not survived the competition with methods introduced more or less at the same time: first, an approach using contrast agents (Belliveau et al. 1991), immediately supplanted by the BOLD method (Ogawa et al. 1992). Not requiring injections, BOLD fMRI was clearly much easier to implement and was also much more sensitive, which left no space for the IVIM method, which was more challenging in terms of image quality. Nevertheless, the application of the IVIM concept to fMRI has been validated later, with an increase of IVIM perfusion parameters in the active brain regions (increased apparent diffusion coefficient, or ADC), and IVIM does provide a way to better understand the different vascular contributions in BOLD fMRI (Song et al. 1996; Gangstead and Song 2002; Jin et al. 2006; Bihan et al. 2018).

Interestingly, IVIM MRI has been also used in the fMRI context in a "negative" way to tackle the BOLD fMRI limitation of intrinsic spatial resolution. If diffusion/IVIM MRI gradient pulses are added to the BOLD MRI sequences, the contribution of the largest vessels (with faster blood flow) to the BOLD signal can be suppressed, leaving only the effect of the smaller vessels and thus decreasing the spatial extension of the vascular areas affected by neuronal activation (Boxerman et al. 1995; Duong et al. 2003; Song and Li 2003; Michelich et al. 2006). The signal of vessels with faster flow decreases rapidly with increasing diffusion weighting values (very low b-values), whereas the smaller vessels with a slower flow can still contribute to the IVIM signal acquired with b-values greater than 200 s/mm^2. Several research groups, even if not always sufficiently in favor of the IVIM concept, have exploited this strategy to improve the spatial functional resolution of BOLD fMRI.

5.2.3. *Diffusion functional MRI*

Another promising direction that emerged later is the possibility of using diffusion MRI itself to detect cerebral activation instead of BOLD. Here, we are not referring anymore to IVIM and perfusion, but rather to the actual diffusion changes that occur in tissues during neuronal activation – a *decrease* in ADC in this case.

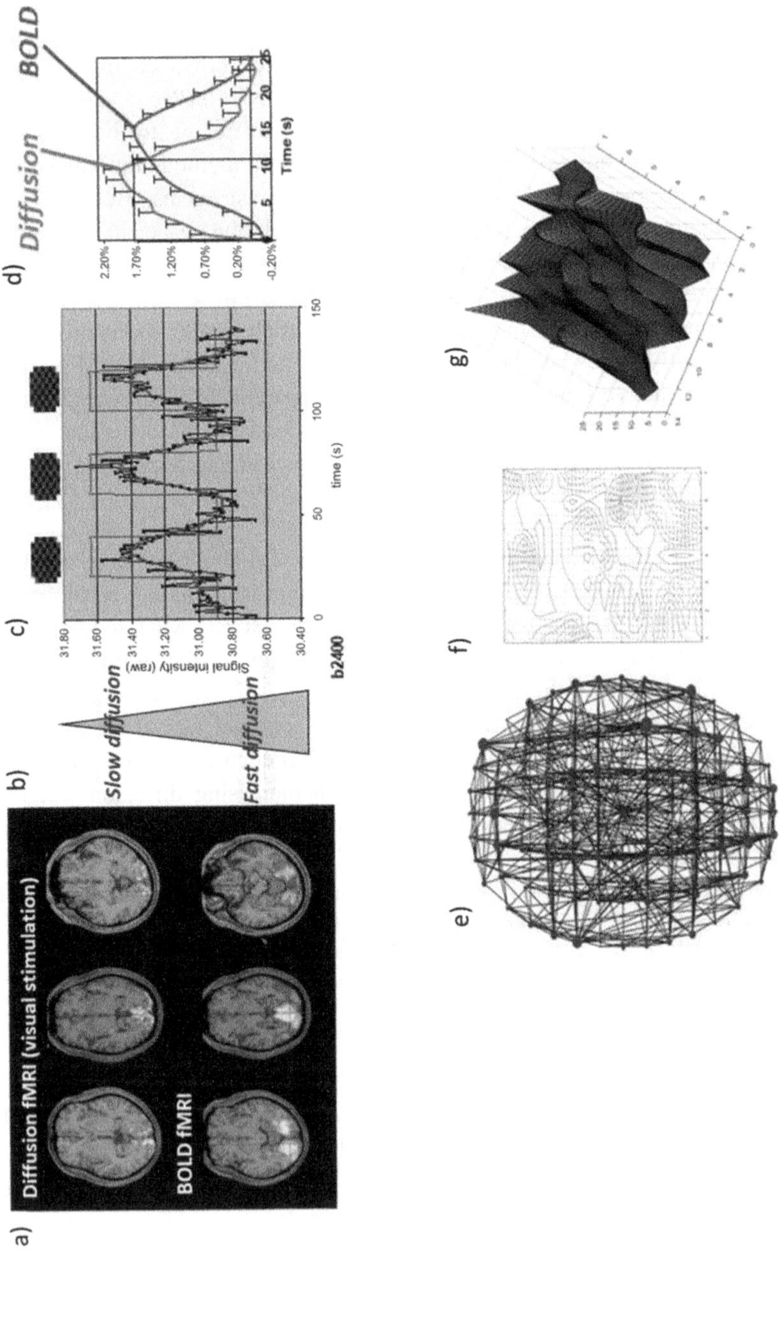

Figure 5.12. *Principles of diffusion fMRI*

COMMENTS ON FIGURE 5.12.– *(a) Non-Gaussian diffusion MRI with high b-values (here, b 2,400 s/mm²) can be used to obtain neuronal activity maps (here, for visual stimulation) (b). The signal increases (decreasing diffusion) in the visual cortex during the stimulation of a shimmering checkboard pattern (c). The supposed principle of diffusion fMRI is the change in neuronal tissue microstructure (neuronal swelling and neuromechanical coupling) concurrent with neuronal activity. The activation pattern seems to be more accurate in time and space (d) than in BOLD fMRI, where it is only indirectly related to neuronal activation via the neurovascular coupling principle. (d) The propagation of neuronal activity along the fiber trajectories (network "edges") between the brain nodes can be modeled in a pseudo-relativistic way in a cerebral 4D space-time with a speed limit c* (e). Each node is characterized by a "mass" that depends on its activity and warps the cerebral space-time (g). The activity flow follows the corresponding geodesics that minimize the distances in the four-dimensional space-time (f). Reciprocally, the activity flow modifies the nodes' activation degree and thus the curvature, which changes dynamically.*

5.2.3.1. *Principles of diffusion fMRI*

Several studies have shown that the responses of DfMRI and BOLD fMRI to different stimuli are different in qualitative and quantitative ways (i.e. in amplitude and temporal evolution of the responses) (Le Bihan et al. 2006; Aso et al. 2009; Albers et al. 2019; De Luca et al. 2019; Nunes et al. 2019, 2021), which suggests that the processes underlying BOLD fMRI and DfMRI must be different, although some doubt that (Miller et al. 2007). While BOLD fMRI is based on the indirect mechanism of NVC (Roy and Sherrington 1890; Ogawa et al. 1992; Logothetis et al. 2001; Schmithorst et al. 2015; O'Herron et al. 2016), the currently hypothesized mechanism of DfMRI is related to the cell swelling triggered by neuronal activation, which is supported by several arguments (Cohen et al. 1968; Andrew and MacVicar 1994).

As described in detail later, many preclinical studies with pharmacological situations interfering with the NVC or cell swelling have confirmed that (1) the responses of DfMRI and BOLD fMRI could be decoupled, confirming the difference in their mechanisms; (2) DfMRI response does not depend on the vascular condition and it is sensitive to the underlying neuronal swelling (Abe et al. 2017a, 2017b); and (3) DfMRI response follows the neuronal activity state more closely and exactly compared to BOLD fMRI, in particular under anesthesia or in the presence of vasoactive medication (Abe et al. 2017b).

Rodent studies have shown that although the BOLD fMRI response is suppressed by blocking the neurovascular response, the DfMRI response persists, which demonstrates that the DfMRI signal does not have a vascular cause and its mechanism is quite different from the BOLD one. In addition, the DfMRI response is faster (in terms of time to reach the activation peak and time to return to baseline) than the hemodynamic BOLD response, as shown by visual stimulation experiments in human subjects and rodents (Le Bihan et al. 2006; Nunes et al. 2021).

Based on several prior studies indicating that the apparent diffusion coefficient (ADC, see Chapter 4) of water decreases in the presence of cellular swelling (although the exact physical mechanisms are still debated, they include the decrease in extracellular space and increase of a layer of bound water with low diffusion, attached to cell membranes (Le Bihan 2014)) and that the neuronal swelling is one of the responses associated with the neuronal activation, the first hypothesis that comes to mind is that the observed decrease in ADC, corresponding to the neuronal responses to stimulation, is due to a dynamic swelling of neurons or parts of neurons in a sort of neuromechanical coupling. This hypothesis is corroborated by the observation via MR microscopy in aplysia neuronal preparations that water diffusion decreases when the cells are exposed to swelling inducers such as hypotonic solution or ouabain (an inhibiter of Na+/K+ pumps) or after neuronal activation induced by dopamine-solution perfusion (Abe et al. 2017a). Interestingly, the decrease in ADC is observed at the tissue level (neuronal ganglion comprising neurons and extracellular space), whereas inside the neurons an intracellular increase of ADC occurs in relation to the cytoplasm dilution induced by the swelling. Furthermore, cellular swelling can be directly shown and quantified via MR and optical microscopy.

Inversely, water diffusion increases in brain regions that have decreased neuronal activity under the effect of anesthesia (observed with LFPs), especially in regions involved in wakefulness (Abe et al. 2017b). In contrast, BOLD signals show nonspecific changes, reflecting the systemic effects of the anesthesia on overall brain hemodynamics status. Electrical stimulation of the central medial thalamus nucleus (CM) exhibiting this anesthesia-induced ADC increase leads the animals to transiently wake up. Infusion in the CM of furosemide, a specific neuronal swelling blocker, leads the water diffusion to further increase locally and increases the current threshold required for awakening the animals under CM electrical stimulation. Oppositely, induction of cell swelling in the CM through the infusion of a hypotonic solution (−80 mOsm aCSF) leads to a local water diffusion decrease and a lower current threshold to wake up the animals. Strikingly, the local water diffusion changes produced by blocking or enhancing cell swelling in the CM were also mirrored remotely in areas functionally connected to the CM, such as the cingulate and somatosensory cortex. Together, those results strongly suggest that neuronal swelling is a significant mechanism underlying DfMRI, as well as the cerebral function at the cellular level.

Therefore, contrary to vascular approaches, DfMRI reflects the changes in intrinsic physical properties of water during brain activation which can be more intimately related to the neuronal activation mechanisms and lead to a better spatial and temporal resolution for fMRI (Figure 5.12(a)). Extensive literature describes the neuronal swelling that happens along with cellular depolarization (Cohen et al. 1968; Ransom et al. 1985; Kusano and Tasaki 1990; MacVicar and Hochman 1991; Andrew and MacVicar 1994; Schwartzkroin et al. 1998; Tasaki 1999; MacVicar et al. 2002; Inoue et al. 2005), in particular in dendritic spines: there are approximately 8,108 synapses/mm^3 in the cortex, 20,000/neuron, with a dendritic length of 10 mm/neuron, that is, 400 m/mm^3 (Schüz and Palm 1989; DeFelipe et al. 1999). It has been determined that water diffusion (measured via MRI or other, more invasive methods) decreases in tissues undergoing cell swelling in pathological, extra physiological and physiological conditions (Zhong et al. 1993; van der Toorn et al. 1996; Buckley et al. 1999; O'Shea et al. 2000; Sotak 2004; Abe et al. 2017a). This suggests that the microstructural effects unveiled by water diffusion behavior during activation could well be an active component of this process because if water homeostasis and motion undoubtedly play a central role in brain physiology, neuronal membranes do not have aquaporin channels, contrarily to the astrocytes which cannot regulate their volume, and are thus directly exposed to transmembranal water flows. What is the contribution to the cerebral tissue function of these rapid "mechanical" changes that have been observed in tissue microstructure (such as the "dance" of dendritic spines reported by Crick (1982))? Since nature laws are usually reversible, could we consider that the neurons act as piezoelectric sensors that depolarize when they "sense" the motion of neighboring cells, in a faster alternative way than in synaptic transmission of information flowing within neuronal clusters? In such a case, diffusion MRI could also help us to understand these mechanisms.

5.2.3.2. *Practical considerations*

A DfMRI scan is implemented exactly like a BOLD fMRI scan, except for the T_2*-weighted EPI MRI sequence used for BOLD fMRI (typically a gradient echo sequence, although a spin echo sequence increases the contribution of small vessels and thus the spatial resolution), which is replaced by a diffusion-weighted spin echo EPI sequence (Le Bihan et al. 2006). By employing very low weighting values (b ~ 0-200 s/mm^2), a diffusion MRI sequence is nothing other than a spin echo BOLD fMRI sequence, although some IVIM effects can be present, as described above. The specific response induced by diffusion appears whenever a strong diffusion weighting is applied (b = 1800 s/mm^2 or greater) (Aso et al. 2009). To completely remove residual BOLD effects, images with low and high b-values can be acquired (ideally, in an interleaved way) to calculate ADC and its temporal evolution, for example, $ADC = ln(S_0/S_{1800})/1800$ with b = 0 and 1800 s/mm^2 for the S_0 and S_{1800} signals, respectively. For completeness, it should be mentioned that a spin echo sequence with double refocusing can be used to completely suppress the effects of local magnetic field gradients created by blood DHb (and thus by the BOLD effect) on the b-values, although these effects are usually completely negligible (Le Bihan et al. 2006).

At this point, one can rightfully ask why DfMRI is not employed more in fMRI given the limitations of BOLD fMRI. These limitations can be acceptable for cognitive human imaging at coarse spatial and temporal resolutions, but they are a great disadvantage for neuroscientific applications at a finer level, which will be achievable by the next ultra-high field MRI systems (Bihan and Schild 2017; Budinger and Bird 2018) or for preclinical models under anesthesia. The main reason for the limited utilization of DfMRI is probably a technical one: the relatively higher noise level encountered in diffusion MRI based on spin echos with a long TE compared to BOLD fMRI, based on gradient echo (the amplitudes of the responses of diffusion and BOLD fMRI are actually very similar), usually requires the signal to be averaged over repeated fMRI acquisitions, which is a potential limitation for human studies. Another possible reason is that the supposed mechanism behind fMRI and its direct link with neuronal activity (i.e. neuromechanical coupling) remains up for debate. This uncertainty should dissolve with time, in the light of experimental facts (Abe et al. 2017b; Nunes et al. 2019, 2021).

5.2.4. *Toward functional tractography: a global diffusion framework within the brain connectome*

Tractography based on DTI (Koch et al. 2002; Le Bihan 2014) (see Chapter 4) is an indispensable tool for interpreting functional MRI data and determining the anatomical connection networks behind cognitive processes. A significant challenge consists in reconstructing the correspondence between the functional connectivity provided by functional MRI (BOLD or diffusion based) and the anatomical connectivity obtained via DTI to determine the human "connectome", a map of the connections in the entire brain (Gong et al. 2009; Biswal 2012). However, at this stage, it should be reminded that tractography estimations are dominated by the large white matter fibers (rather than the smaller intracortical connections) and, most of all, that there is no indication regarding the directionality and functional status of the information flow along these fibers. Certainly, for the time being, being able to visualize the activity flow along axons in a non-invasive way at the scale of an entire brain remains out of reach. In the future, detailed knowledge of the anatomical connections (in terms of fiber length and size, which can be obtained via diffusion tensor measurements) could also yield estimations of the propagation time between active regions (nodes) and, thereby, provide indirect indications regarding the temporal behavior of the activation in each node of a network. This kind of information is fundamental for exploring the connections' dynamics, the state of synchronizations between cortical regions and, therefore, what is done during cerebral activity or even consciousness.

In this regard, the diffusion process can again be used for modeling the dynamics of brain connections, similarly to the modeling of blood microcirculation as a pseudo-diffusion process in IVIM MRI, but this time considering the flow of action potentials within the brain connectome (Le Bihan 2020). However, difficulties arise when it is realized that the propagation speed of action potentials has a finite limit.

As a result, the "present" and "simultaneity" concepts are ill-defined in the brain connectome and, besides diffusion, these concepts are borrowed from Einstein's special and general relativity theories where relevant (Le Bihan 2020). In particular, as in the universe, time and space can be considered to be inseparable in the connectome, such that the functional and structural features of the brain could be unified into a combined cerebral "space-time". This four-dimensional cerebral space-time obeys a sort of relativist principle, with a functional curvature caused by cerebral activity in the same way as the gravitational masses warp the four-dimensional space-time of the universe. This coherent physical and biological view of the whole brain enables a fusion between the "activity" of gray matter and the "transmission" of the white matter into a unique framework to describe the way in which neuronal activity flows in the cerebral connectome. The space-time is warped by the activity or energy ("mass") in the brain nodes composed of gray matter clusters. The activity generated by these nodes flows along the connections following "cerebral lines" with a geodesic shape (the shortest path in four dimensions) in the warped brain's space-time. In other words, the geodesic lines representing the activity flow in the brain follow specific connections deriving from activity potential in the continuously changing cerebral space-time landscape underpinning our mental activity (Figure 5.12(b)).

The theoretical framework can already clarify the functional features of a typical brain, such as attention, and some dysfunctional phenotypes (clinical expression of symptoms) observed in some neuropsychiatric disorders, such as the voices heard by people with schizophrenia (Le Bihan 2020). Among that which remains, this new approach has to be validated and we should investigate its capability of "explaining" or modeling brain functioning in typical or pathological conditions. For this purpose, we need to gather data on the anatomical connectivity (using diffusion-based tractography, which today is the only available approach) and functional data (using BOLD or DfMRI, or even EEG or MEG) at the resolution and scale required for this context, until a kind of "functional tractography" will become available (Deslauriers-Gauthier et al. 2019). It is hoped that ultra-high magnetic field MRI (Bihan and Schild 2017) will provide such data.

5.3. Conclusion

By now, diffusion tensor imaging and functional MRI are well-established modalities in the biomedical imaging landscape, recently joined by DfMRI. While T_1 and T_2 relaxation, magnetic susceptibility, magnetization contrast, etc., exist only due to the presence of the magnetic field in an MRI system, diffusion is not in itself an "MRI parameter". MRI is simply a sophisticated tool for measuring diffusion in the body in a local and non-invasive way. Water is fundamental for life and its molecular diffusion naturally occurs outside MRI magnets. Indeed, all biological processes require interaction between molecules, either for DNA or RNA duplication, protein transcription, protein and enzyme activity, transmembranal transport, neurotransmission, etc. In addition, to be able to interact, the molecules must first meet with an intrinsic rhythm, which makes diffusion a sort of universal process exploited by Mother Nature (and evolution) for that purpose. More than an imaging modality, diffusion MRI should be considered a powerful and original multidisciplinary concept available to us for studying cellular physiology and life. Thus, let us keep our eyes open as diffusion MRI might well reserve other surprises for explaining the functioning of our brains and, above all, allow us to repair it when necessary.

5.4. References

Abe, Y., Van Nguyen, K., Tsurugizawa, T., Ciobanu, L., Le Bihan, D. (2017a). Modulation of water diffusion by activation-induced neural cell swelling in Aplysia Californica. *Scientific Reports*, 7(1), 6178.

Abe, Y., Tsurugizawa, T., Le Bihan, D. (2017b). Water diffusion closely reveals neural activity status in rat brain loci affected by anesthesia. *PLoS Biology*, 15(4), e2001494.

Albers, F., Wachsmuth, L., Schache, D., Lambers, H., Faber, C. (2019). Functional MRI readouts from BOLD and diffusion measurements differentially respond to optogenetic activation and tissue heating. *Frontiers in Neuroscience*, 13, 1104.

Andrew, R.D. and MacVicar, B.A. (1994). Imaging cell volume changes and neuronal excitation in the hippocampal slice. *Neuroscience*, 62(2), 371–383.

Aso, T., Urayama, S., Poupon, C., Sawamoto, N., Fukuyama, H., Le Bihan, D. (2009). An intrinsic diffusion response function for analyzing diffusion functional MRI time series. *NeuroImage*, 47(4), 1487–1495.

Belliveau, J.W., Kennedy, D.N., McKinstry, R.C., Buchbinder, B.R., Weisskoff, R.M., Cohen, M.S., Vevea, J.M., Brady, T.J., Rosen, B.R. (1991). Functional mapping of the human visual cortex by magnetic resonance imaging. *Science (New York, N.Y.)*, 254(5032), 716–719.

Belloy, M.E., Shah, D., Abbas, A., Kashyap, A., Roßner, S., Van der Linden, A., Keilholz, S.D., Keliris, G.A., Verhoye, M. (2018). Quasi-periodic patterns of neural activity improve classification of Alzheimer's disease in mice. *Scientific Reports*, 8(1), 10024.

Bhandari, R., Kirilina, E., Caan, M., Suttrup, J., De Sanctis, T., De Angelis, L., Keysers, C., Gazzola, V. (2020). Does higher sampling rate (multiband + SENSE) improve group statistics – An example from social neuroscience block design at 3T. *NeuroImage*, 213, 116731.

Biswal, B.B. (2012). Resting state fMRI: A personal history. *NeuroImage*, 62(2), 938–944.

Biswal, B.B., Yetkin, F.Z., Haughton, V.M., Hyde, J.S. (1995). Functional connectivity in the motor cortex of resting human brain using echo-planar MRI. *Magnetic Resonance in Medicine*, 34(4), 537–541.

Boxerman, J.L., Bandettini, P.A., Kwong, K.K., Baker, J.R., Davis, T.L., Rosen, B.R., Weisskoff, R.M. (1995). The intravascular contribution to fMRI signal change: Monte Carlo modeling and diffusion-weighted studies in vivo. *Magnetic Resonance in Medicine*, 34(1), 4–10.

Buckley, D.L., Bui, J.D., Phillips, M.I., Zelles, T., Inglis, B.A., Plant, H.D., Blackband, S.J. (1999). The effect of ouabain on water diffusion in the rat hippocampal slice measured by high resolution NMR imaging. *Magnetic Resonance in Medicine*, 41(1), 137–142.

Budinger, T.F. and Bird, M.D. (2018). MRI and MRS of the human brain at magnetic fields of 14T to 20T: Technical feasibility, safety, and neuroscience horizons. *NeuroImage*, 168, 509–531.

Buxton, R.B., Wong, E.C., Frank, L.R. (1998). Dynamics of blood flow and oxygenation changes during brain activation: The balloon model. *Magnetic Resonance in Medicine*, 39(6), 855–864.

Calhoun, V.D., Miller, R., Pearlson, G., Adali, T. (2014). The chronnectome: Time-varying connectivity networks as the next frontier in fMRI data discovery. *Neuron*, 84(2), 262–274.

Cao, M., Huang, H., Peng, Y., Dong, Q., He, Y. (2016). Toward developmental connectomics of the human brain. *Frontiers in Neuroanatomy*, 10, 25.

Cheng, Y., van Zijl, P.C.M., Hua, J. (2015). Measurement of parenchymal extravascular R_2* and tissue oxygen extraction fraction using multi-echo vascular space occupancy MRI at 7 T. *NMR in Biomedicine*, 28(2), 264–271.

Cohen, L.B., Keynes, R.D., Hille, B. (1968). Light scattering and birefringence changes during nerve activity. *Nature*, 218(5140), 438–441.

Cohen, A.D., Jagra, A.S., Yang, B., Fernandez, B., Banerjee, S., Wang, Y. (2021). Detecting task functional MRI activation using the multiband multiecho (MBME) echo-planar imaging (EPI) sequence. *Journal of Magnetic Resonance Imaging: JMRI*, 53(5), 1366–1374.

Crick, F. (1982). Do dendritic spines twitch? *Trends in Neurosciences*, 5, 44–46.

De Luca, A., Schlaffke, L., Siero, J.C.W., Froeling, M., Leemans, A. (2019). On the sensitivity of the diffusion MRI signal to brain activity in response to a motor cortex paradigm. *Human Brain Mapping*, 40(17), 5069–5082.

DeFelipe, J., Marco, P., Busturia, I., Merchán-Pérez, A. (1999). Estimation of the number of synapses in the cerebral cortex: Methodological considerations. *Cerebral Cortex*, 9(7), 722–732.

Degiorgis, L., Karatas, M., Sourty, M., Faivre, E., Lamy, J., Noblet, V., Bienert, T., Reisert, M., von Elverfeldt, D., Buée, L. et al. (2020). Brain network remodelling reflects tau-related pathology prior to memory deficits in Thy-Tau22 mice. *Brain: A Journal of Neurology*, 143(12), 3748–3762.

Deisseroth, K. (2011). Optogenetics. *Nature Methods*, 8(1), 26–29.

Demetriou, L., Kowalczyk, O.S., Tyson, G., Bello, T., Newbould, R.D., Wall, M.B. (2018). A comprehensive evaluation of increasing temporal resolution with multi-band-accelerated protocols and effects on statistical outcome measures in fMRI. *NeuroImage*, 176, 404–416.

Deslauriers-Gauthier, S., Lina, J.M., Butler, R., Whittingstall, K., Gilbert, G., Bernier, P.M., Deriche, R., Descoteaux, M. (2019). White matter information flow mapping from diffusion MRI and EEG. *NeuroImage*, 201, 116017.

Du, Y., Pearlson, G.D., Yu, Q., He, H., Lin, D., Sui, J., Wu, L., Calhoun, V.D. (2016). Interaction among subsystems within default mode network diminished in schizophrenia patients: A dynamic connectivity approach. *Schizophrenia Research*, 170(1), 55–65.

Duong, T.Q., Yacoub, E., Adriany, G., Hu, X., Ugurbil, K., Kim, S.G. (2003). Microvascular BOLD contribution at 4 and 7 T in the human brain: Gradient-echo and spin-echo fMRI with suppression of blood effects. *Magnetic Resonance in Medicine*, 49(6), 1019–1027.

Einstein, A. (1905). Über die von der molekularkinetischen Theorie der Wärme geforderte Bewegung von in ruhenden Flüssigkeiten suspendierten Teilchen. *Annalen der Physik*, 322, 549–560.

Fornito, A., Zalesky, A., Breakspear, M. (2015). The connectomics of brain disorders. *Nature Reviews. Neuroscience*, 16(3), 159–172.

Fox, M.D. and Raichle, M.E. (2007). Spontaneous fluctuations in brain activity observed with functional magnetic resonance imaging. *Nature Reviews. Neuroscience*, 8(9), 700–711.

Friston, K. (2005). A theory of cortical responses. *Philosophical Transactions of the Royal Society of London. Series B, Biological Sciences*, 360(1456), 815–836.

Gangstead, S.L. and Song, A.W. (2002). On the timing characteristics of the apparent diffusion coefficient contrast in fMRI. *Magnetic Resonance in Medicine*, 48(2), 385–388.

Gil, R., Fernandes, F.F., Shemesh, N. (2021). Neuroplasticity-driven timing modulations revealed by ultrafast functional magnetic resonance imaging. *NeuroImage*, 225, 117446.

Gong, G., He, Y., Concha, L., Lebel, C., Gross, D.W., Evans, A.C., Beaulieu, C. (2009). Mapping anatomical connectivity patterns of human cerebral cortex using in vivo diffusion tensor imaging tractography. *Cerebral Cortex*, 19(3), 524–536.

Grandjean, J., Preti, M.G., Bolton, T.A.W., Buerge, M., Seifritz, E., Pryce, C.R., Van De Ville, D., Rudin, M. (2017). Dynamic reorganization of intrinsic functional networks in the mouse brain. *NeuroImage*, 152, 497–508.

Greicius, M.D., Srivastava, G., Reiss, A.L., Menon, V. (2004). Default-mode network activity distinguishes Alzheimer's disease from healthy aging: Evidence from functional MRI. *Proceedings of the National Academy of Sciences of the United States of America*, 101(13), 4637–4642.

Guo, W., Liu, F., Zhang, J., Zhang, Z., Yu, L., Liu, J., Chen, H., Xiao, C. (2014). Abnormal default-mode network homogeneity in first-episode, drug-naive major depressive disorder. *PLoS One*, 9(3), e91102.

Gusnard, D.A. and Raichle, M.E. (2001). Searching for a baseline: Functional imaging and the resting human brain. *Nature Reviews. Neuroscience*, 2(10), 685–694.

Gutierrez-Barragan, D., Basson, M.A., Panzeri, S., Gozzi, A. (2019). Infraslow state fluctuations govern spontaneous fMRI network dynamics. *Current Biology: CB*, 29(14), 2295–2306.

Havlicek, M., Ivanov, D., Poser, B.A., Uludag, K. (2017). Echo-time dependence of the BOLD response transients – A window into brain functional physiology. *NeuroImage*, 159, 355–370.

Howarth, C., Mishra, A., Hall, C.N. (2021). More than just summed neuronal activity: How multiple cell types shape the BOLD response. *Philosophical Transactions of the Royal Society of London. Series B, Biological Sciences*, 376(1815), 20190630.

Huber, L.R, Handwerker, D.A., Jangraw, D.C., Chen, G., Hall, A., Stüber, C., Gonzalez-Castillo, J., Ivanov, D., Marrett, S., Guidi, M. et al. (2017). High-resolution CBV-fMRI allows mapping of laminar activity and connectivity of cortical input and output in human M1. *Neuron*, 96(6), 1253–1263.

Huber, L.R., Poser, B.A., Kaas, A.L., Fear, E.J., Dresbach, S., Berwick, J., Goebel, R., Turner, R., Kennerley, A.J. (2021). Validating layer-specific VASO across species. *NeuroImage*, 237, 118195.

Huettel, S.A., Song A.W., McCarthy, G. (2014). *Functional Magnetic Resonance Imaging.* Sinauer Associates, Sunderland.

Inoue, H., Mori, S.I., Morishima, S., Okada, Y. (2005). Volume-sensitive chloride channels in mouse cortical neurons: Characterization and role in volume regulation. *The European Journal of Neuroscience*, 21(6), 1648–1658.

Iraji, A., Deramus, T.P., Lewis, N., Yaesoubi, M., Stephen, J.M., Erhardt, E., Belger, A., Ford, J.M., McEwen, S., Mathalon, D.H. et al. (2019). The spatial chronnectome reveals a dynamic interplay between functional segregation and integration. *Human Brain Mapping*, 40(10), 3058–3077.

Jin, T., Zhao, F., Kim, S.G. (2006). Sources of functional apparent diffusion coefficient changes investigated by diffusion-weighted spin-echo fMRI. *Magnetic Resonance in Medicine*, 56(6), 1283–1292.

Jones, D.T., Vemuri, P., Murphy, M.C., Gunter, J.L., Senjem, M.L., Machulda, M.M., Przybelski, S.A., Gregg, B.E., Kantarci, K., Knopman, D.S. et al. (2012). Non-stationarity in the "resting brain's" modular architecture. *PLoS One*, 7(6), e39731.

Jung, W.B., Im, G.H., Jiang, H., Kim, S.G. (2021). Early fMRI responses to somatosensory and optogenetic stimulation reflect neural information flow. *Proceedings of the National Academy of Sciences of the United States of America*, 118(11), e2023265118.

Kahn, I., Desai, M., Knoblich, U., Bernstein, J., Henninger, M., Graybiel, A.M., Boyden, E.S., Buckner, R.L., Moore, C.I. (2011). Characterization of the functional MRI response temporal linearity via optical control of neocortical pyramidal neurons. *Journal of Neuroscience*, 31(42), 15086–15091.

Kim, S.G. and Bandettini, P.A. (2010). Principles of functional MRI. In *BOLD fMRI: A Guide to Functional Imaging for Neuroscientists*, Faro, S.H. and Mohamed, F.B. (eds). Springer, New York.

Kim, S.G. and Ogawa, S. (2012). Biophysical and physiological origins of blood oxygenation level-dependent fMRI signals. *Journal of the International Society of Cerebral Blood Flow and Metabolism*, 32(7), 1188–1206.

Koch, M.A., Norris, D.G., Hund-Georgiadis, M. (2002). An investigation of functional and anatomical connectivity using magnetic resonance imaging. *NeuroImage*, 16(1), 241–250.

Komaki, Y., Debacker, C., Djemai, B., Ciobanu, L., Tsurugizawa, T., Le Bihan, D. (2020). Differential effects of aquaporin-4 channel inhibition on BOLD fMRI and diffusion fMRI responses in mouse visual cortex. *PLoS One*, 15(5), e0228759.

Kusano, K. and Tasaki, I. (1990). Mechanical changes associated with synaptic transmission in the mammalian superior cervical ganglion. *Journal of Neuroscience Research*, 25(2), 243–248.

Le Bihan, D.L. (2014). Diffusion MRI: What water tells us about the brain. *EMBO Molecular Medicine*, 6(5), 569–573.

Le Bihan, D.L. (2020). On time and space in the brain: A relativistic pseudo-diffusion framework. *Brain Multiphysics*, 1, 100016.

Le Bihan, D.L. and Breton, E. (1985). In vivo magnetic resonance imaging of diffusion. *Comptes rendus des séances de l'Académie des Sciences Série 2*, 301(15), 1109–1112.

Le Bihan, D.L. and Schild, T. (2017). Human brain MRI at 500 MHz, scientific perspectives and technological challenges. *Superconductor Science and Technology*, 30(3), 033003.

Le Bihan, D.L., Breton, E., Lallemand, D., Grenier, P., Cabanis, E., Laval-Jeantet, M. (1986). MR imaging of intravoxel incoherent motions: Application to diffusion and perfusion in neurologic disorders. *Radiology*, 161(2), 401–407.

Le Bihan, D.L., Breton, E., Lallemand, D., Aubin, M.L., Vignaud, J., Laval-Jeantet, M. (1988). Separation of diffusion and perfusion in intravoxel incoherent motion MR imaging. *Radiology*, 168(2), 497–505.

Le Bihan, D.L., Urayama, S., Aso, T., Hanakawa, T., Fukuyama, H. (2006). Direct and fast detection of neuronal activation in the human brain with diffusion MRI. *Proceedings of the National Academy of Sciences of the United States of America*, 103(21), 8263–8268.

Le Bihan, D.L., Federau, M.I.C., Sigmund, E.E. (2018). *Intravoxel Incoherent Motion (IVIM) MRI*. Routledge, London.

Logothetis, N.K. (2002). The neural basis of the blood-oxygen-level-dependent functional magnetic resonance imaging signal. *Philosophical Transactions of the Royal Society of London. Series B, Biological Sciences*, 357(1424), 1003–1037.

Logothetis, N.K. and Wandell, B.A. (2004). Interpreting the BOLD signal. *Annual Review of Physiology*, 66, 735–769.

Logothetis, N.K., Pauls, J., Augath, M., Trinath, T., Oeltermann, A. (2001). Neurophysiological investigation of the basis of the fMRI signal. *Nature*, 412(6843), 150–157.

MacVicar, B.A. and Hochman, D. (1991). Imaging of synaptically evoked intrinsic optical signals in hippocampal slices. *The Official Journal of the Society for Neuroscience*, 11(5), 1458–1469.

MacVicar, B.A., Feighan, D., Brown, A., Ransom, B. (2002). Intrinsic optical signals in the rat optic nerve: Role for K(+) uptake via NKCC1 and swelling of astrocytes. *Glia*, 37(2), 114–123.

Mandino, F., Vrooman, R.M., Foo, H.E., Yeow, L.Y., Bolton, T.A.W., Salvan, P., Teoh, C.L., Lee, C.Y., Beauchamp, A., Luo, S. et al. (2021). A triple-network organization for the mouse brain. *Molecular Psychiatry*, 27, 865–872.

Menon, R.S., Ogawa, S., Tank, D.W., Uğurbil, K. (1993). Tesla gradient recalled echo characteristics of photic stimulation-induced signal changes in the human primary visual cortex. *Magnetic Resonance in Medicine*, 30(3), 380–386.

Michelich, C.R., Song, A.W., Macfall, J.R. (2006). Dependence of gradient-echo and spin-echo BOLD fMRI at 4 T on diffusion weighting. *NMR in Biomedicine*, 19(5), 566–572.

Miller, K.L., Bulte, D.P., Devlin, H., Robson, M.D., Wise, R.G., Woolrich, M.W., Jezzard, P., Behrens, T.E.J. (2007). Evidence for a vascular contribution to diffusion FMRI at high b value. *Proceedings of the National Academy of Sciences of the United States of America*, 104(52), 20967–20972.

Mingoia, G., Wagner, G., Langbein, K., Maitra, R., Smesny, S., Dietzek, M., Burmeister, H.P., Reichenbach, J.R., Schlösser, R.G.M., Gaser, C. et al. (2012). Default mode network activity in schizophrenia studied at resting state using probabilistic ICA. *Schizophrenia Research*, 138(2/3), 143–149.

Nunes, D., Ianus, A., Shemesh, N. (2019). Layer-specific connectivity revealed by diffusion-weighted functional MRI in the rat thalamocortical pathway. *NeuroImage*, 184, 646–657.

Nunes, D., Gil, R., Shemesh, N. (2021). A rapid-onset diffusion functional MRI signal reflects neuromorphological coupling dynamics. *NeuroImage*, 231, 117862.

O'Herron, P., Chhatbar, P.Y., Levy, M., Shen, Z., Schramm, A.E., Lu, Z., Kara, P. (2016). Neural correlates of single-vessel haemodynamic responses in vivo. *Nature*, 534(7607), 378–382.

O'Shea, J.M., Williams, S.R., van Bruggen, N., Gardner-Medwin, A.R. (2000). Apparent diffusion coefficient and MR relaxation during osmotic manipulation in isolated turtle cerebellum. *Magnetic Resonance in Medicine*, 44(3), 427–432.

Ogawa, S., Lee, T.M., Kay, A.R., Tank, D.W. (1990). Brain magnetic resonance imaging with contrast dependent on blood oxygenation. *Proceedings of the National Academy of Sciences of the United States of America*, 87(24), 9868–9872.

Ogawa, S., Tank, D.W., Menon, R., Ellermann, J.M., Kim, S.G., Merkle, H., Ugurbil, K. (1992). Intrinsic signal changes accompanying sensory stimulation: Functional brain mapping with magnetic resonance imaging. *Proceedings of the National Academy of Sciences of the United States of America*, 89(13), 5951–5955.

Park, H.J. and Friston, K. (2013). Structural and functional brain networks: From connections to cognition. *Science*, 342(6158), 1238411.

Pauling, L. and Coryell, C.D. (1936). The magnetic properties and structure of hemoglobin, oxyhemoglobin and carbonmonoxyhemoglobin. *Proceedings of the National Academy of Sciences of the United States of America*, 22(4), 210–216.

Poser, B.A. and Norris, D.G. (2009). Investigating the benefits of multi-echo EPI for fMRI at 7 T. *NeuroImage*, 45(4), 1162–1172.

Posse, S. (2012). Multi-echo acquisition. *NeuroImage*, 62(2), 665–671.

Pradier, B., Wachsmuth, L., Nagelmann, N., Segelcke, D., Kreitz, S., Hess, A., Pogatzki-Zahn, E.M., Faber, C. (2021). Combined resting state-fMRI and calcium recordings show stable brain states for task-induced fMRI in mice under combined ISO/MED anesthesia. *NeuroImage*, 245, 118626.

Raichle, M.E. (2011). The restless brain. *Brain Connectivity*, 1(1), 3–12.

Raichle, M.E. (2015). The restless brain: How intrinsic activity organizes brain function. *Philosophical Transactions of the Royal Society of London. Series B, Biological Sciences*, 370(1668), 20140172.

Raichle, M.E., MacLeod, A.M., Snyder, A.Z., Powers, W.J., Gusnard, D.A., Shulman, G.L. (2001). A default mode of brain function. *Proceedings of the National Academy of Sciences of the United States of America*, 98(2), 676–682.

Ransom, B.R., Yamate, C.L., Connors, B.W. (1985). Activity-dependent shrinkage of extracellular space in rat optic nerve: A developmental study. *The Journal of Neuroscience*, 5(2), 532–535.

Roy, C.S. and Sherrington, C.S. (1890). On the regulation of the blood-supply of the brain. *The Journal of Physiology*, 11(1/2), 85–158.

Schmithorst, V.J., Vannest, J., Lee, G., Hernandez-Garcia, L., Plante, E., Rajagopal, A., Holland, S.K., CMIND Authorship Consortium (2015). Evidence that neurovascular coupling underlying the BOLD effect increases with age during childhood. *Human Brain Mapping*, 36(1), 1–15.

Schüz, A. and Palm, G. (1989). Density of neurons and synapses in the cerebral cortex of the mouse. *The Journal of Comparative Neurology*, 286(4), 442–455.

Schwalm, M., Schmid, F., Wachsmuth, L., Backhaus, H., Kronfeld, A., Aedo Jury, F., Prouvot, P.H., Fois, C., Albers, F., van Alst, T. et al. (2017). Cortex-wide BOLD fMRI activity reflects locally-recorded slow oscillation-associated calcium waves. *eLife*, 6, e27602.

Schwartzkroin, P.A., Baraban, S.C., Hochman, D.W. (1998). Osmolarity, ionic flux, and changes in brain excitability. *Epilepsy Research*, 32(1/2), 275–285.

Song, A.W. and Li, T. (2003). Improved spatial localization based on flow-moment-nulled and intra-voxel incoherent motion-weighted fMRI. *NMR in Biomedicine*, 16(3), 137–143.

Song, A.W., Wong, E.C., Tan, S.G., Hyde, J.S. (1996). Diffusion weighted fMRI at 1.5 T. *Magnetic Resonance in Medicine*, 35(2), 155–158.

Sotak, C.H. (2004). Nuclear magnetic resonance (NMR) measurement of the apparent diffusion coefficient (ADC) of tissue water and its relationship to cell volume changes in pathological states. *Neurochemistry International*, 45(4), 569–582.

Tasaki, I. (1999). Rapid structural changes in nerve fibers and cells associated with their excitation processes. *The Japanese Journal of Physiology*, 49(2), 125–138.

Ter-Minassian, A. (2006). Cerebral metabolism and brain injury. *Annales françaises d'anesthésie et de réanimation*, 25(7), 714–721.

van der Toorn, A., Syková, E., Dijkhuizen, R.M., Voríšek, I., Vargova, L., Skobisová, E., van Lookeren Campagne, M., Reese, T., Nicolay, K. (1996). Dynamic changes in water ADC, energy metabolism, extracellular space volume, and tortuosity in neonatal rat brain during global ischemia. *Magnetic Resonance in Medicine*, 36(1), 52–60.

Tsurugizawa, T., Abe, Y., Le Bihan, D. (2017). Water apparent diffusion coefficient correlates with gamma oscillation of local field potentials in the rat brain nucleus accumbens following alcohol injection. *Journal of Cerebral Blood Flow and Metabolism*, 37(9), 3193–3202.

Turner, R., Jezzard, P., Wen, H., Kwong, K.K., Le Bihan, D., Zeffiro, T., Balaban, R.S. (1993). Functional mapping of the human visual cortex at 4 and 1.5 tesla using deoxygenation contrast EPI. *Magnetic Resonance in Medicine*, 29(2), 277–279.

Uludağ, K. and Blinder, P. (2018). Linking brain vascular physiology to hemodynamic response in ultra-high field MRI. *NeuroImage*, 168, 279–295.

Uludağ, K., Müller-Bierl, B., Uğurbil, K. (2009). An integrative model for neuronal activity-induced signal changes for gradient and spin echo functional imaging. *NeuroImage*, 48(1), 150–165.

Van Dijk, K.R., Hedden, T., Venkataraman, A., Evans, K.C., Lazar, S.W., Buckner, R.L. (2010). Intrinsic functional connectivity as a tool for human connectomics: Theory, properties, and optimization. *Journal of Neurophysiology*, 103(1), 297–321.

Varela, F., Lachaux, J.P., Rodriguez, E., Martinerie, J. (2001). The brainweb: Phase synchronization and large-scale integration. *Nature Reviews Neuroscience*, 2(4), 229–239.

Yang, J., Huber, L., Yu, Y., Bandettini, P.A. (2021). Linking cortical circuit models to human cognition with laminar fMRI. *Neuroscience & Biobehavioral Reviews*, 128, 467–478.

Zhong, J., Petroff, O.A., Prichard, J.W., Gore, J.C. (1993). Changes in water diffusion and relaxation properties of rat cerebrum during status epilepticus. *Magnetic Resonance in Medicine*, 30(2), 241–246.

6

Vascular Imaging: Flow and Perfusion

Sylvain MIRAUX[1], Frank KOBER[2] and Emmanuel Luc BARBIER[3,4]

[1] *CRMSB, CNRS, Université de Bordeaux, France*

[2] *CRMBM, CNRS, Université Aix-Marseille, France*

[3] *GIN, Inserm, Université Grenoble Alpes, France*

[4] *IRMaGe, CNRS, Inserm, CHUGA, Université Grenoble Alpes, France*

6.1. Introduction

Tissue vascularization presents itself as a branched network starting from large vessels (~1 cm in diameter in humans) and finishing with capillaries (~6 μm in diameter). Capillaries are where the exchanges between blood and tissues occur. Two main types of vascular imaging exist: flow and perfusion imaging. This is not a biological distinction; it is related to spatial resolution. For example, let us consider a 1 mm pixel:

– In flow imaging, the blood flow is coherent within the pixel(s) in terms of motion direction. Such flow imaging, which is also called angiography, detects the circulation of blood directed toward (artery) or from (vein) tissues. This topic is addressed in section 6.3.

– In perfusion imaging, the pixel size is greater than the vessel size. Therefore, the pixel contains several capillaries with different orientations and the blood motion is incoherent within the pixel. This topic is addressed in section 6.4.

For a color version of all the figures in this chapter, see www.iste.co.uk/ratiney-beuf/challenges.zip.

The Challenges of MRI,
coordinated by Hélène RATINEY and Olivier BEUF.

In vascular imaging, it is common to use contrast agents, similar to the colorants used to track water in rivers. The properties of contrast agents are detailed in section 6.2. In order to understand their use, let us recall a few basic physiological notions.

Blood contains cells and plasma. The percentage of red cells is called the hematocrit. It is approximately 15% lower in capillaries than in large vessels. Blood cells and plasma do not circulate at the same speed. In other words, blood is not a homogeneous liquid, and contrast agents circulate like plasma.

Blood circulation can be represented as vascular loops that start from the heart and return to the heart: for example, the heart–brain, right arm–heart or heart–heart loops. At the end of each loop, there is a capillary network. Blood flow is not uniform along the loop. For instance, it varies from about 50 cm/s in the aorta (in reality a very variable speed, due to the cardiac pulsations) to 0.1 cm/s in the capillaries, and up to 30 cm/s on average in the veins that reach the heart. Venous blood arriving at the heart is then directed toward the lungs, where it becomes oxygenated, returns to the heart and leaves it again via the aorta, the largest arterial trunk in the body.

6.2. Contrast agents

6.2.1. *Biological behavior*

Contrast agents must modify the MRI signal but not the physiology. Therefore they consist of chemically and biologically inert molecules that do not modify the blood behavior (so-called tracers). A very low volume (about 10–20 mL of solution), compared to the blood volume, is typically injected into an arm vein. To allow the contrast agent to reach the organs in the most compact way and in the shortest time (a bolus), a physiological serum is injected after the contrast agent to quickly push the latter from the arm vein to the vena cava. After the small circulation (heart–lung–heart), it is ejected into the aorta at physiological pressure. A first pass of contrast agent occurs in each organ. Due to the branching of the vascular network at the end of each loop, the contrast agent becomes more diluted when flowing through an organ. Furthermore, the contrast agent gradually leaves the vascular bed: it is extracted at the kidneys and liver and, if its hydrodynamic diameter is sufficiently small (the molecule's diameter, including its hydration layer) and if the vessel walls are permeable, it also spreads in tissues. After some minutes, the contrast agent concentration in the blood gradually decreases, typically over several hours. This slow decrease is characterized by the plasmatic half-life of the contrast agent. It should be noted that the vast majority of vessels are permeable to contrast agents, except in a healthy brain where the vessel walls constitute a barrier, called the blood–brain barrier (BBB).

6.2.2. *Diamagnetism, paramagnetism and superparamagnetism*

Since MRI detects protons of water, several preclinical experiments have investigated the delivery of contrast agents using other nuclei, such as fluorine. In practice, chemistry and the need for specific equipment are not favorable for their routine usage in clinics. Therefore, clinical settings employ agents that influence the water signal.

The matter's behavior inside a magnetic field is characterized by magnetic susceptibility, denoted as χ. Water and biological tissues are usually diamagnetic: when they are placed into a magnetic field, they produce very weak magnetization that opposes the magnetic field. Their magnetic susceptibility is negative and very low (water: -9.05×10^{-6}; human tissues: between -11×10^{-6} and -7×10^{-6}) (Schenck 1996). Conversely, contrast agents are paramagnetic or superparamagnetic: when placed inside a magnetic field, they produce a magnetization oriented along the magnetic field. Their magnetic susceptibility is positive, with the susceptibility of superparamagnetic agents greater than that of paramagnetic agents. All contrast agents produce two types of effects on the MRI signal, a relaxivity effect and a susceptibility one.

6.2.3. *Relaxivity effect*

Paramagnetic or superparamagnetic contrast agents accelerate the spin-spin (T_2) and spin-lattice (T_1) relaxation processes. At a molecular level, thermal oscillations of the contrast agent produce small and rapid local fluctuations of the magnetic field. The frequency component that corresponds to the magnetic resonance of water molecules accelerates the relaxation of water located in the hydration layer of the contrast agent. For a given condition of the magnetic field, temperature and biological environment, the relaxation power or relaxivity of a contrast agent is characterized by two values: r_1 and r_2. For a homogenous liquid, this can be written as:

$$T_{1AC} = 1/T_{10} + r_1[AC]\ T_{2AC} = 1/T_{20} + r_2[AC] \qquad [6.1]$$

where T_{1AC} (respectively, T_{2AC}) is the T_1 (respectively, T_2) in the presence of a contrast agent, T_{10} (respectively, T_{20}) is the T_1 (respectively, T_2) in the absence of a contrast agent, r_1 (respectively, r_2) is the relaxivity ($mMol^{-1} \cdot s^{-1}$) and [AC] is the contrast agent concentration in mMol.

Some generic observations on the relaxivity effects should be highlighted: if the membranes hinder the water molecules' motion, the relaxivity effect is reduced. The greater the magnetic field intensity, the lower the relaxivity effect. The larger the hydrodynamic diameter of the contrast agent, the stronger the relaxivity effect. Moreover, T_1 and T_2 effects are opposite: when T_1 decreases, the signal level usually increases; when T_2 decreases, the opposite occurs. Thus, for a spin echo sequence, the relationship between the signal and the contrast agent concentration follows a bell-shaped curve: at low concentrations, the T_1 effect is dominant and the signal amplitude increases with the concentration. At higher concentrations, the T_2 effect becomes dominant and the signal amplitude decreases with the concentration. The bell-shaped curve of signal level as a function of concentration is not bijective and leads to quantification difficulties.

6.2.4. *Susceptibility effect*

The magnetic susceptibility effect is based on the perturbation of the magnetic field lines in the vicinity of the contrast agent. Since the magnetic field around the contrast agent is non-uniform, the spins of hydrogen atoms situated nearby gradually dephase and the magnitude of the vector sum of these spins – the magnetization – becomes lower than in the absence of a contrast agent. This effect, related to T_2* (non-uniformity of the magnetic field at a microscopic level), is distinctly visible in gradient echo images and less visible with spin echo sequences.

Some generic observations on the susceptibility effect can be made: the membranes have no impact on this effect. Moreover, the stronger the magnetic field, the greater the susceptibility effect. Finally, the larger the contrast agent's diameter, the greater the susceptibility effect (one may consider that the effect extends over a distance equivalent to the diameter of the contrast agent). Therefore, contrast agent molecules that are gathered in the same biological compartment (capillary, cell, vesicle) will have a greater susceptibility effect than if they were relatively uniformly distributed in the same volume of tissue. The inverse phenomenon occurs for the relaxivity effect: it will be maximum if the contrast agent is uniformly distributed in the biological tissue. Superparamagnetic contrast agents have a larger diameter and lead to greater susceptibility effects than paramagnetic contrast agents. However, today, their clinical use in humans is not approved, because their benefit compared to existing contrast agents has not been demonstrated.

6.3. Angiography

Numerous MRI sequences exist for visualizing large vessels (veins and arteries). Typically, they are adapted to the type of investigated vessels and their location and can be divided into three large categories:

– white-blood techniques based on the "time-of-flight" (TOF) principle or on the injection of a contrast agent with T_1 contrast;

– approaches based on phase contrast;

– black-blood methods.

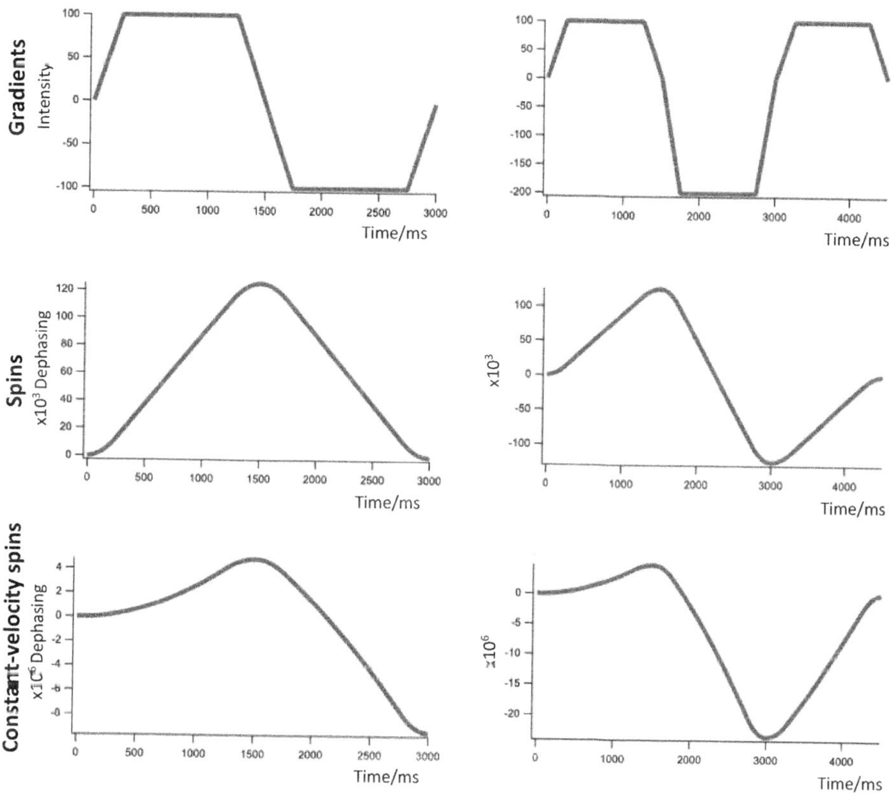

Figure 6.1. *Gradient waveforms (1; (– 1)) and (1; (– 2); 1) and plots showing the accumulated phase as a function of time for stationary spins and spins with a constant velocity*

We shall describe the physical principle of each method with their advantages and disadvantages and show images of examples. Finally, we shall mention the most recent time-resolved techniques that not only detect the location of the blood vessels but also visualize the blood motion in these vessels.

As a foreword, we shall tackle the principle of gradients and flow compensation (Simonetti et al. 1991; Parker et al. 2003). This gradient pattern is almost always employed in angiography sequences (TOF, phase and sometimes even with T_1 contrast agents) and dynamic angiography.

Figure 6.1 illustrates the principle of flow compensation via gradients. In a standard gradient echo sequence (1;(– 1) pattern), only the stationary spins are rephased at the end of the gradient pattern. Conversely, moving spins are dephased, which consequently causes a decrease or even absence of their signal. To address this problem, patterns such as 1;(– 2);1 can be used to rephase moving spins. All of this can only be done at the price of a longer TE in the sequence. A 1;(– 2);5;(– 2);1 pattern can be also used to compensate for the dephasing of spins with a constant acceleration.

6.3.1. *White-blood imaging*

6.3.1.1. *"Time-of-flight" imaging*

White-blood and "time-of-flight" (Laub 1995) imaging sequences are basic slice-selective gradient echo sequences. However, they include the feature of flow compensation. Today, these sequences are mostly used in three dimensions for angiography applications. For this reason, they employ very short repetition times *TR* (<25 ms) compared to the longitudinal spin relaxation time T_1 in order to keep the acquisition time of a volume short. Most of all, however, the usage of short *TR* causes the attenuation of the signal from stationary spins due to the "saturation" or "partial saturation" effect. This effect becomes more pronounced as the TR/T_1 ratio decreases. In the case of a 3D volume with slice selection, stationary spins (i.e. spins in muscle tissues and gray and white matter) are directly affected by this phenomenon and exhibit a strongly attenuated signal.

Conversely, blood spins, that is, moving spins, exhibit no or only partial effect of the saturation phenomenon as they are not always present in the imaging slice during the entire scan. This mechanism is described with the name "flow-related enhancement" or "entry slice phenomenon". It increases with flow velocity, the vessel's orthogonal orientation with respect to the slice, and decreases with slice thickness (Figure 6.2).

In practice, TOF angiography imaging is performed for vessels in the brain (visualization of the Willis polygon) and in the neck (carotid arteries).

In the brain, the MOTSA (multiple overlapping thin slab acquisition) (Davis et al. 1994) or sequential 3D TOF technique is used. By acquiring three or four small volumes, it maximizes the flow-related enhancement effect while reducing the scan time. The sequence is flow-compensated and employs the parameters described below (at 3 T). This type of sequence becomes more efficient at higher magnetic fields. As stationary spins' T_1 is longer at 3 T than at 1.5 T, these spins are more saturated. The TOF phenomenon, on the other hand, is less sensitive to the magnetic field intensity.

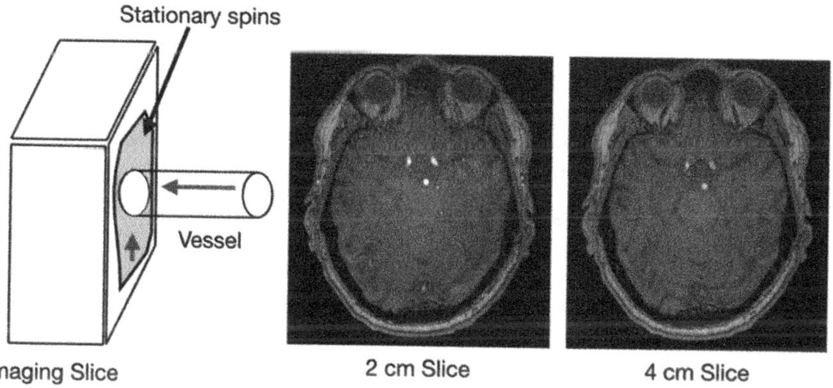

Figure 6.2. *Schematic of the "time-of-flight" principle. The images are extracted from a 3D volume with a selection of slices of 2 cm and 4 cm thickness. The "time-of-flight" effect highlights vessels with a strong signal (red arrows). It is more prominent when the slice thickness is smaller. Some vessels visible on the 2 cm slice are not visible any longer on the 4 cm slice (dashed arrows)*

To increase the quality of TOF images, in particular in terms of contrast, several blocks can be used at the beginning of the sequence (magnetization transfer, fat suppression; Atkinson et al. 1994). To reduce the saturation phenomenon at the end of the slice, radiofrequency pulses with variable flip angles can be employed (TONE; Saib et al. 2019).

ACQUISITION PARAMETERS FOR A TOF SEQUENCE AT 3 T.– FLASH 3D sequence with four adjacent selective slices of 2 cm: TE/TR = 3.42/21 ms; flip angle: 18°; field of view: 200 × 181 mm; resolution: 0.3 × 0.3 × 0.5 mm; phase acceleration factor: 2; in-slice partial Fourier: 7/8; acquisition time: 5:33 min.

6.3.1.2. *Contrast agent imaging*

The goal of contrast agents used in angiography is to modify the relaxation times of the blood (Prince 1994). The most employed contrast agent is gadolinium in a chelated form (Weinmann et al. 1984). An injector is used to accurately control the dose and speed during the injection.

Similar to TOF imaging, 3D gradient echo sequences are used. Contrary to the former method, no specific slice positioning is necessary. Indeed, the signal enhancement is uniform within the vessels. However, the acquisition speed is the most important criterion to be taken into account. Sequences with large receive bandwidths, short *TR* (<10 ms), partial Fourier acquisition and parallel imaging techniques are employed. One of the challenges of this type of method is the synchronization of the acquisition with the first pass of a contrast agent inside the arterial system. Often, a 2D sequence combined with a pre-bolus with a small volume is used to determine the optimum timing of the 3D acquisition. In these approaches, the center of the k-space must be acquired at the moment of the contrast agent's first pass in the arterial system such that the acquisition is not "contaminated" by the signal from the venous system. Elliptical acquisitions that start from the k-space center are used (Wilman et al. 1998). Advancements in the domain of parallel imaging enable dynamic image acquisitions with a coarser spatial resolution that show and confirm the first pass. By combining these techniques with advanced reconstruction methods, it is possible to reconstruct high-resolution images of the first pass a posteriori. The venous system visualization, in contrast, presents fewer constraints in terms of acquisition time and high-resolution images can be acquired in this case (Farb et al. 2003).

ACQUISITION PARAMETERS WITH CONTRAST AGENT.– 3D FLASH sequence: TE/*TR* = 1.2/4.4 ms; flip angle: 20°; field of view: 160 × 160 mm; resolution: 0.5 × 0.5 × 0.5 mm; phase acceleration factor: 2; in-slice partial Fourier: 7/8; elliptical centric phase-encoding; acquisition time: 54.8 s.

6.3.1.3. *White-blood imaging limitations*

The main difficulty in white-blood imaging is the lack of a positive signal. Its main possible cause is a too-slow blood velocity in the vessels in TOF imaging. In particular, this occurs in pathologies such as aneurysms, where the blood's circulation velocity is decreased. In these conditions, a contrast agent is added to compensate for the reduced signal.

Intra-voxel dephasing is also a cause of low blood signal in TOF imaging due to turbulent flows with variable velocity.

In contrast-agent imaging, the main cause of the lack of signal lies in a poor synchronization of the bolus injection with the readout of the k-space center. The T_2* effect caused by adding contrast agents at high concentrations can also lead to signal loss, which can be compensated by reducing the TE of the sequence.

6.3.2. *Phase contrast imaging*

Phase contrast imaging was introduced in 1982 by Moran (1982) and its 3D version by Dumoulin et al. (1989). The goal of this method is to acquire images of spin circulation by applying flow-encoding gradients.

In phase imaging, velocity encoding gradients translate flow velocity into phase values. In practice, a bipolar gradient is applied during a gradient echo sequence. The gradient applies a phase to the magnetization that is linearly proportional to the velocity. This gradient is called the "velocity encoding gradient". The axis along which the gradient is applied determines the direction of flow sensitivity. Such gradients can be added to a gradient echo sequence along three spatial directions.

In practical implementations, two sets of images are acquired with the same parameters, except for the first moment of the bipolar gradients. The two images are then subtracted pixel by pixel.

This method provides images where the pixel's intensity is directly related to the flow velocity. Generally, flow is displayed with a positive sign when it has the same direction as the bipolar gradient and a negative sign when it has the opposite orientation. Stationary spins have an average signal (gray) with a zero phase. To obtain a flow image without direction information, the absolute value is obtained from the combination of the phase images of the three orthogonal flow-encoding directions; this represents a "velocity" image. The amount of velocity encoding is defined by the variation in the moment between two bipolar gradients. To quantify this, the VENC (Velocity ENCoding, expressed in cm/s) parameter is introduced in phase imaging, and its value is determined before the scan by the operator. This value is positive and inversely proportional to the difference of the first gradient moments according to the following equation:

$$VENC = \frac{\pi}{|\gamma \Delta m_1|} \qquad [6.2]$$

where Δm_1 is the variation of the first moment of the bipolar velocity gradient (when the gradient waveform is executed).

6.3.2.1. *Limitations of phase contrast imaging*

Contrary to TOF and contrast agent methods, the phase contrast imaging technique is not often used. The reason lies in the relatively long acquisition time for this method due to the need to combine several images. However, this approach is compatible with parallel acquisition techniques, and its acquisition time can be significantly reduced in such a way.

6.3.2.2. *Usage*

The phase contrast technique is mainly used for intracranial angiography. However, although it was initially developed for acquiring images of blood vessels, phase-based techniques are widely employed in other applications (measurements of motion, temperature imaging, CSF flow imaging, etc.).

SEQUENCE ACQUISITION PARAMETERS.– Phase contrast 3D sequence (EG) with VENC 40 cm/s and four slices of 2 cm: TE/*TR* = 6.49/44.2 ms; flip angle: 10°; field of view: 240 × 180 mm; resolution: 0.5 × 0.5 × 0.9 mm; phase acceleration factor: 2; in-slice partial Fourier: 7/8; acquisition time: 3:59 min.

6.3.3. *Black-blood imaging*

Black- (or dark-)blood imaging is another type of angiography technique. As indicated by the name, the principle underlying these methods is to suppress the blood signal and thereby visualize its location with respect to stationary tissues by observing a negative effect in blood vessels. Such methods must strongly attenuate the blood signal while preserving the signal from surrounding stationary tissues.

Diminishing or suppressing the blood signal is achieved via sequences exploiting the "exit slice" effect. This phenomenon is found in most standard spin echo methods, whether accelerated (RARE) or not (conventional spin echo). As illustrated in Figure 6.3, while stationary spins are subjected to the effect of a 90° pulse followed by a refocusing 180° pulse to generate a spin echo, moving spins are subjected to only one of the two pulses. Therefore, their signal is almost non-existent in the images. This effect becomes more prominent as the spin velocity increases. In practice, a saturation slice can be used before the image acquisition to suppress the signal from slowly moving spins in an even more efficient way.

Other sequences can be employed to suppress the blood signal, such as inversion recovery (Mayo et al. 1989) or double inversion recovery (Simonetti et al. 1996) sequences.

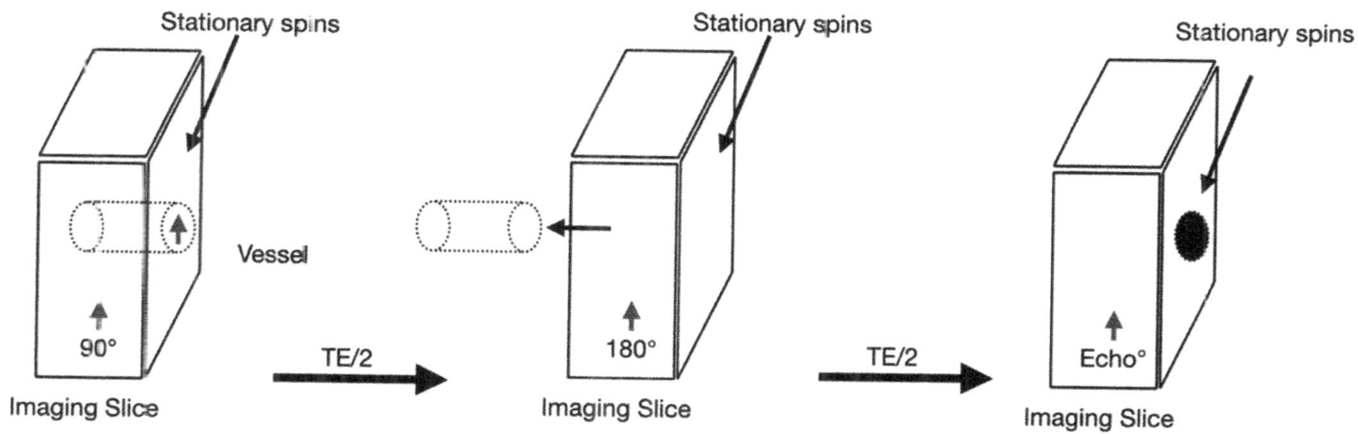

Figure 6.3A. *Principle of black-blood imaging using a spin echo sequence*

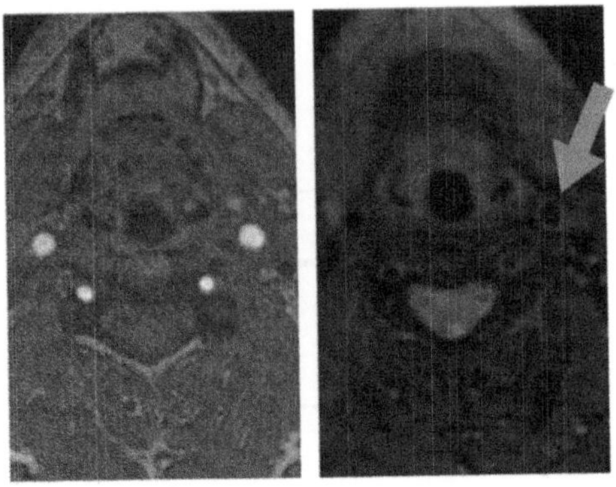

Figure 6.3B. *Images obtained in the same volunteer with white-blood and black-blood methods to visualize the carotid arteries (pink arrow)*

Black-blood sequences are typically used for imaging of the heart or vessel walls (e.g. in carotid vessels) to better detect stenosis or atheromatous plaques. In the case of cardiac imaging, the sequences are synchronized with the electrocardiogram (ECG) signal. In such conditions, the sequence has to be perfectly synchronized to acquire the images during the most static phase of the heart while efficiently suppressing the blood signal.

Acquisition parameters for a T_2 black-blood sequence at 3 T are the following: 2D spin echo sequence; TE/*TR* = 123/1,300 ms; flip angle: 10°; field of view: 220 × 171 mm; voxel size: 0.9 × 0.9 × 0.9 mm; phase acceleration factor: 2; in-slice partial Fourier: 6/8; enabled fat suppression; acquisition time: 5:17 min.

An alternative to black-blood sequences consists of using the T_2* of the deoxyhemoglobin in the blood. Such an approach is called SWI imaging, or susceptibility-weighted imaging, and it produces a black blood venogram.

In practice, a 3D volume is acquired with a gradient echo sequence with a long TE (> 15 ms at 3 T). Magnitude and phase images are reconstructed from the same raw k-space data. Phase images are filtered with a high-pass filter to remove any phase that is not due to local susceptibility variations. Since phase images are more sensitive to variations than magnitude images, they are used to calculate an image mask which is multiplied by the magnitude image (Haacke et al. 2004). Figure 6.4 (right) shows an SWI image of a volunteer's brain.

In black-blood imaging, contrary to TOF imaging, turbulent flows represent an advantage. This is especially the case in areas with a complex flow such as stenoses, where TOF imaging can prove inefficient, while black-blood angiography can enable pathology detection with better specificity.

The main inconvenience of black-blood sequences is their low SNR, as well as the difficulty in applying them in three dimensions for high-resolution imaging. SWI imaging, on the other hand, is by definition very sensitive to susceptibility effects, which can lead to a lot of artifacts that make image interpretation impossible.

6.3.4. *Other techniques*

Several other angiographic techniques have been developed that are neither white-blood, black-blood nor contrast agent techniques. This research area is very active, as MRI is a very good alternative to Angio-X methods thanks to its harmlessness. Among these techniques, fresh blood imaging (Miyazaki et al. 2000) provides images of the extremities with very good contrast. Balanced SSFP (Fan et al. 2009) or quiescent-interval single-shot (QISS) (Edelman et al. 2010) sequences are also employed for lower limb imaging. Finally, spin marking approaches can prove as efficient as invasive catheter-based methods (Grist et al. 2012).

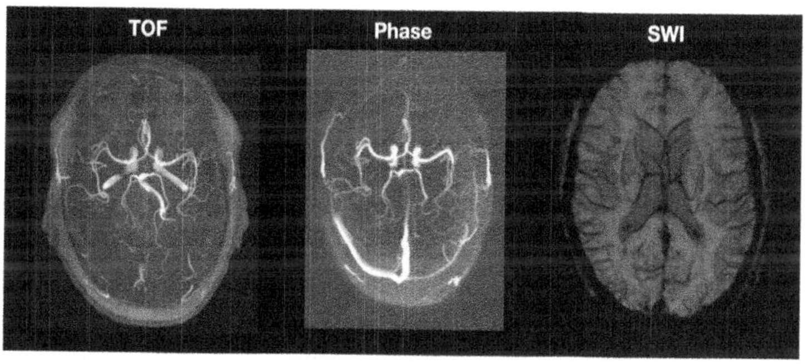

Figure 6.4. *Brain angiography of the same volunteer with a 3D TOF, 3D phase contrast and SWI sequence. The visualization is done using maximum intensity projection (MIP) and minimum Intensity Projection (mIP) algorithms for white-blood and black-blood imaging, respectively*

6.3.5. *Dynamic angiography*

Today, thanks to advances in hardware, in particular with parallel imaging, it is possible to acquire time-resolved angiographic images, whether with or without contrast agents and even with phase imaging (Markl et al. 2012). These methods are typically based on the utilization of acceleration techniques such as keyhole, compressed sensing or alternative methods such as VIPR (radial 3D Vastly undersampled Isotropic PRojection) (Mistretta 2009). These methods acquire less spatially resolved images than anatomical angiographic techniques. Nevertheless, the obtained information makes them an alternative to invasive fluoroscopy methods. Becoming established in the clinical routine is a long and tedious process. This is due to the long acquisition time and the complex processing techniques that need to be implemented.

6.4. Perfusion imaging

6.4.1. *Dynamic susceptibility contrast*

As described by the method's name, the dynamic susceptibility contrast (DSC) approach is based on the susceptibility effect of a paramagnetic contrast agent. This is injected in the form of a bolus and MRI acquisition is done dynamically to capture the first pass of the contrast agent in the blood circulation. This approach is particularly suitable for the brain: due to the BBB, the contrast agent remains confined to the vessels. In this context, the central volume principle, a mathematical model, relates the measurement of the contrast agent's concentration evolution to the estimation of physiological parameters that characterize perfusion.

In DSC, T_2* weighted sequences are typically used since they are sensitive to susceptibility effects. To obtain a temporal resolution of about 1.5 s and good spatial coverage, gradient echo EPI sequence is mainly utilized. It is recommended that approximately 30 s of signal is acquired to obtain a robust estimation of the baseline signal (the signal before the appearance of the contrast agent). The entire scan typically lasts between 1 and 2 minutes. Its goal is to properly sample the first pass of the contrast agent and, if possible, some time afterward. In the case of vascular anomalies (e.g. cerebral stroke), a 2 min acquisition is recommended. Due to the spatial coverage and time resolution constraints, spatial resolution is typically between 2 and 4 mm. Initially obtained with segmented acquisitions and thus shorter *TR* than the temporal resolution indicated above, these acquisitions used to be sensitive to T_1 variations (relaxivity effects). Today, parallel imaging approaches (e.g. SENSE) enable non-segmented acquisitions and thus reduce these T_1 effects by employing long *TR*. Multi-band acquisitions (simultaneous excitation of several slices) offer new perspectives to make the scans even more robust to T_1 effects via the acquisition of several echoes for measuring the T_2* effect and compensating for it during the analysis. Finally, some groups use spin echo EPI sequences, hence T_2 weighted, to achieve higher sensitivity to small vessels, although the signal-to-noise ratio is lower than in gradient echo sequences. We shall come back to this aspect in section 6.4.3.

In the 1990s, numerical simulations and mathematical models explored the relationship between MRI signal variations and the changes in contrast agent concentration. These approaches were based on strong hypotheses, such as a uniform distribution of the vessels' directions (i.e. without a preferential orientation), a unique vessel diameter, absence of interactions between the contributions from the different vessels, small blood volume and a constant difference in magnetic susceptibility between intra- and extra-vascular compartments (this difference is caused by the contrast agent concentration and the employed magnetic field).

In 1994, Yablonskiy and Haacke (1994) published a set of equations that demonstrated a linear relationship between the volume occupied by the vessels and the variation of the gradient echo signal due to the magnetic susceptibility effect. In 1995, Boxerman et al. (1995) published numerical simulations investigating the MRI signal change induced by a given contrast agent concentration. They have studied the signal variation for gradient echo sequences – characterized by ΔR_2*, that is, the difference between $R_2*=1/T_2*$ with and without contrast agent – and spin echo sequences. If the above-mentioned hypotheses are true, ΔR_2* is proportional to the contrast agent concentration. Several elements should be highlighted here:

– If the contrast agent exits the vessels, then (i) the hypotheses of the model for estimating perfusion parameters are no longer valid, and (ii) the relationship between the MRI signal and the contrast agent concentration does not hold. Indeed, the susceptibility effect is no longer dominant and a significant relaxivity effect appears. In the brain, this situation can become a source of errors in the case of BBB alteration.

– If the voxel contains mainly blood (e.g. more than 20% blood), then the relationship between the MRI signal and the contrast agent concentration is not the same. The case of large vessels (100% of the voxel) has been investigated by van Osch et al. (2018). They have shown that a quadratic relationship between the signal and the contrast agent concentration exists and that using the signal's phase is more robust.

– If the spin echo is acquired instead of gradient echo, then the measurement does not have the same sensitivity for all vascular diameters. In particular, Boxerman et al. (1995) have shown that the smaller vessels have a larger contribution.

Two main approaches are used for signal analysis: the oldest consists of an analysis of the curve features and its most recommended version employs the arterial input function (AIF) to obtain data that is well-quantified as possible via a sensitive deconvolution step (Willats and Calamante 2013). Actually, up to the current day, it is not possible to extract absolute quantitative maps of blood flow or volume. Due to this fact, there is no clear consensus on the best analysis method.

In the classic approach, the following formula is calculated:

$$\Delta R_2^* = -1/TE \times ln(S(t)/S_{baseline}) \quad [6.3]$$

where TE is the echo time, $S(t)$ is the gradient echo signal and $S_{baseline}$ is the average signal before the appearance of the contrast agent.

The area under the curve provides an estimation of the blood volume V. The cerebral blood flow F can then be estimated as $F = V/MTT$, where MTT is the mean transit time required for the contrast agent to move through the voxel. This approach is only robust under the hypothesis that all the tracer enters the voxel at the same time. In practice, this is not the case: the AIF should be taken into account (Willats and Calamante 2013). However, if we consider that the AIF is identical for all the pixels, then the bias is also constant and relative measurements are possible. The measurement of the AIF is typically obtained from a few pixels located at the periphery of the large arteries with an orthogonal orientation to the magnetic field (maximum susceptibility effect), such as the middle cerebral artery for the brain. Examples of signals, images and maps of V and MTT are shown in Figure 6.5.

As mentioned above, in the case of extravasation of the contrast agent, both the relationship signal versus concentration and the model hypotheses are no longer valid. This leads to an underestimation of the blood volume and blood flow. To avoid this effect, some authors have proposed performing a pre-injection.

The most recommended analysis consists of deconvoluting the concentration–time curve measured at a voxel with the AIF. The latter depends on parameters such as injection duration, cardiac frequency, state of pulmonary circulation or arteries along the heart–organ path. Deconvolution is very sensitive to noise and greatly benefits from a robust baseline (30 s are recommended in humans).

Cerebral perfusion measurement is used to characterize brain tumors. In the case of malignant tumors, angiogenesis occurs and blood volume increases.

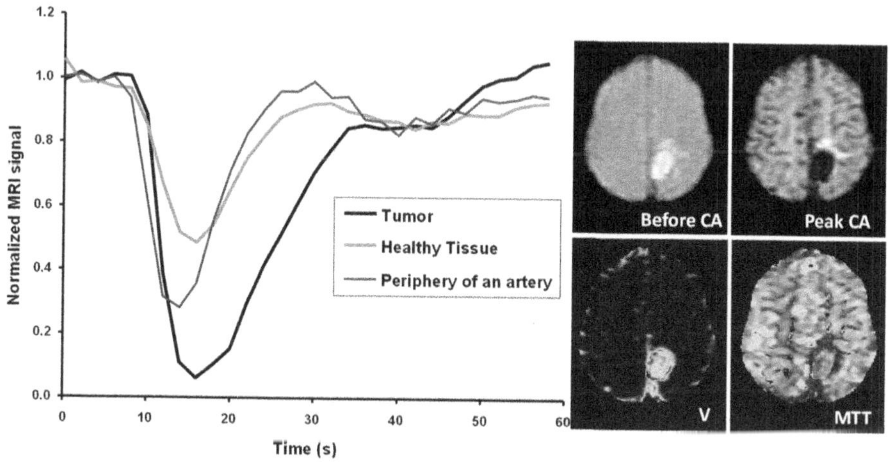

Figure 6.5. *Example of signals obtained in a patient during the pass of a gadolinium bolus. The black and white images were obtained before (before CA) and at the peak (peak CA) of the contrast agent concentration. The parametric maps correspond to the blood volume (V) and to the mean transit time (MTT). The curves are extracted from the regions of interest inside the tumor, healthy tissue and an artery's periphery. Data: IRMaGe*

6.4.2. *Dynamic contrast-enhanced*

The dynamic contrast-enhanced (DCE) approach is based on the T_1 relaxivity effect of a paramagnetic contrast agent. Contrary to the DSC approach, the phenomena of blood flow and extravasation of the contrast agent are taken into account (Tofts et al. 1999; Barbier et al. 2001). In the heart, DCE is a standard method for quantifying tissue blood flow and the extracellular volume (ECV), since the DSC approach is challenging due to heart movements and the rapid flow of ventricular blood. The DCE technique can also characterize vascular permeability and tissue properties such as the ECV, which is of interest when studying lesions, such as tumors, in different organs. The DCE approach is therefore very complementary to the DSC approach. In DCE, rapid T_1-weighted sequences (e.g. FLASH) are typically used because of their sensitivity to longitudinal relaxivity effects.

To measure permeability, the temporal resolution requirement is less strong than in DSC and it is common to acquire data with a temporal resolution of several tens of seconds. Because of that, the scans may be performed with a better spatial resolution than with DSC. The acquisition duration in humans is limited by the exam duration to a few minutes, although at least 10 min would be preferable for investigating low permeability situations. The aid of parallel imaging and multi-band techniques (see Chapter 3) offers perspectives in terms of quantification, by separating the relaxivity effects from the susceptibility effects that can occur, in particular during the first pass. More recently, the use of the MR Fingerprinting approach (see Chapter 10) has improved the quantification in permeability imaging.

On the other hand, to measure myocardial blood flow, higher temporal resolutions are employed, because the durations of bolus transit in the capillary system are shorter than the characteristic membrane diffusion time. Due to the cardiac motion, each image is acquired within a few hundred milliseconds in synchronization with an ECG. Most commonly, snap-shot FLASH or bSSFP sequences are used with a presaturation pulse. Each image is reconstructed and displayed in real-time, enabling the visualization of the arrival of the bolus into the left ventricle (LV), starting from when the subject can be instructed to stop breathing for the maximum possible time (typically 20–30 s). The acquisition continues for approximately 1 min. Due to ECG synchronization, temporal resolution is limited to the duration of a heartbeat. Figure 6.6 shows a typical behavior of the signal in the LV and a region of myocardial tissue during this scan.

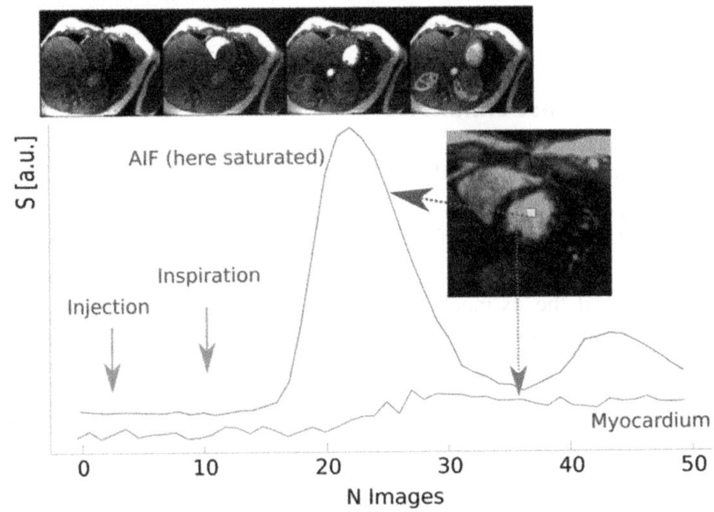

Figure 6.6. *Signal behavior after intravenous injection of gadolinium in a human in two regions of interest (red: myocardium, blue: LV chamber). The bolus arrival is visible in the LF, as well as its spreading in the myocardium. The images above illustrate the different key moments after injection, from left to right: pre-injection, arrival of the bolus into the right and left ventricles and diffusion in the myocardium. Data: CRMBM*

The analysis of tissue blood flow and volume is performed similarly to the DSC analysis in the brain: tissue signal is converted into CA concentration, deconvoluted using AIF measured in the blood of the LV and/or adjusted (via different models) to quantify the blood volume and flow. This analysis is done pixel by pixel or simply in predefined regions of interest.

For permeability measurement analysis, several approaches exist. The signal-time curve can directly provide different kinds of information: peak time, area under the curve and maximum signal enhancement. These parameters can be extracted in a robust way and they are sufficiently representative of the underlying physiologic conditions (Cheng 2009), with the area under the curve providing an approximation of permeability. The pharmacokinetic approach uses a two-compartment model or an extended Tofts et al.'s (1999) model. This model is described by the following equation:

$$C_{voxel}(t) = V \cdot AIF(t) + V_e \cdot k_{pe} \int_0^{\infty} AIF(\tau) \cdot exp[-k_{ep}(t-\tau)]d\tau \qquad [6.4]$$

where V is the plasmatic volume, $AIF(t)$ is the arterial input function, V_e is the extravascular ECV, and k_{pe} and k_{ep} are the exchange rates between the two compartments. PS, the product of permeability by vascular surface, equals k_{pe} x V. It is worth noting that F and PS are expressed in the same units: they are both flows. A similitude with water flowing in a leaking tube can be made: F is the flow inside the tube and PS is the flow through the holes of the tube.

These analyses can be done by using the MRI signals directly or by converting the evolution of the signal into that of the contrast agent concentration. For this purpose, a reference T_1 map has to be obtained before injecting the contrast agent. The signal evolution is converted into T_1 evolution and further into concentration variations by means of the contrast agent's relaxivity at the employed magnetic field, with the hypothesis that the agent is uniformly distributed. The challenge of estimating the AIF is also present in DCE. Once again, analyzing the signal's phase proves to be more robust in the brain.

In terms of result interpretation, if $F < PS$, then F is a limiting factor (with an exaggeration, it is not possible to know if the tube is leaking in the case of an absence of flow inside the tube) and PS can be underestimated. If $F > PS$, the conditions are propitious for a robust estimation of PS.

In the end, for long times (>10 min) after injection, the contrast agent with potential extravasation reduces the tissue relaxation time and thus provides a way to estimate the ECV. The comparison between T_1 before injection and late after injection yields a map of the ECV fraction and therewith the proportion of fibrosis in the tissue, even when the fibrosis is distributed in a diffuse way:

$$ECV = (1 - hct) \, [\, (1/T_1{}^{post}{}_{myo} - 1/T_1{}^{pre}{}_{myo}) \, / \, (1/T_1{}^{post}{}_{blood} - 1/T_1{}^{pre}{}_{blood}) \,] \qquad [6.5]$$

where *hct* is the hematocrit ratio; the exponents and indices indicate the origin of the T_1 values: pre- and post-injection, in myocardium and blood.

Thanks to its simplicity, this quantification is performed quite often in routine cardiovascular MRI.

In practice, in both DSC and DCE methods, a sequence of images is acquired after the injection of a contrast agent bolus. The quality of the quantification depends on the accuracy of the models and on the correct execution of these steps. One of the main difficulties, in any organ, consists of measuring or modeling the AIF: for the brain, this requires T_2* weighted images of the signal in the periphery of the main cerebral arteries that remain small compared to the resolution. For the heart, the AIF can be easily obtained from the blood signal in the LV, but the contrast/concentration relationship is strongly nonlinear for the high contrast agent concentrations present in the blood briefly after injection. A second injection at a low dose or a special sequence (a recent example is presented in (Milidonis et al. 2021)) with double T_1 weighting is required to quantify the AIF (and perfusion) in the heart. Besides, clinical applications are interested in the variation of perfusion under stress conditions (CO_2 for the brain, pharmacological vasodilators for the heart), and thus employ a second scan with an injection that increases the complexity of this technique.

In summary, all these considerations illustrate the relative complexity of quantitative perfusion mapping via DSC/DCE. Consequently, still to this day, quantitative perfusion methods are rarely used in routine clinical work, and most clinical centers settle for qualitative or semi-quantitative evaluations, based on parameters such as up-slope integral, time-to-peak and others.

Section 6.4.3 presents the ASL technique, an alternative MRI method for mapping the blood flow in tissues without using a contrast agent, for which quantification is, in theory, simpler, although it is limited to the measurement of capillary blood flow. Its usefulness is also hindered by its low sensitivity to tissues with high blood flow.

6.4.3. *Arterial spin labeling (ASL)*

The main advantage of the arterial spin labeling (ASL) approach is that it does not require any contrast agent. This method can thus be used when a contrast agent is contraindicated for a patient or to perform repeated measurements in a healthy subject within the same scan session.

ASL methods are based on the subtraction of two images acquired in two different conditions: an image acquired after inverting the blood's magnetization upstream from the slice and a control image, without inversion. The blood spins whose magnetization was inverted perfuse into the slice. The difference between an image "perfused" by blood with equilibrium magnetization (control image) and an image "perfused" by blood with inverted magnetization (labeled image) is proportional to the blood flow (Figure 6.7) (Detre et al. 1992).

Several ASL methods exist, and they are typically divided into "continuous" ASL methods (Williams et al. 1992), "pulsed" ASL (Kim 1995), or those based on the blood's velocity, "velocity-encoded" ASL (Guo et al. 2016). Here, we shall describe in more detail the method with the most consensus, the "pseudo-continuous" approach or pCASL (Alsop et al. 2015). One of the difficulties in inverting the arterial blood's magnetization is its variable velocity: due to the cardiac pulsation, the blood velocity varies between 0 and 50 cm/s. pCASL employs an elegant strategy of flow-driven adiabatic blood inversion (Dixon et al. 1986). Continuous inversion is replaced by a sequence (more than a thousand) of very short and close pulses (e.g. 400 μs every 800 μs) and the continuous magnetic field gradient also becomes segmented. On the one hand, this enables the selection of the labeling plane, and, on the other hand, it ensures that the induced phase evolution is either adiabatic (labeled image) or without any effect on the magnetization (control image). The labeling module typically lasts several seconds. Finally, a delay – the post-labeling delay – allows the blood to move toward tissues and thus attenuates the differences in arrival time of the labeled blood through the slice (Alsop and Detre 1996). In pCASL, perfusion quantification is performed via:

$$F = \frac{\lambda \cdot (SI_{control} - SI_{label}) e^{PLD/T_{1b}}}{2 \cdot \alpha \cdot T_{1b} \cdot SI_{PD}\left(1 - e^{\tau/T_{1b}}\right)} \qquad [6.6]$$

where λ is the brain-blood partition coefficient for water (0.9 mL/g; Herscovitch and Raichle 1985), the signal intensity (SI) corresponds to the intensities of the MRI signal for the control condition (control), labeled condition (label) and the proton-density-weighted condition (PD), the post-labeling delay (PLD) is the delay between the end of labeling and the image acquisition, τ is the labeling duration, T_{1b} is the T_1 of blood, and α is the inversion efficiency of the labeling RF pulse.

To improve ASL quantification, an alternative consists of acquiring several images by varying the delay, in order to acquire maps of the arrival time and to take into account this value in the calculation of the flow maps. This approach is called time-encoded ASL (van Osch et al. 2018). In addition, ASL enables vascular territory mapping (Bokkers et al. 2016).

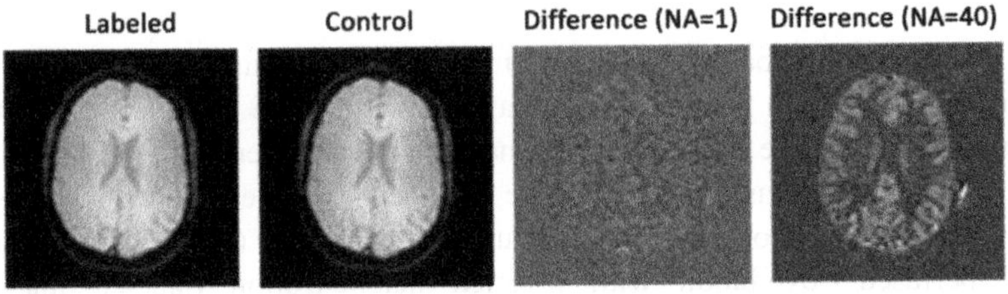

Figure 6.7. *Example of pCASL imaging at 3 T. The difference between a labeled image and a control image (number of accumulations (NA = 1) has a signal-to-noise ratio that is too low. After several averages (NA = 40), the cerebral perfusion image becomes readable*

In humans, SAR becomes a limiting factor for pCASL approaches. At higher fields, SAR increases (Hirschler et al. 2020), and inverting the magnetization in a robust way is more difficult (B_0 inhomogeneities).

ASL is successfully used in the kidneys and heart, where capillary blood flows are generally high. The main advantage for clinical cardiovascular applications lies in the repeatability of the technique under different physiological conditions (rest/stress). It should be noted that contrast agents are contraindicated for a high percentage of patients with cardiovascular diseases. From the technical point of view, the pCASL version cannot be used in the thorax region due to large cardiac and breathing movements, and due to the pulsating flow in coronary vessels that supply the heart muscle. Many studies have employed the FAIR-bSFFP method with different motion synchronization solutions (Poncelet et al. 1999; Zun et al. 2009; Aramendía-Vidaurreta et al. 2020), although other approaches have been proposed, such as steady-pulsed ASL (Troalen et al. 2013; Capron et al. 2015; Lee et al. 2020) for increasing sensitivity. Thanks to very high blood flow in rodents, cardiac ASL is routinely used, while its routine usage in humans is still prevented by the lack of robustness.

Figure 6.8 shows an illustration of some examples of regional blood flow maps for different experimental configurations.

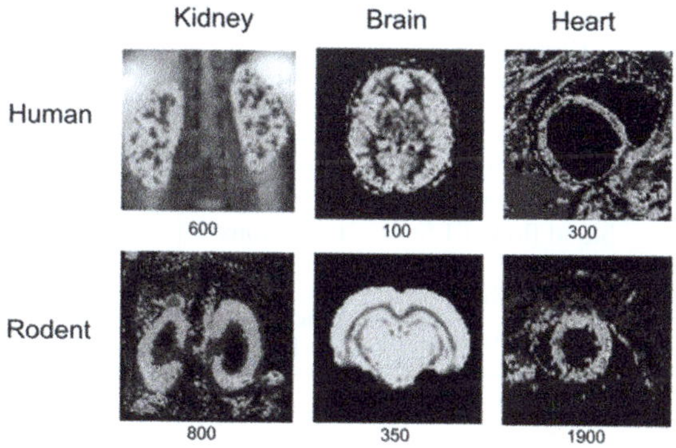

Figure 6.8. *Examples of tissue blood flow obtained via ASL in healthy subjects (humans and rodents, kidney: mouse, brain: rat, heart: rat under adenosine stress). Color scales: rainbow from blue to red, with the number under each image indicating the scale's maximum in mL/100 g/min. Images: Courtesy of E. Barbier, J. Warnking, GIN Grenoble (brain), F. Kober, T. Troalen, CRMBM Marseille (heart), G. Duhamel, V. Prevost, CRMBM Marseille (mouse kidney; Prevost et al. 2015). Human kidney: extracted with a license from Nery et al. (2018)*

6.4.4. *Experimental approaches*

The approaches presented above are all usable in clinical MRI scanners. From the experimental point of view, other methods have been developed. The oldest is the IVIM approach, which provides information on the rapid incoherent motion (blood) and the slow incoherent motion (water diffusion) by means of diffusion gradients of variable intensity (see Chapter 4). From the perfusion point of view, IVIM quantification remains challenging.

By taking advantage of the difference between the evolution of the spin echo and gradient echo signals acquired simultaneously after injecting a contrast agent, several methods have been developed to characterize the average microvascular diameter (vessel size index) or the microvascular density (Lemasson et al. 2013). These methods can work based on a DSC type of approach with multi-echos (e.g. a gradient echo and a spin echo) or based on the so-called "equilibrium" approach where the measurements are performed before and after injecting a contrast agent. These equilibrium approaches require contrast agents with a certain vascular persistence, achieved via greater hydrodynamic diameters. Ultrasmall superparamagnetic iron oxide particles (USPIO) are suitable for these techniques.

	Parameters	Organs	Commentaries
DSC	Blood flow, blood volume, average transit time, Tmax	Brain	Bolus injection of a contrast agent, T_2* or T_2 effect
DCE	Vascular permeability, blood volume, blood flow, EES	All organs, cerebral lesions	Bolus injection of a contrast agent, T_1 effect
ASL	Blood flow, arrival time	Brain, heart, eye, kidney	No contrast agent; difficult in humans > 3T (SAR problem)
IVIM	Rapid and slow incoherent motion	All organs	No contrast agent (diffusion gradient)
VSI	Microvascular diameter and density	All organs	Contrast agent injection. T_2 and T_2* effects
StO_2, qBOLD	Tissue oxygen saturation, oxygen extraction fraction	All organs	May use an injection of a contrast agent to estimate blood volume. T_2 and T_2* effects
Vasoreactivity	Vasoreactivity	Brain, heart	Requires a vascular challenge: gaseous or pharmacologic

Table 6.1. *Measurable physiologic parameters and measurement methods*

By quantifying the BOLD effect, that is, the difference between T_2 and T_2*, via the estimation of blood volume, it is eventually possible to map the tissue oxygen saturation (using approaches such as qBOLD (Yablonskiy et al. 2013) or StO_2 (Christen et al. 2014)).

Gaseous vascular stress (via hypercapnia) or a pharmacological stress can lead to a measurement of cerebral reserves (or cerebral vasoreactivity), thanks to approaches that do not require contrast agents, such as BOLD (see Chapter 5) or ASL methods. The coronary reserves can be determined by inducing stress (Dobutamine) or a general (Adenosine) or selective (Regadenoson) vasodilation.

6.5. Considerations for imaging in humans and small animals

The most advantageous methods and, sometimes, strategies for angiography or perfusion MRI present significant differences between preclinical and clinical studies. This can be explained by considering some vascular properties, the typical values of which (order of magnitude) are summarized in Table 6.2.

There are considerable differences in proportions between small animals, large animals and humans.

Property	Human	Rat*	Mouse*
Body weight	80 kg	0.3 kg	0.03 kg
Total blood volume	5 L	18 mL	1.8 mL
Cardiac end-diastolic volume	180 mL	300 µL	50 µL
Heart rate	80 bpm	300 bpm	600 bpm
Cardiac output	5 L/min	150 mL/min	20 mL/min
Re-circulation time	1 min	7 s	5 s
Diameter of the aorta	33 mm	3.5 mm	1.4 mm
Peak velocity of blood ejected in the aorta	100 cm/s	200 cm/s	300 cm/s
Breath rate	12 bpm	70 bpm	110 bpm
Myocardial perfusion	1 mL/g/min	5 mL/g/min	7 mL/g/min
Cerebral tissue perfusion	0.5 mL/g/min	0.8 mL/g/min	1.1 mL/g/min

Table 6.2. *Order of magnitude of some physiological parameters in humans, rats and mice. *Anesthetized with isoflurane*

The first difference is related to the blood flow delivered by the heart in proportion to the body weight. This flow determines the total volume of blood exchanged in the body per unit of time and the blood's circulation velocity in the arteries. The relative cardiac flow is 10 times greater in rodents than in humans. On the other hand, the relative total blood volume is comparable between species shown in Table 6.2. As a result, the high flow in rodents is achieved with very high relative circulation velocities in large vessels and high flow and regional blood volume in tissues. The time between the ejection of a unit of blood volume from the heart and its return into the LV via the venous system and the lungs is approximately 10 times shorter in rodents than in humans.

The second major difference lies in the microvascularization density, characterized by the regional blood volume, among other contributors. Its value reaches 5% in the heart of a rat, and 10% in the heart of a mouse. In most tissues, very high values of regional blood flow are observed in small animals.

Such differences have implications regarding the design and choice of angiographic MRI and perfusion mapping methods in rodents.

6.5.1. *Angiography in rodents*

Flow velocities are high in large vessels and they are indeed comparable to those observed in humans in much larger vessels. As a result, there are more constraints on the duration of the gradients used in imaging sequences. For this reason it is difficult to, for example, map flow velocities in the thorax region using bipolar encoding in combination with gradient echo sequences, because the slice selection and rephasing gradients already provide high flow sensitivity. On the other hand, the very short transit times in rodents are of great benefit for the contrast in TOF methods.

6.5.2. *Perfusion MRI in rodents*

In rodents, regional blood flows are high, thereby providing a great benefit for ASL methods that are also advantageous at the high magnetic fields used in preclinical MRI scanners where blood's T_1 is longer. Thanks to the very short transit times, continuous or pseudo-continuous ASL methods perform particularly well. However, it should be noted that a volume transmit coil is required for pulsed ASL sequences. These invert the magnetization of all the blood that might enter the slices of interest (e.g. the entire heart must be covered even when only the brain is investigated). Finally, the short timings and high velocities of the circulation become major constraints for techniques that dynamically follow a bolus. Advanced acceleration methods and/or low spatial resolutions are, therefore, necessary for bolus tracking.

6.6. References

Alsop, D.C. and Detre, J.A. (1996). Reduced transit-time sensitivity in noninvasive magnetic resonance imaging of human cerebral blood flow. *Journal of Cerebral Blood Flow & Metabolism*, 16(6), 1236–1249.

Alsop, D.C., Detre, J.A., Golay, X., Gu, M., Hendrikse, J., Hernandez-Garcia, L., Lu, H., MacIntosh, B.J., Parkes, L.M., Smits, M. et al. (2015). Recommended implementation of arterial spin-labeled perfusion MRI for clinical applications: A consensus of the ISMRM Perfusion Study Group and the European Consortium for ASL in dementia. *Magnetic Resonance in Medicine*, 73, 102–116.

Aramendía-Vidaurreta, V., Echeverría-Chasco, R., Vidorreta, M., Bastarrika, G., Fernández-Seara, M.A. (2020). Quantification of myocardial perfusion with vasodilation using arterial spin labeling at 1.5T. *Journal of Magnetic Resonance Imaging: JMRI*, 53(3), 777–788.

Atkinson, D., Brant-Zawadzki, M., Gillan, G., Purdy, D., Laub, G. (1994). Improved MR angiography: Magnetization transfer suppression with variable flip angle excitation and increased resolution. *Radiology*, 190(3), 890–894.

Barbier, E.L., Lamalle, L., Décorps, M. (2001). Methodology of brain perfusion imaging. *Journal of Magnetic Resonance Imaging*, 13(4), 496–520.

Bokkers, R.P.H., De Cocker, L.J., van Osch, M.J.P., Hartkamp, N.S., Hendrikse, J. (2016). Selective arterial spin labeling: Techniques and neurovascular applications. *Topics in Magnetic Resonance Imaging*, 25(2), 73–80.

Boxerman, J.L., Hamberg, L.M., Rosen, B.R., Weisskoff, R.M. (1995). MR contrast due to intravascular magnetic susceptibility perturbations. *Magnetic Resonance in Medicine*, 34(4), 555–566.

Capron, T., Troalen, T., Robert, B., Jacquier, A., Bernard, M., Kober, F. (2015). Myocardial perfusion assessment in humans using steady-pulsed arterial spin labeling. *Magnetic Resonance in Medicine*, 74(4), 990–998.

Cheng, H.L.M. (2009). Improved correlation to quantitative DCE-MRI pharmacokinetic parameters using a modified initial area under the uptake curve (mIAUC) approach. *Journal of Magnetic Resonance Imaging*, 30(4), 864–872.

Christen, T., Bouzat, P., Pannetier, N., Coquery, N., Moisan, A., Lemasson, B., Thomas, S., Grillon, E., Detante, O., Rémy, C. et al. (2014). Tissue oxygen saturation mapping with magnetic resonance imaging. *Journal of Cerebral Blood Flow & Metabolism*, 34(9), 1550–1557.

Davis, W.L., Blatter, D.D., Harnsberger, H.R., Parker, D.L. (1994). Intracranial MR angiography: Comparison of single-volume three-dimensional time-of-flight and multiple overlapping thin slab acquisition techniques. *AJR: American Journal of Roentgenology*, 163(4), 915–920.

Detre, J.A., Leigh, J.S., Williams, D.S., Koretsky, A.P. (1992). Perfusion imaging. *Magnetic Resonance in Medicine*, 23(1), 37–45.

Dixon, W.T., Du, L.N., Faul, D.D., Gado, M., Rossnick, S. (1986). Projection angiograms of blood labeled by adiabatic fast passage. *Magnetic Resonance in Medicine*, 3(3), 454–462.

Dumoulin, C.L., Souza, S.P., Walker, M.F., Wagle, W. (1989). Three-dimensional phase contrast angiography. *Magnetic Resonance in Medicine*, 9(1), 139–149.

Edelman, R.R., Sheehan, J.J., Dunkle, E., Schindler, N., Carr, J., Koktzoglou, I. (2010). Quiescent-interval single-shot unenhanced magnetic resonance angiography of peripheral vascular disease: Technical considerations and clinical feasibility. *Magnetic Resonance in Medicine*, 63(4), 951–958.

Fan, Z., Sheehan, J., Bi, X., Liu, X., Carr, J., Li, D. (2009). 3D noncontrast MR angiography of the distal lower extremities using flow-sensitive dephasing (FSD)-prepared balanced SSFP. *Magnetic Resonance in Medicine*, 62(6), 1523–1532.

Farb, R.I., Scott, J.N., Willinsky, R.A., Montanera, W.J., Wright, G.A., Terbrugge, K.G. (2003). Intracranial venous system: Gadolinium-enhanced three-dimensional MR venography with auto-triggered elliptic centric-ordered sequence-initial experience. *Radiology*, 226(1), 203–209.

Grist, T.M., Mistretta, C.A., Strother, C.M., Turski, P.A. (2012). Time-resolved angiography: Past, present, and future. *Journal of Magnetic Resonance Imaging: JMRI*, 36(6), 1273–1286.

Guo, J., Buxton, R.B., Wong, E.C. (2016). Wedge-shaped slice-selective adiabatic inversion pulse for controlling temporal width of bolus in pulsed arterial spin labeling. *Magnetic Resonance in Medicine*, 76(3), 838–847.

Haacke, E.M., Xu, Y., Cheng, Y.C.N., Reichenbach, J.R. (2004). Susceptibility weighted imaging (SWI). *Magnetic Resonance in Medicine*, 52(3), 612–618.

Herscovitch, P. and Raichle, M.E. (1985). What is the correct value for the brain-blood partition coefficient for water? *Journal of Cerebral Blood Flow & Metabolism*, 5(1), 65–69.

Hirschler, L., Collomb, N., Voiron, J., Köhler, S., Barbier, E.L., Warnking, J.M. (2020). SAR comparison between CASL and pCASL at high magnetic field and evaluation of the benefit of a dedicated labeling coil. *Magnetic Resonance in Medicine*, 83(1), 254–261.

Kim, S.G. (1995). Quantification of relative cerebral blood flow change by flow-sensitive alternating inversion recovery (FAIR) technique: Application to functional mapping. *Magnetic Resonance in Medicine*, 34(3), 293–301.

Laub, G.A. (1995). Time-of-flight method of MR angiography. *Magnetic Resonance Imaging Clinics of North America*, 3(3), 391–398.

Lee, N.G., Javed, A., Jao, T.R., Nayak, K.S. (2020). Numerical approximation to the general kinetic model for ASL quantification. *Magnetic Resonance in Medicine*, 84(5), 2846–2857.

Lemasson, B., Valable, S., Farion, R., Krainik, A., Rémy, C., Barbier, E.L. (2013). In vivo imaging of vessel diameter, size, and density: A comparative study between MRI and histology. *Magnetic Resonance in Medicine*, 69(1), 18–26.

Markl, M., Frydrychowicz, A., Kozerke, S., Hope, M., Wieben, O. (2012). 4D flow MRI. *Journal of Magnetic Resonance Imaging: JMRI*, 36(5), 1015–1036.

Mayo, J.R., Culham, J.A., MacKay, A.L., Aikins, D.G. (1989). Blood MR signal suppression by preexcitation with inverting pulses. *Radiology*, 173(1), 269–271.

Milidonis, X., Franks, R., Schneider, T., Sánchez-González, J., Sammut, E.C., Plein, S., Chiribiri, A. (2021). Influence of the arterial input sampling location on the diagnostic accuracy of cardiovascular magnetic resonance stress myocardial perfusion quantification. *Journal of Cardiovascular Magnetic Resonance*, 23(1), 35.

Mistretta, C.A. (2009). Undersampled radial MR acquisition and highly constrained back projection (HYPR) reconstruction: Potential medical imaging applications in the post-Nyquist era. *Journal of Magnetic Resonance Imaging: JMRI*, 29(3), 501–516.

Miyazaki, M., Sugiura, S., Tateishi, F., Wada, H., Kassai, Y., Abe, H. (2000). Non-contrast-enhanced MR angiography using 3D ECG-synchronized half-Fourier fast spin echo. *Journal of Magnetic Resonance Imaging: JMRI*, 12(5), 776–783.

Moran, P.R. (1982). A flow velocity zeugmatographic interlace for NMR imaging in humans. *Magnetic Resonance Imaging*, 1(4), 197–203.

Nery, F., Gordon, I., Thomas, D.L. (2018). Non-invasive renal perfusion imaging using arterial spin labeling MRI: Challenges and opportunities. *Diagnostics (Basel, Switzerland)*, 8(1), E2.

van Osch, M.J., Teeuwisse, W.M., Chen, Z., Suzuki, Y., Helle, M., Schmid, S. (2018). Advances in arterial spin labelling MRI methods for measuring perfusion and collateral flow. *Journal of Cerebral Blood Flow & Metabolism*, 38(9), 1461–1480.

Parker, D.L., Goodrich, K.C., Roberts, J.A., Chapman, B.E., Jeong, E.K., Kim, S.E., Tsuruda, J.S., Katzman, G.L. (2003). The need for phase-encoding flow compensation in high-resolution intracranial magnetic resonance angiography. *Journal of Magnetic Resonance Imaging: JMRI*, 18(1), 121–127.

Poncelet, B.P., Koelling, T.M., Schmidt, C.J., Kwong, K.K., Reese, T.G., Ledden, P., Kantor, H.L., Brady, T.J., Weisskoff, R.M. (1999). Measurement of human myocardial perfusion by double-gated flow alternating inversion recovery EPI. *Magnetic Resonance in Medicine*, 41(3), 9–510.

Prevost, V.H., Girard, O.M., Callot, V., Cozzone, P.J., Duhamel, G. (2015). Fast imaging strategies for mouse kidney perfusion measurement with pseudocontinuous arterial spin labeling (pCASL) at ultra high magnetic field (11.75 tesla). *Journal of Magnetic Resonance Imaging: JMRI*, 42(4), 999–1008.

Prince, M.R. (1994). Gadolinium-enhanced MR aortography. *Radiology*, 191(1), 155–164.

Saib, G., Gras, V., Mauconduit, F., Boulant, N., Vignaud, A., Brugières, P., Le Bihan, D., Le Brusquet, L., Amadon, A. (2019). Time-of-flight angiography at 7T using TONE double spokes with parallel transmission. *Magnetic Resonance Imaging*, 61, 104–115.

Schenck, J.F. (1996). The role of magnetic susceptibility in magnetic resonance imaging: MRI magnetic compatibility of the first and second kinds. *Medical Physics*, 23(6), 815–850.

Simonetti, O.P., Wendt, R.E., Duerk, J.L. (1991). Significance of the point of expansion in interpretation of gradient moments and motion sensitivity. *Journal of Magnetic Resonance Imaging: JMRI*, 1(5), 569–577.

Simonetti, O.P., Finn, J.P., White, R.D., Laub, G., Henry, D.A. (1996). "Black blood" T_2-weighted inversion-recovery MR imaging of the heart. *Radiology*, 199(1), 49–57.

Tofts, P.S., Brix, G., Buckley, D.L., Evelhoch, J.L., Henderson, E., Knopp, M.V., Larsson, H.B., Lee, T.Y., Mayr, N.A., Parker, G.J. et al. (1999). Estimating kinetic parameters from dynamic contrast-enhanced T(1)-weighted MRI of a diffusable tracer: Standardized quantities and symbols. *Journal of Magnetic Resonance Imaging: JMRI*, 10(3), 223–232.

Troalen, T., Capron, T., Cozzone, P.J., Bernard, M., Kober, F. (2013). Cine-ASL: A steady-pulsed arterial spin labeling method for myocardial perfusion mapping in mice. Part I. Experimental study. *Magnetic Resonance in Medicine*, 70(5), 1389–1398.

Weinmann, H.J., Brasch, R.C., Press, W.R., Wesbey, G.E. (1984). Characteristics of gadolinium-DTPA complex: A potential NMR contrast agent. *AJR: American Journal of Roentgenology*, 142(3), 619–624.

Willats, L. and Calamante, F. (2013). The 39 steps: evading error and deciphering the secrets for accurate dynamic susceptibility contrast MRI. *NMR in Biomedicine*, 26(8), 913–931.

Williams, D.S., Detre, J.A., Leigh, J.S., Koretsky, A.P. (1992). Magnetic resonance imaging of perfusion using spin inversion of arterial water. *Proceedings of the National Academy of Sciences of the United States of America*, 89(1), 212–216.

Wilman, A.H., Riederer, S.J., Huston, J., Wald, J.T., Debbins, J.P. (1998). Arterial phase carotid and vertebral artery imaging in 3D contrast-enhanced MR angiography by combining fluoroscopic triggering with an elliptical centric acquisition order. *Magnetic Resonance in Medicine*, 40(1), 24–35.

Yablonskiy, D.A. and Haacke, E.M. (1994). Theory of NMR signal behavior in magnetically inhomogeneous tissues: The static dephasing regime. *Magnetic Resonance in Medicine*, 32(6), 749–763.

Yablonskiy, D.A., Sukstanskii, A.L., He, X. (2013). Blood oxygenation level-dependent (BOLD)-based techniques for the quantification of brain hemodynamic and metabolic properties – Theoretical models and experimental approaches: Cerebral hemodynamics and metabolism. *NMR in Biomedicine*, 26(8), 963–986.

Zun, Z., Wong, E.C., Nayak, K.S. (2009). Assessment of myocardial blood flow (MBF) in humans using arterial spin labeling (ASL): Feasibility and noise analysis. *Magnetic Resonance in Medicine*, 62(4), 975–983.

7

Quantitative Biomechanical Imaging via Magnetic Resonance Elastography

Olivier BEUF[1], Philippe GARTEISER[2], Kevin TSE VE KOON[1] and Jonathan VAPPOU[3]

[1] *CREATIS, CNRS, Inserm, INSA Lyon, Université Claude Bernard Lyon 1, France*
[2] *Centre de recherche sur l'inflammation, Inserm, Paris, France*
[3] *ICUBE, CNRS, Université de Strasbourg, France*

7.1. Fundamentals of magnetic resonance elastography

7.1.1. *Introduction*

Many pathologies affect the tissue structure and composition at different levels, including cellular modifications and the interactions between cells and their close surroundings, from the extracellular matrix up to the entire organ. Since the tissue structure and its composition determine how these tissues deform in response to an applied force, there is a correlation between the mechanical properties and the pathologic tissue alterations.

Due to this fact, the measurement of mechanical tissue properties or "elastography" has been proposed as a quantitative marker of pathological or healthy conditions. Several development works have been dedicated to imaging methods that would be capable of measuring the mechanical properties in a clinical setting.

The Challenges of MRI,
coordinated by Hélène RATINEY and Olivier BEUF.

Historically, ultrasound elastography was the first instance of virtual palpation. Magnetic resonance imaging was later adopted as an imaging tool to develop magnetic resonance elastography (MRE). Regardless of the underlying imaging method, all elastography approaches are based on three aspects: the application of a static or dynamic constraint, the measurement of the induced deformation and the reconstruction of mechanical properties. In the case of MRE, these elements consist of the generation and propagation of a shear wave, a phase-contrast MRI sequence and a quantitative reconstruction starting from the estimation of the shear modulus.

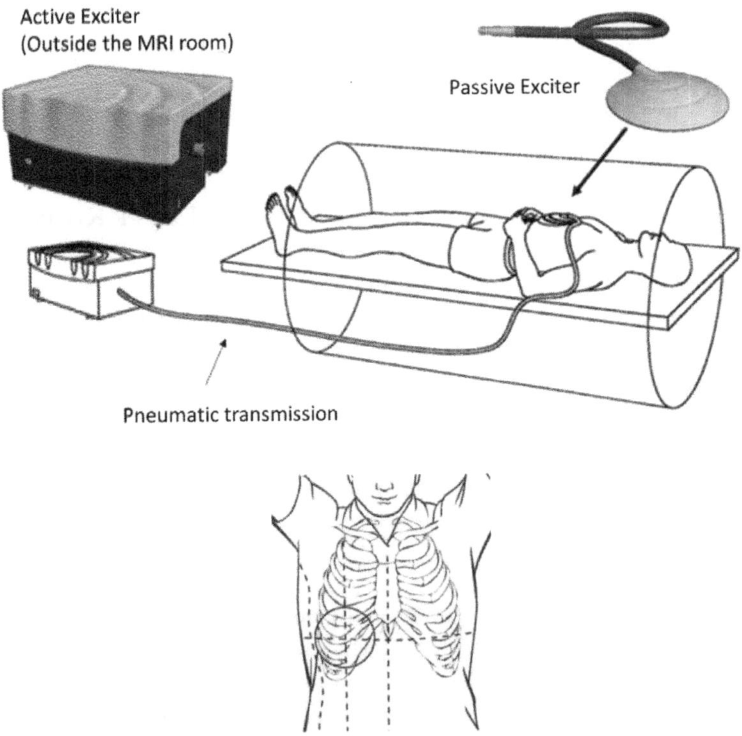

Figure 7.1. *Schematics of a pneumatic transducer employed in a clinical setting. The passive transducer is placed upon the thorax to transmit shear waves to the liver. Image from Resoundant (Rochester, MN, USA)*

Frequencies in the order of 50 Hz are typically used in clinics or even higher frequencies, in particular in preclinical scanners, where higher spatial resolutions are required. Several driver technologies are employed to produce shear waves in the region of interest. The most common approach in clinical settings is pneumatic excitation: a loudspeaker located outside the MRI room delivers acoustic vibration via a semi-rigid tube to a passive transducer made of a chamber with a membrane that vibrates in contact with the patient's skin (Venkatesh et al. 2013), as illustrated in Figure 7.1. Mechanical excitation can also be generated by an electromechanical or piezoelectric transducer and can be transmitted as a rigid motion to the MRI room, delivered directly to the actuator (Tse et al. 2009) or obtained from the rotation of an axis with an eccentric mass at its end in contact with the patient (Runge et al. 2019).

In such practical conditions, which are the most common ones, the displacement induced in tissues by the external transducer can be considered to be well represented by a harmonic plane shear wave. This hypothesis enables applying well-established wave propagation equations to estimate local mechanical properties. The equation of a propagating wave in a linear viscoelastic medium is given by:

$$-\rho\omega^2 u = \mu\Delta u + i\omega\eta.\Delta u \qquad [7.1]$$

where ρ is the tissue density, ω is the angular frequency of the wave and u is the displacement field (and Δ is its Laplacian). Here, the mechanical properties are composed of a real part μ corresponding to the elasticity of the tissue and of an imaginary part $\omega\eta$ corresponding to its viscosity that together can be represented as a complex shear modulus G:

$$G = \mu + i\omega\eta \qquad [7.2]$$

The real part of G is the storage modulus, sometimes denoted as G', and corresponds to the elasticity of the tissue, whereas the imaginary part, or loss modulus G'', is related to its viscosity. The magnitude of G and the damping ratio $G''/2G'$, derived from the representation of the complex value G in polar coordinates, are sometimes employed. In this way, we obtain the fundamental equation that relates the displacement induced by the wave to the mechanical properties of the medium in which it propagates:

$$-\rho\omega^2 u = G.\Delta u \qquad [7.3]$$

To visualize the waves generated via the different vibration devices mentioned above, motion-sensitive imaging sequences have to be used. For this purpose, encoding gradients are added to standard sequences such as gradient echo or spin echo sequences. The employed encoding gradients are designed to create a phase change in the signal that is proportional to the displacement (Lewa 1991). In order to solve equation [7.3], instantaneous tissue displacement has to be detected. This is achieved by temporally synchronizing the encoding gradients ($\vec{G}_{MEG}$ in equation [7.4]) with the mechanical vibration and repeating the measurement for different phase offsets between the encoding gradient and the mechanical vibration. The obtained phase can be expressed in terms of the time profile of the gradients and the tissue displacement at a point $\vec{\boldsymbol{r}}$ in the image:

$$\phi = \gamma \int_{t_0}^{t_0+\tau_G} \vec{\boldsymbol{G}}_{MEG}(t).\vec{\boldsymbol{u}}(\vec{\boldsymbol{r}}.t)dt \qquad [7.4]$$

In practice, most often, gradients (typically with a sinusoidal or trapezoidal shape) that oscillate at the same frequency as the mechanical wave are used. Tissue displacement can also be described as sinusoidal motion whose frequency is imposed by the transducer and whose amplitude and phase vary within the sample. When required, the different spatial components of displacement can be estimated by consecutively encoding the motion with gradients oriented along the three spatial directions.

Once the phase images are obtained, phase unwrapping followed by a conversion from radians to micrometers is performed to obtain the displacement field $\vec{\boldsymbol{u}}$. The compression displacement component is then removed (using one of the several available methods) to obtain the complete shear displacement field (typically as amplitude and phase data in the acquired image domain). The latter is then used to perform a local inversion of equation [7.3], thus leading to an estimation of G over the entire image or on an area of the image where both wave propagation and sufficient signal-to-noise ratio (SNR) are obtained.

7.1.2. *MRE signal encoding*

If we consider a (plane) shear wave that propagates in the y-direction with displacement motion along the z-direction, the displacement field can be expressed as:

$$\vec{\boldsymbol{u}}(\vec{\boldsymbol{r}},t) = Asin(\omega t - k.y + \theta_0)\vec{\boldsymbol{u}_z} \qquad [7.5]$$

A represents the amplitude of this wave, ω is its frequency, k is the wave vector, oriented here along the y-direction, and θ_0 is the initial phase of the wave which for now we consider equal to zero. Equation [7.4] shows that in order to encode this wave displacement into the phase of the MRI signal, the gradient $\vec{\boldsymbol{G}}_{MEG}(t)$ has to have at least one component parallel to the direction of tissue displacement (z in equation [7.5]). Ideally, to maximize the encoding, $\vec{\boldsymbol{G}}_{MEG}(t)$ is chosen such that:

$$\vec{\boldsymbol{G}}_{MEG}(t) = G_0(t)\vec{\boldsymbol{u}}_z \qquad [7.6]$$

where $G_0(t)$ is a periodic function (often with the same period as the wave). Figures 7.2(A)–(C) illustrate the phase encoding in a relatively simple case of a plane wave generated by a vibrating plate with a frequency of 50 Hz and amplitude of 25 µm described by equation [7.5] and a trapezoidal gradient with the same frequency of 50 Hz and an amplitude of 40 mT/m.

Figure 7.2(B) shows the displacement obtained at four separate points along the direction of propagation as well as the phase variation (according to equation [7.4]) when the motion encoding gradient is applied for one period. Figure 7.2(C) represents the final phase value depending on the position along the direction of propagation. As we can see, the phase provides an image of the displacement field. Other images at different instants of the wave propagation are required; this is achieved by repeating the acquisition with a delay between the motion and the application of the encoding gradient. Usually, at least four different sequential acquisitions are performed.

By observing the obtained encoded phase in Figure 7.2(C), it can be noted that its absolute value is greater than π. In MRI, the signal's phase is bounded between $-\pi$ and π and this means that the acquired phase image will exhibit phase wraps, which can be easily unwrapped in the present example. However, phase continuity between the different acquisitions must be ensured as well, and in the case of more complex or noisy displacement fields, the phase unwrapping step can be quite difficult.

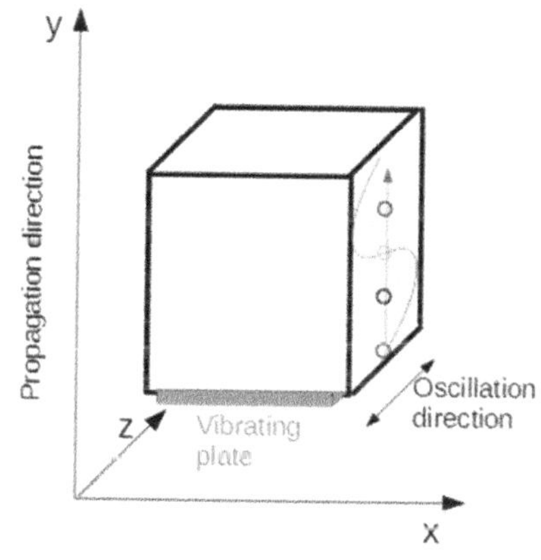

Figure 7.2A. *Schematics illustrating a device for generating shear waves within a phantom*

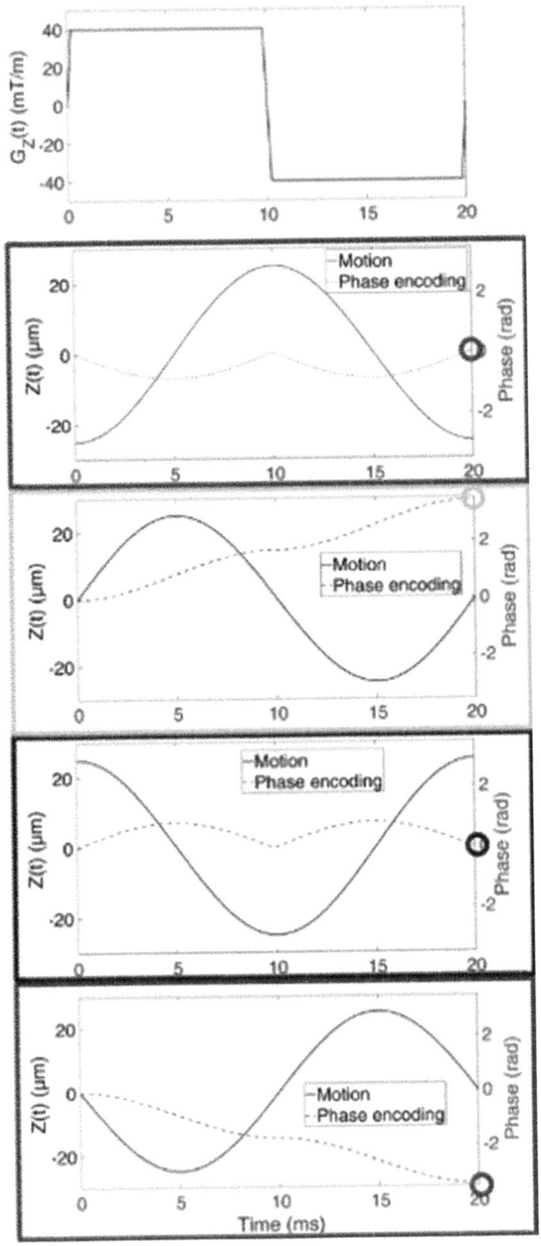

Figure 7.2B. *Motion-encoding gradient (40 mT/m amplitude, 50 Hz frequency) as a function of time, wave (25 µm amplitude and 50 Hz frequency) and phase encoding obtained at four equidistant points along the propagation direction during one period*

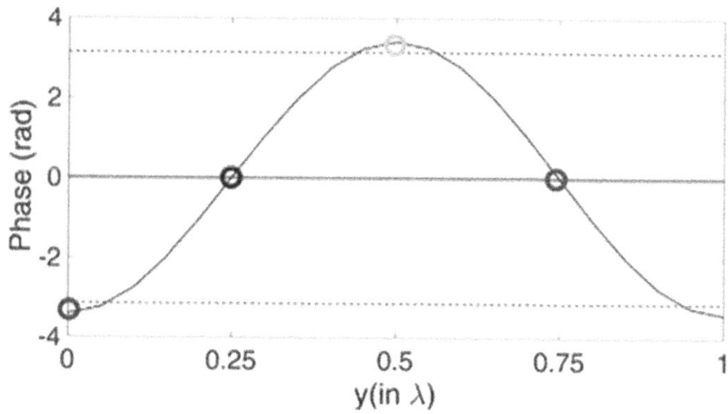

Figure 7.2C. *Phase accumulated after one period at different points along the direction of propagation. For a color version of the three parts of this figure, see www.iste.co.uk/ratiney-beuf/challenges.zip*

However, the phase of the acquired MRI signal is affected by other physical phenomena that are static most of the time, that is, constant over time. The most common effect is related to the non-uniformities of the static magnetic field B_0, which translates into a static phase ϕ_s in the acquired images. In order to remove these undesirable effects in MRE, two acquisitions are performed with opposite polarities of the motion-encoding gradients, and the phase signal of interest is retrieved by subtracting the phase images of the two acquisitions. However, since phase images can exhibit different wraps that are not necessarily well localized, the phase related to the wave is typically extracted from complex images:

$$\begin{matrix} \phi_{acq1} = \phi_s + \phi_{wave} \\ \phi_{acq2} = \phi_s - \phi_{wave} \end{matrix} \Rightarrow \quad \phi_{wave} = \frac{1}{2} Arg\left(\frac{e^{i\phi_{acq1}}}{e^{i\phi_{acq2}}}\right) \qquad [7.7]$$

Phase encoding by means of encoding gradients can be added to any kind of MRI sequence. Such gradients are executed after the excitation pulse and before the signal readout gradients, which, as a consequence, increases the echo time. Figure 7.3 represents the case of a gradient echo sequence where motion encoding is performed along the slice direction. Encoding the motion along the other directions is possible as well; displacement fields are commonly acquired in a sequential way along the three orthogonal spatial directions in advanced scans, or even along oblique directions by exploiting the simultaneous application of several gradient directions in order to maximize the effective gradient amplitude. The sequence chronogram in Figure 7.3 additionally shows that motion is triggered before the encoding gradients are applied, such that a stationary state of the shear wave is achieved. In some cases, motion is continuously induced, but this requires choosing a TR of the sequence equal to an integer number of motion periods and ensuring the absence of any time drift between the different clocks intervening in a scan (the MRI system clock and vibration device). The accumulation of small delays over several consecutive TRs yields an increasingly negative impact over the scan's duration. In order to probe different instants of the wave propagation, a phase offset φ is introduced between the wave and the motion-encoding gradient. Four acquisitions (corresponding to four different values of φ) are usually performed with a constant phase offset over the interval $[0, 2\pi[$, referred to as different phase steps.

The employed frequency of the shear wave is chosen depending on the targeted organ or tissue and on the achievable spatial resolution. Since the wave attenuation increases with increasing frequencies, it is important to choose an appropriate frequency that enables sufficient penetration into the investigated region. Thus, in most clinical MRI scans, the employed frequencies vary between 20 Hz and 200 Hz. The lower frequency boundary is related to the corresponding wavelength. Although a local wavelength measurement is sought (from which to extract the shear speed or shear modulus), it is necessary that the reconstruction step be performed with wavelengths shorter than the size of the targeted organ. Because of this, small-animal applications employ higher frequencies, varying from 200 Hz to approximately 1 kHz.

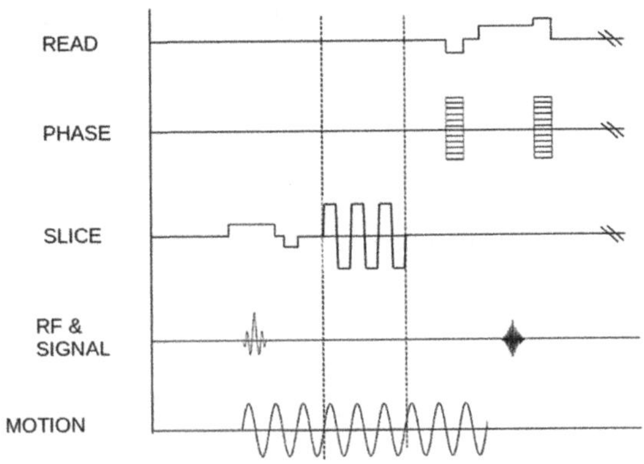

Figure 7.3. *Chronogram of a magnetic resonance elastography sequence based on a gradient echo sequence and an encoding gradient with a duration of three periods along the slice direction*

One last aspect to be taken into account is related to the acquisition matrix in the slice plane. The resulting image should provide a visualization of the wave propagating inside the region of interest, which defines the maximum pixel size in the image plane. On the other hand, the minimum size is imposed by the resulting SNR of the image. A general rule is to choose a pixel size such that a wavelength covers the equivalent of about ten pixels while ensuring an SNR greater than 10.

7.1.3. *MRE data reconstruction*

7.1.3.1. *Fundamentals*

Once the displacement field has been encoded into the phase of the MRI signal, the last step is the reconstruction of the mechanical properties. Overall, the various reconstruction methods can be classified into three categories:

1) Local frequency estimation methods (LFE): these methods are based on the estimation of spatial frequencies in the wave image, leading to a mapping of the wavelength and thus of the local elasticity. This reconstruction method is employed in approved clinical MRE products and we will describe its principle in detail below.

2) Direct inversion methods, where the wave equation is inverted, are also common and widely used by several research groups. In a purely elastic linear medium, the wave propagation equation [7.1] can be written as:

$$\mu = -\rho\omega^2 \frac{u_i}{\Delta u_i} \qquad [7.8]$$

It is thus possible to determine the shear modulus μ by discretizing the above equation. This apparently simple method does however have the major disadvantage of being sensitive to noise. We shall see how some conditioning steps such as frequency filtering can significantly improve the robustness of this method.

3) Iterative methods: such methods exploit the simulation of displacement fields u_{sim} via direct approaches, for example, using finite difference or finite elements. The goal of these methods is to minimize the error between a simulated displacement field u_{sim} and the experimentally measured displacement field u_{exp} (Van Houten et al. 1999). Such methods can potentially be powerful as they are capable of extracting the parameters of rather complex models, such as those describing tissue anisotropy, but they are demanding in terms of computation time.

7.1.3.2. *Pre-processing/conditioning*

Before any inversion algorithm is applied, the first step is to unwrap the phase. The latter is obtained as the arctangent of the ratio between the imaginary part and the real part of the MRI signal, hence it is confined between -π and π. From a physical point of view, there is no reason for the phase to be restricted only to this range and an unwrapping step is often required to retrieve the actual phase. A second step that is widely employed in MRE, including in clinical MRE, is filtering based on the temporal Fourier transform (TFT). Applying the TFT is much more than a simple pre-processing step, since it leads to direct implications regarding the MRI scan: for example, the N phase steps required for the TFT (typically, $N = 4$) usually imply N different acquisitions and a scan time multiplied by the same factor. For each voxel of the region of interest, the TFT is applied to the N measurements, thereby selecting the displacement occurring at the frequency of mechanical excitation while filtering out the other frequency components. This step significantly improves the robustness of the reconstruction.

7.1.3.3. *LFE method: local frequency estimation*

The LFE method is rather complex and our goal here is to illustrate its main aspects. The reader can find detailed explanations in Manduca et al. (2003) as well as in the original article by Knutsson et al. (1994) about radar signals, which is the foundation for the LFE method in MRE. This method is based on processing steps following a spatial Fourier transform of the wave image. Clearly, spatial frequencies ν (and thus, indirectly, shear wavelengths λ from λ =1/ν) are located in the Fourier space, although without any information on their localization in space. The LFE method enables localizing the spatial frequencies of the Fourier domain in space. For this purpose, it can be shown that the local spatial frequency ν of a signal S can be found by applying lognormal filters R_i and R_j with central frequencies ν_i and ν_j, respectively:

$$\nu = \sqrt{\nu_i \nu_j} Re\left(\frac{r_j \times S}{r_i \times S}\right) \quad [7.9]$$

with r_i and r_j the inverse Fourier transforms of R_i and R_j, respectively. In summary, the LFE algorithm is composed of the following steps:

– spatial FT of the wave image, displaying the spatial frequency peaks (corresponding to the different wavelengths and thus to elasticity in the image) in the Fourier domain;

– filtering via pairs of lognormal filters with central frequencies chosen a priori;

– calculation of the ratio between the filtered signals, providing the radial spatial frequency;

– combination of radial and directional filters to extend the method to a 2D image.

Once these operations have been performed, a map of spatial frequencies $v(x,y) = 1/\lambda(x,y)$ is obtained, and hence the shear modulus $\mu(x,y)$ is retrieved with the hypothesis of a purely elastic and incompressible medium via $\mu = \rho.\lambda^2.f^2$, where f is the excitation frequency. Figure 7.4 represents the three steps required to perform an MRE acquisition.

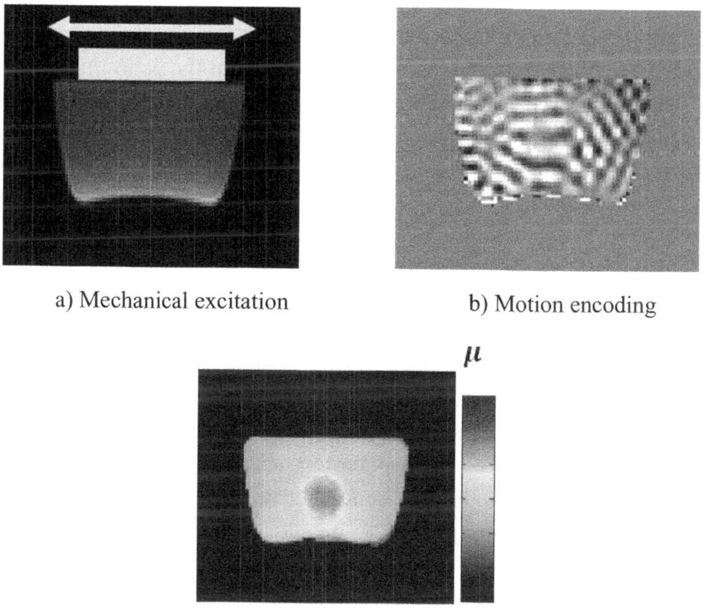

a) Mechanical excitation

b) Motion encoding

c) Reconstruction

Figure 7.4. *Illustration of the three steps of an MRE acquisition. (a) Generation and transmission of a shear wave in the region of interest, (b) visualization of the motion on the phase images of an MRE scan and (c) mapping of the mechanical properties by means of reconstruction algorithms. Data obtained in a gel made up of 2.5% gelatine with a stiffer inclusion (4% gelatine). For a color version of this figure, see www.iste.co.uk/ratincy-beuf/challenges.zip*

7.2. MRE sequences

The way to encode the MRE signal has evolved significantly since the first sequence was proposed (Muthupillai et al. 1995). Each modification has sought to perform faster scans, increase the amount of information acquired or decrease the echo time to increase the SNR. Some of such sequences are non-exhaustively described in this section.

7.2.1. *Fractional encoding*

One of the characteristic MRE limitations is related to the duration of the motion-encoding gradients. Since they are applied after the excitation pulse of the imaging sequence, their duration leads to an increase in the echo time causing a loss of signal. This is further reinforced at lower mechanical frequencies. The goal of fractional encoding is to remove this undesired coupling between the applied mechanical frequency and the available signal at the price of reduced sensitivity to motion.

The idea is based on the fact that, according to equation [7.4], it is possible to obtain a non-zero phase accumulation even when the gradient shape is different to the case illustrated in Figure 7.2(B). In practice, encoding gradients are executed with a frequency higher than the mechanical frequency. This enables a decreased echo time, thanks to the shorter duration of the motion-encoding gradients, and, hence, a gain in signal. Such a strategy can become advantageous in particular in organs such as the liver, where some pathologies are characterized by a strong loss of signal. On the other hand, the difference between the mechanical frequency and the encoding gradient frequency leads to a reduced accumulation of phase, all the more so as a smaller fraction of the mechanical vibration cycle is exploited for the encoding. The ratio q between the duration of the encoding τ_G and the period of the mechanical oscillation T (or, equivalently, between the mechanical frequency and the encoding frequency), $q = \frac{\tau_G}{T} = \frac{\omega}{\omega_G}$, then represents a characteristic variable in the sequence. By integrating equation [7.4], in which the gradient shape is replaced by a sinusoidal signal with a pulsation ω_G (period T_G) and an amplitude G_{MEG}, the accumulated phase ϕ over a given encoding duration T_G is expressed with respect to the ratio q as:

$$\phi = \frac{\gamma \cdot G_{\mathrm{MEG}} \cdot A \cdot T_G}{\pi} \cdot \frac{sin(\pi q)}{1 - q^2} \qquad [7.10]$$

In typical conditions, where the aim is to obtain echo times shorter than the mechanical period, T_G will have to be maximized to maintain as high a sensitivity as possible. This kind of encoding can be exploited for simultaneously acquiring several multiples of the base mechanical frequency, by means of a transducer capable of generating arbitrary mechanical waveforms (Garteiser et al. 2013).

7.2.2. *Multidirectional encoding*

In order to retrieve the mechanical properties of anisotropic tissues, displacements induced along the three orthogonal spatial directions have to be measured. This can be done by sequentially applying the motion-encoding gradients along the three directions, at the expense of the acquisition time being multiplied by three. Klatt et al. (2013) have proposed a method that enables simultaneous acquisitions of the three spatial directions in the case of a mono-frequential shear wave.

The underlying principle consists of applying an encoding gradient first in phase with the wave and then with an increasing phase offset. In the case when a single period of a sinusoidal encoding gradient is employed with a frequency equal to the wave frequency, following equation [7.4], the encoded phase is given by:

$$\phi(t_0) = \frac{\gamma G_0 A}{2f} \vec{u}_G . \vec{u}_u cos(2\pi f t_0 + \theta) \qquad [7.11]$$

The simultaneous application of gradients along the three spatial directions (i = 1, 2, and 3, for the directions x, y, and z, respectively) with different initial execution times $t_{0i,n}$ (and thus different phase offsets) and a sampling of at least eight phases (N = 8) described by:

$$\Delta t_i = \frac{i}{N.f}$$
$$t_{0i,n} = n\,\Delta t_i, n = 0,1,\dots,N-1 \qquad [7.12]$$

results in the nth encoded phase being the sum of the encoding obtained from the three gradients:

$$\phi_n = \sum_{i=1}^{3} \frac{\gamma G_{0,i} A}{2f} \vec{u}_{G,i} . \vec{u}_u \ cos\left(2\pi \frac{i.n}{N} + \theta_i\right) \qquad [7.13]$$

In these conditions, equation [7.13] shows that the phase encoding of each direction translates into a different apparent frequency in the temporal evolution of ϕ_n. The encoding of x, y and z directions is obtained by applying the Fourier transform and by retrieving first, second and third harmonics, respectively. This method, called SLIM-MRE (SampLe Interval Modulation), has another version where the initial phase of the encoding is changed (Kearney et al. 2017).

7.2.3. *Diffusion MRE*

Due to the common requirement of applying encoding gradients, the elastography and diffusion techniques are similar in terms of acquisition methods. In fact, similar to diffusion-encoding gradients employed in diffusion-weighted sequences, the motion-encoding gradients used in MRE introduce a dephasing, with a greater effect in more mobile water molecules. The decrease in signal amplitude detected in such a way can be exploited to estimate the apparent or average diffusion coefficient via the methods described originally by Stejskal and Tanner (see Chapter 4). The feasibility of this approach has been established in an experimental phantom (Yin et al. 2014) and in a mouse brain (Yin et al. 2017b). The simultaneous encoding of incoherent motion related to diffusion in the image magnitude and periodic motion related to the acoustic wave in the phase image leads to an advantageous reduction of the acquisition time, compared to a consecutive execution of a diffusion scan and an MRE scan. Besides, spatial co-registration between elastography and diffusion data is automatic in the simultaneous approach. On the downside, undesired interactions between the two modalities can often occur when the wave amplitude reaches sufficiently high levels to affect the magnitude image due to intravoxel phase dispersion (Glaser et al. 2003).

7.2.4. *Optimal control MRE*

Most motion-encoding techniques for MRE are based on motion-encoding gradients. However, it is also possible to encode motion during the generation of the transverse magnetization. For this purpose, a gradient has to be applied, which can be constant (and not oscillating) while the excitation pulse selects the slice and encodes the motion into the phase of the signal. Computing such a pulse is not a trivial matter and is achieved using optimal control.

Optimal control is a method that determines a control that has to be applied to bring a dynamic system from an initial state to a final state for a given optimality criterion defined via a cost function. From a mathematical point of view, this method is based on Pontryagin's maximum principle (Pontryagin et al. 1963). An analytical solution can be found in the case of low-dimensional problems, while in other cases it requires numerical solvers (Khaneja et al. 2005). In NMR and MRI, the dynamic system is composed of different isochromats[1] that have to be controlled and whose evolution can be described by Bloch equations (or by using quantum formulations). The applied control, whose duration has to be specified beforehand, is done by the RF pulse, which brings the dynamic system from an initial state, which in this case corresponds to the thermodynamic equilibrium state, to a target state, whose formulation below provides phase encoding similarly to the one obtained in MRE with an oscillating gradient:

$$\vec{M}_i^{\perp} = M_0 \begin{bmatrix} \cos(\pi.\cos\left(\dfrac{2\pi(i-1)}{N_{iso}}\right)) \\ \sin(\pi.\cos\left(\dfrac{2\pi(i-1)}{N_{iso}}\right)) \end{bmatrix} \quad [7.14]$$

$i \in [1\ ;\ N_{iso}]$ where N_{iso} represents the number of isochromats to be controlled along a wavelength as illustrated in Figure 7.5 ($N_{iso} = 10$). The target state regards only the transverse magnetization, whose two components defined by equation [7.14] provide the desired phase of the MRI signal while targeting a maximized modulus of the transverse magnetization and, hence, maximized signal amplitude.

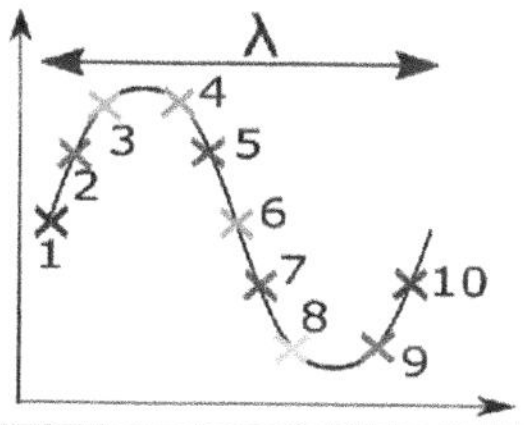

Figure 7.5. *Discretization of the wavelength for Ni$_{so}$ = 10 isochromats. For a color version of this figure, see www.iste.co.uk/ratiney-beuf/challenges.zip*

In order to calculate the RF field to be applied, the controlled system has to be described as precisely as possible. This is done using Bloch equations (by taking into account the relaxation time constants T_1 and T_2 during the execution of the RF pulse) and including the effect of a constant gradient applied while the shear wave is propagating. For the system described in Figure 7.2, to obtain a slice in the yOx plane, a constant gradient will have to be applied along the z-direction.

1 An isochromat is defined as an ensemble of nuclear spins that are exposed to the same static magnetic field and behave in a similar way.

Displacement generated by the wave (equation [7.5]) leads in such cases to a variation of the B_0 field given by:

$$\Delta B_0(y,z,t) = G_z\left(z + A.\sin\left(\omega t - \frac{2\pi.y}{\lambda}\right)\right) \quad [7.15]$$

where z represents the position in the direction of application of the constant gradient. In the case of 2D imaging, the fact that the isochromats have a resting position (in the absence of a shear wave) different from $z = 0$ has to be taken into account. Equation [7.15] describes the variation of the B_0 field that would be perceived by an isochromat at position z due to the simultaneous application of the G_z gradient and shear wave. A slice with a thickness Δz_{in} will correspond to a bandwidth (in Hz):

$$BW_{in} = \gamma G_z.\Delta z_{in} \quad [7.16]$$

Thus, for the optimization problem and the associated cost function, a certain number of isochromats within the desired slice has to be defined. This number has to be sufficiently large for the applied control to be robust such that the isochromats located within the control intervals follow the same dynamics as the controlled ones. However, a large number would considerably increase the computation time and the risk of the algorithm's non-convergence. Moreover, the spatial selectivity of the pulse has to be ensured by guaranteeing that the executed pulse does not affect the isochromats outside the selected slice. This is achieved by considering a certain number of isochromats located outside the slice thickness that should remain in the thermal equilibrium state. If Δz_{out} is the spatial location of these isochromats, this condition can be written as:

$$\vec{M_j} = \begin{pmatrix} 0 \\ 0 \\ M_0 \end{pmatrix}, \nabla j | Z_j \in \Delta z_{out} \quad [7.17]$$

Figure 7.6 represents the magnitude of such a pulse (the phase is set to 0). It can be noted that the magnitude has an upper bound of 94 µT, which corresponds to one of the optimization criteria that have to be defined beforehand to comply with the specifications of the employed transmit coil.

This MRE acquisition method presents advantages and disadvantages which should be mentioned. The advantages include a better SNR for a given phase encoding efficiency (Van Reeth et al. 2018), the use of a constant, and not oscillating, gradient, which reduces the requirements regarding the gradients system, the possibility of acquiring signals with extremely short echo times and thus of targeting tissues with a short T_2, and the possibility of creating pulses that simultaneously encode several frequencies (Sango et al. 2020). The main constraints consist of the current impossibility of encoding displacements in other directions than the slice selection, the specific absorption rates considerations, since the executed pulses are more efficient when their amplitudes are higher, the need for precise knowledge of the experimental system (gradient amplitude, motion frequency, relaxation times T_2), although it is possible to take into account possible non-uniformities of B_0, and, finally, the computation time which can be rather long (in the order of several days) without a guarantee of satisfactory convergence. However, once the pulse is calculated, it can be used without any constraint whenever the experimental conditions correspond to the optimization criteria used in the optimization process.

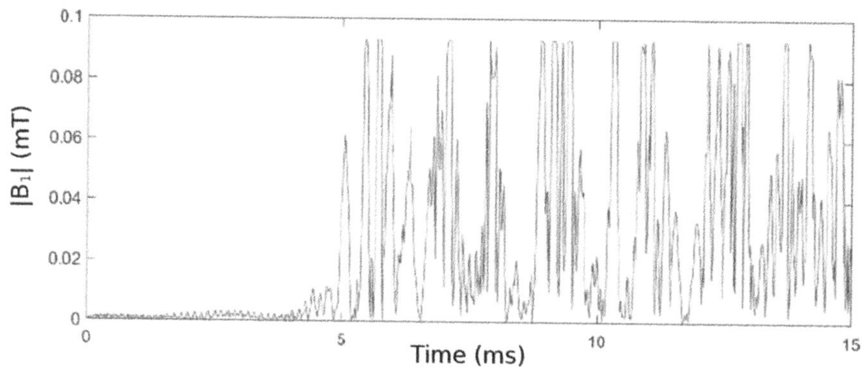

Figure 7.6. *Example of the magnitude (the phase is set to 0) of a pulse calculated via optimal control for MRE*

7.3. Main targeted organs and applications

7.3.1. *Liver MRE*

The liver is a preferential MRE target. Respiratory motion is a challenge, but it can be mitigated via breath-hold acquisitions. As it is located relatively close to the body surface, transmitting acoustic waves within its volume from one or two external sources is simple. Moreover, specific coils and long-established MRI scans are widely available and common in imaging centers. Finally, the measurement of the hepatic mechanical properties can be of great interest to several clinical diagnostic approaches.

Above all, liver MRE has been used for the diagnosis of fibrosis. In this pathological condition, which can have viral (in particular, hepatitis B and C), alcoholic or metabolic causes (non-alcoholic hepatic diseases such as non-alcoholic steatohepatitis), the presence of even small quantities of collagen fibers, whose stiffness is several orders of magnitude greater than a healthy liver's stiffness, leads to a significant increase in measured mechanical properties, even at earlier disease stages. Since the mechanical properties increase with the degree of fibrosis, as illustrated in Figure 7.7, threshold stiffness values can be determined to stage the patients' fibrosis class before resorting to a biopsy, which is the universally recognized reference method in clinical practice. The latter, although it is the only acknowledged technique for fibrosis diagnostics, is associated with low intraobserver repeatability, a very small analyzed volume that can lead to sampling biases, and a non-zero risk of complications for the patient. Besides, it is not suitable for repeated examinations required for monitoring or therapeutic follow-up.

Several studies have quantified in detail the performance of MRE for the diagnostics of fibrosis. This technique is now considered to be a useful examination for fibrosis diagnostics in patients with non-alcoholic hepatic diseases (Chalasani et al. 2018) and the viscoelastic parameters of biomarkers have been validated in this context. Although inflammation that accompanies fibrosis can lead to greater mechanical properties, this increase is not sufficient to exploit stiffness as a clear inflammation marker. Other parameters obtained via MRE are being evaluated regarding their sensitivity to inflammation or other associated disorders such as ballooning. The viscoelastic ratio (Yin et al. 2017a) could eventually provide indications regarding these other hepatic diseases. Some works also measure the mechanical properties at several mechanical excitation frequencies, either to make the measurement more robust (Tzschätzsch et al. 2016) or to use the frequency dispersion coefficients as additional biomarkers (Asbach et al. 2010).

In its more advanced form, fibrosis can worsen into cirrhosis, the most severe fibrosis stage in pathological classifications. In cirrhosis, the amount of collagen is very large for any degree of severity, but in some patients this pathology is accompanied by varying degrees of hypertension in the hepatic and abdominal vascular systems, such as in the spleen. This hypertension progresses into esophagus varicose veins with a risk of bleeding. For cirrhosis patients, MRE can be performed both in the liver and spleen to evaluate portal hypertension due to the relationship between the vascular pressure in these two abdominal organs and their mechanical properties (Ronot et al. 2014).

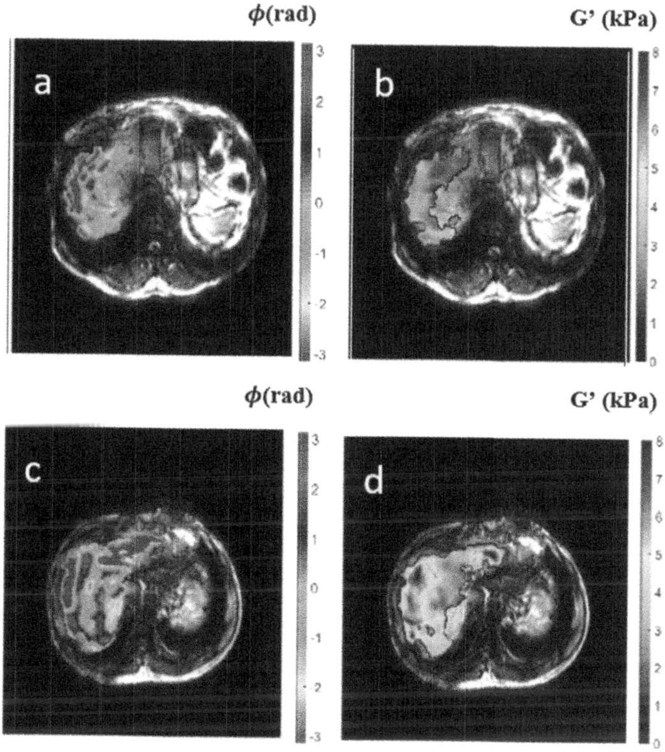

Figure 7.7. *Illustration of the MRE in the context of hepatic fibrosis. (a and b) Phase images illustrating the wave propagation and maps of the shear modulus (average: 2.4 ± 0.5 kPa), respectively, for a patient without fibrosis (METAVIR score F0). (c and d) Phase images illustrating the wave propagation and maps of the shear modulus (average: 4.4 ± 1.4 kPa), respectively, for a patient diagnosed with stage-F3 fibrosis. For a color version of this figure, see www.iste.co.uk/ratiney-beuf/challenges.zip*

MRE is also suitable for the mechanical characterization of cancerous hepatic lesions. The different tumor types encountered in the liver can differ in extracellular matrix composition, vascularization implications or degree of cellularity and necrosis. However, in the context of cancerous lesions, precaution is required concerning MRE. In fact, the application of spatial filters, or the calculation of spatial derivatives required for most reconstructions can negatively affect the images via a point-spread function whose width can be similar to the lesion size. This problem is naturally exacerbated in the case of small tumors, that is, smaller than 8 mm (Bohte et al. 2013).

7.3.2. *Brain MRE*

MRE of the brain is particularly interesting in the sense that assessing this organ via ultrasound elastography methods is very difficult due to the attenuation of the ultrasound in the skull. Several studies have investigated different pathologies and their effect on the elasticity of cerebral tissue measured via MRE.

7.3.2.1. *MRE and neuro-oncology*

About a dozen studies have performed MRE on different types of brain tumors (Bunevicius et al. 2020). Overall, glioblastomas have been reported as being softer than healthy parenchyma (Streitberger et al. 2014) and the elastic modulus of gliomas seems to decrease with increasing glioma grade. The elastic modulus of meningiomas seems to be more variable and heterogeneous than in other tumors. Globally, the discrimination of different tumor types using the elasticity parameter is restricted and it can hardly be sufficient for diagnosis, although it represents complementary information in addition to other MRI acquisitions.

7.3.2.2. *MRE and pathologies affecting the global elasticity of brain tissue*

Overall, neurodegenerative diseases are correlated with a decrease in the elastic modulus. Alzheimer's and Parkinson's diseases and Lewy body dementia seem to lead to a significantly decreased stiffness of cerebral tissue (ElSheikh et al. 2017).

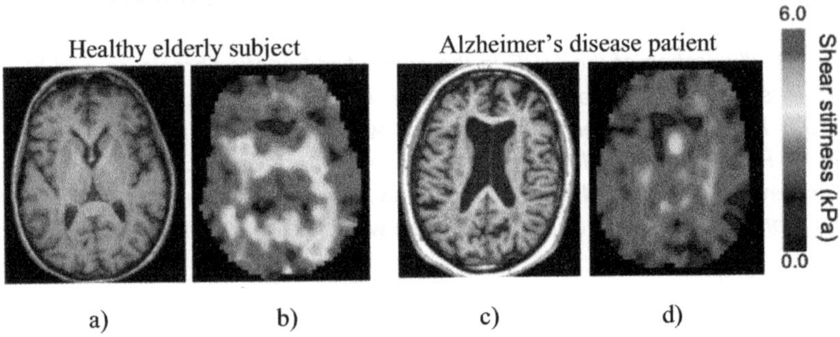

Figure 7.8. *Illustration of MRE of the brain in Alzheimer's disease. (a and c) Anatomical images; (b and d) maps of the shear modulus. For a color version of this figure, see www.iste.co.uk/ratiney-beuf/challenges.zip*

In a similar way, multiple sclerosis tends to induce a decrease in elastic modulus of cerebral tissue (Wuerfel et al. 2010) and the viscoelastic parameters seem capable of predicting the progression of this disease (Streitberger et al. 2012).

7.3.2.3. *MRE and pre-operatory planning in neurosurgery*

It is important to underline that the mechanical properties of cerebral tissue are also very important for pre-operatory planning. In particular, the adherence of the tumor to the surrounding tissue represents valuable information that can help neurosurgeons plan a resection procedure. Discontinuities of displacement fields measured by MRE have been proposed as markers for predicting this adherence, with a good correlation with the adherence estimated during interventions on meningiomas and vestibular schwannomas (Yin et al. 2017c).

7.3.3. *MRE and other organs*

Several other organs are worth investigating using MRE. However, the fact that this is not currently the case is essentially related to the intrinsic difficulties in applying MRE to these organs. Such challenges are related to the design of the mechanical wave-generating device and its validation for clinical use, the MRI data acquisition required for the elastogram reconstruction, or the reconstruction of elastograms in tissues where the usual hypotheses (isotropy, local homogeneity) are not valid. The three examples below illustrate such cases.

7.3.3.1. *MRE of the breast*

Breast cancer is the most common cancer in females and its screening methods are either invasive in the case of biopsies or ionizing in the case of mammography. Therefore, there is a great need for alternative detection and staging, all the more so as mortality is mostly due to the resulting metastases rather than primary tumors. MRI is not a primary tool for breast cancer screening. Breast MRI scans require a prone position of the patient with a dedicated multichannel receive coil surrounding each breast. The wave-generating device then has to be integrated into the receive coil, which excludes any large or stand-alone device. Some research groups have developed functional solutions that provide images with good quality (Plewes et al. 2000; Sinkus et al. 2005). An MRE examination has to be performed covering the entire breast and with a sufficient spatial resolution for precise demarcation of tumor areas. Currently, this can be done in slightly more than 10 min, which, although promising, is still too long to be included in a clinical protocol. At the present time, in terms of results, the shear modulus obtained via MRE alone does not allow tumor staging and detection of lesions with the highest probability of metastasis. However, the retrieved information is valuable and complementary to that obtained via other imaging methods (in particular, with contrast-agent dynamic MRI). A detailed and recent review of MRE applications for breast cancer screening has been compiled by Bohte et al. (2018).

7.3.3.2. *MRE of the muscles*

Since the muscles are organized into fiber fascicles, at a local scale, they exhibit properties of transverse isotropy and not three-dimensional isotropy, which is an assumption required for many reconstruction algorithms and for LFE in particular (see section 7.1.3.2). A transversely isotropic medium is characterized by two shear moduli, which in the case of muscles correspond to the parallel and transverse orientation with respect to the fiber direction. Characterizing these two moduli requires a priori knowledge of the fiber orientation, which can be obtained via diffusion MRI. However, few studies have been published so far in this direction, and researchers have mostly made different choices ranging from simplified hypotheses of isotropic medium to mono-directional mechanical excitations or spatial filtering to isolate a single wave component.

In terms of devices, most studies have used a pneumatic or electromechanical transducer with a surface coil placed as close as possible to the investigated muscles. The latter are essentially muscles of the thigh and calf or biceps muscles. The results (Dresner et al. 2001) show a growing linear correlation between the muscular contractions for different applied loads and the shear modulus representing the muscular stiffness. These stiffness variations between resting and contraction states are the basis for extracting parameters to characterize muscular disorders, especially in the case of Duchenne muscular dystrophy (Bensamoun et al. 2015).

7.3.3.3. *MRE of the heart*

Cardiovascular diseases are the primary cause of death in Western countries and their early detection is of major importance. Characterizing the myocardium contractility is fundamental in many cardiac pathologies and MRE is quite relevant in this case since the shear modulus could be directly related to the intracardiac pressure (Elgeti et al. 2008). However, MRE of the heart presents several specific aspects that strongly hinder its exploration. The main difficulties are as follows: (1) the heart is a muscle with a myocardium fiber architecture that is even more complex than the one in skeletal muscles; (2) the biomechanical properties of the myocardium have to be characterized at different instants of the cardiac cycle which implies a constraining synchronization of the acquisitions, especially as arrhythmias are present in some pathologies, hence leading to long and repeated scans; (3) the heart is located within the thoracic cage and surrounded by other organs. Consequently, transmitting a shear wave using an external device is not simple. Most of the performed studies have employed very low excitation frequencies.

7.3.4. *Other applications*

As illustrated before, MRE has been mainly developed for diagnostic applications. However, the versatility of this technique offers several opportunities that extend beyond this objective. Here, we shall illustrate two particularly novel applications: on the one hand, MRE as a biomechanical characterization method and, on the other hand, MRE as a guidance method for thermal ablations in interventional MRI.

7.3.4.1. *MRE as a biomechanical characterization tool*

Knowing the mechanical behavior of biological tissue is fundamental in many research and engineering fields. This knowledge is mainly based on experimental results obtained in vitro for reasons that are related to experimental protocols. This is a real limitation in the sense that the biomechanical behavior of tissues can exhibit significant differences between the living and *post-mortem* states. In general, elastography methods have the theoretical potential of characterizing the mechanical properties of tissues in their normal condition in vivo. However, they were originally developed for the purpose of quantitative biomechanical characterization. Our goal here is to illustrate how the MRE technique can be adapted to this particularly original objective.

Diagnostic elastography is essentially based on the hypothesis of purely elastic linear behavior. Clearly, the biomechanical behavior of tissues is much more complex: biological tissue can typically be viscoelastic, with a nonlinear and anisotropic behavior, among other properties. Some of these properties can be characterized via MRE methods.

Viscoelastic properties were historically the first ones to be investigated. Since the early 2000s, some methods for inverting the wave equation have been adapted to characterize not only the elasticity but also the viscosity of biological tissues, essentially for diagnostic purposes. One of the goals of these studies was to investigate biomarkers other than just elasticity and to quantify their sensitivity to some pathologies (Sinkus et al. 2005). In a viscoelastic medium, the shear modulus G is complex and equation [7.2] can be rewritten by simply decomposing G into a real part and an imaginary part: $G = G' + iG''$. G′ is called the storage modulus and represents purely elastic behavior. G″ is called the loss modulus and represents the viscous behavior of tissue. This representation in terms of G′, G″ and their frequency dependence are very common in biomechanics and rheology for viscoelastic characterizations. By inverting the wave equation with the hypothesis of a complex wave number, it is thus possible to characterize G′ and G″ as well as their dynamic behavior, for example, using different mechanical excitation frequencies. This approach has been applied to different organs to model them with different rheological models (Guo et al. 2012; Testu et al. 2017). This kind of novel data represents a major contribution in the field of biomechanics. As an example, until the 2000s, there was a considerable variation in the viscoelastic properties of brain tissue reported in the literature, spanning a range of two orders of magnitude (Chatelin et al. 2010). This variation was mainly due to the specificity of in vitro protocols. For the first time, MRE allowed the viscoelastic behavior of in vivo brain tissue to be established in its normal state (Sack et al. 2008; Vappou et al. 2008).

In addition to their viscoelastic behavior, some tissues have a strong mechanical anisotropy. This is the case of tissues in muscles or the brain. MRE is particularly suitable for characterizing this anisotropy due to the possibility of encoding the three displacement components with the same quality and precision. From an experimental point of view, this approach is rather powerful as it provides an in vivo characterization, whereas an in vitro measurement requires sample preparation, for example, by cutting the sample along different directions before characterizing them. Finally, we can also mention the characterization of the poroelastic properties of tissues (Perriñez et al. 2010). This behavior is characterized by the presence of a liquid phase within a solid matrix. When subjected to deformation, the fluid circulation and its interaction with the solid phase give the tissue a certain resistance, which is particularly difficult to characterize in vitro. Once again, MRE has overcome this major barrier for applications in organs such as the brain (Weaver et al. 2012).

Beyond the contribution of these methods to biomechanics, using more complex models than a simple linear elastic model also brings with it diagnostic opportunities in terms of novel biomarker propositions, which are currently employed in several clinical studies as mentioned throughout section 7.3.

7.3.4.2. *MRE for thermal therapy monitoring*

In this section, we describe how MRE can aid in monitoring thermal therapies. Although it is certainly a minor application, this example helps illustrate how some methodological MRE adaptations can unlock novel applications.

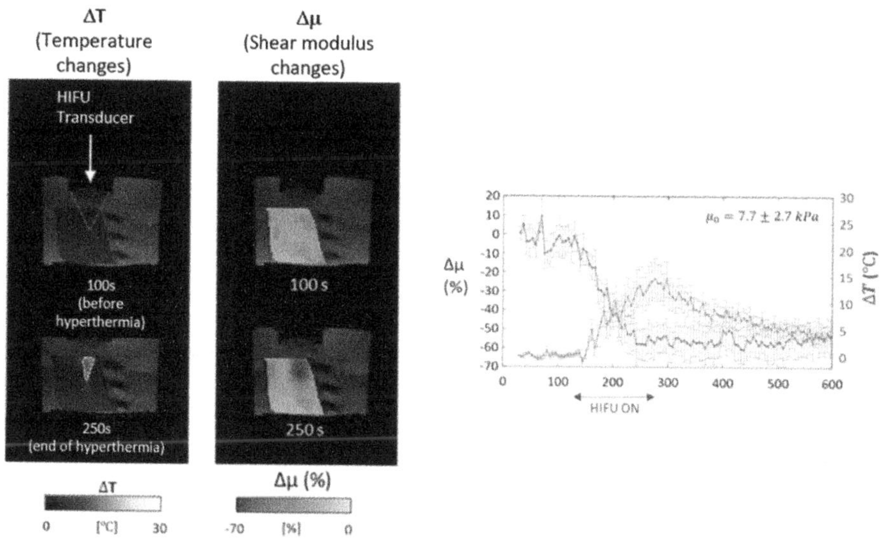

Figure 7.9. *Illustration of MRE for monitoring hyperthermia induced by high-intensity focused ultrasound (HIFU) using simultaneous elastography and thermometry in pig muscle in vitro. Here, moderate hyperthermia (~15°C) is associated with a considerable and permanent decrease in shear modulus. For a color version of this figure, see www.iste.co.uk/ratiney-beuf/challenges.zip*

Minimally invasive thermal ablations have emerged in recent decades as a safe, efficient, and less complicated alternative to traditional surgery in numerous applications. The safety and efficiency of these therapies are, nevertheless, based on real-time guidance and monitoring via medical imaging modalities. Among the latter, MRI offers several advantages, such as intrinsic contrast in soft tissues and the possibility of monitoring the temperature in real time via MR thermometry. However, one of the major challenges in this field consists of obtaining new biomarkers that are sensitive and specific to the structural integrity of the tissue during its ablation. In theory, the mechanical properties of tissues can play this role, as has been shown in some studies that used ultrasound elastography for monitoring thermal ablations (Mariani et al. 2014). Some MRE studies have also found differences between elasticity before and after thermal ablation (Chen et al. 2014). Nonetheless, traditional MRE techniques are still unsuitable for real-time monitoring due to the associated acquisition times. In this context, several research teams have sought to adapt MRE to the interventional context, in particular, to obtain biomechanical information in a real-time fashion for monitoring ablations. Corbin et al. (2016) have developed a percutaneous interventional MRE method based, on the one hand, on direct wave generation by means of the interventional needle, without resorting to an additional external transducer, and, on the other hand, on a fast acquisition/reconstruction method (fractional encoding, number of phase steps reduced to 3, sliding window) providing elastograms at a timescale of seconds. In addition, without additional acquisitions, this method estimates the temperature via PRFS (Proton Resonance Frequency Shift) thermometry. For this purpose, two acquisitions are performed using MEGs with opposite polarities. The difference between these two images helps to retrieve the contribution of the displacements due to the wave propagation, whereas, on the contrary, the sum of these two images helps to detect the changes of phase due to temperature variations.

Other methods have been developed specifically for monitoring thermal ablations via high-intensity focused ultrasound (HIFU). In this case, displacements are produced directly by the ultrasound transducer by means of the acoustic radiation force, which makes an additional external transducer unnecessary (Souchon et al. 2008; Vappou et al. 2018).

7.4. Conclusion

MRE is a multidisciplinary technique. Above all else, it requires the generation of shear waves within the tissue to be investigated and, thus, appropriate devices have to be developed and optimized for the targeted application. Being an MRI technique in its own right, it requires good knowledge of magnetic resonance physics concepts. The reconstruction of maps can mean solving a complex inverse problem, all the more so as MRE is turning to applications in organs with more complex geometry and structure than the originally considered liver. Regarding this topic, some research groups have made their reconstruction software available:

1) LFE by the Mayo Clinic in Rochester (United States): www.mayo.edu/research/labs/advanced-medical-imaging-technology/focus-areas;

2) MDEV (an inversion algorithm for multifrequency wave equations) by Charité in Berlin (Germany): https://bioqic.de/bioqic-server/.

In terms of clinical applications, the contribution of MRE in the diagnostics of hepatic fibrosis is undeniable. In about 20 years, it has become a renowned method for a global examination of the organ, which cannot be done using the reference biopsy method. Another clinical application that is attracting much interest is the brain. Here, again, no other modality can provide measurements of the mechanical properties with such a large coverage. However, research is ongoing to bring brain MRE to the same level as liver MRE, either by focusing on the generation and transmission of waves inside the brain or on the reconstruction of the mechanical properties of the brain. The wide scope of research in this domain is supported by the growing number of scientific articles over the last 20 years, which have seen MRE transitioning from the stage of a novel MRI technique to the stage of a well-established diagnostic modality in clinical routine.

7.5. Acknowledgments

The authors are deeply thankful to Lucie Hiscox for the clinical illustrations of brain MRE provided.

7.6. References

Asbach, P., Klatt, D., Schlosser, B., Biermer, M., Muche, M., Rieger, A., Loddenkemper, C., Somasundaram, R., Berg, T., Hamm, B. et al. (2010). Viscoelasticity-based staging of hepatic fibrosis with multifrequency MR elastography. *Radiology*, 257(1), 80–86.

Bensamoun, S.F., Charleux, F., Debernard, L., Themar-Noel, C., Voit, T. (2015). Elastic properties of skeletal muscle and subcutaneous tissues in Duchenne muscular dystrophy by magnetic resonance elastography (MRE): A feasibility study. *IRBM*, 36(1), 4–9.

Bohte, A.E., Garteiser, P., De Niet, A., Groot, P.F., Sinkus, R., Stoker, J., Nederveen, A.J. (2013). MR elastography of the liver: Defining thresholds for detecting viscoelastic changes. *Radiology*, 269(3), 768–776.

Bohte, A.E., Nelissen, J.L., Runge, J.H., Holub, O., Lambert, S.A., de Graaf, L., Kolkman, S., van der Meij, S., Stoker, J., Strijkers, G.J. et al. (2018). Breast magnetic resonance elastography: A review of clinical work and future perspectives. *NMR Biomed.*, 31(10), e3929.

Bunevicius, A., Schregel, K., Sinkus, R., Golby, A., Patz, S. (2020). Review: MR elastography of brain tumors. *NeuroImage Clin.*, 25, 102109.

Chalasani, N., Younossi, Z., Lavine, J.E., Charlton, M., Cusi, K., Rinella, M., Harrison, S.A., Brunt, E.M., Sanyal, A.J. (2018). The diagnosis and management of nonalcoholic fatty liver disease: Practice guidance from the American Association for the Study of Liver Diseases. *Hepatology*, 67(1), 328–357.

Chatelin, S., Constantinesco, A., Willinger, R. (2010). Fifty years of brain tissue mechanical testing: From in vitro to in vivo investigations. *Biorheology*, 47(5/6), 255–276.

Chen, J., Woodrum, D.A., Glaser, K.J., Murphy, M.C., Gorny, K., Ehman, R. (2014). Assessment of in vivo laser ablation using MR elastography with an inertial driver. *Magn. Reson. Med.*, 72, 59–67.

Corbin, N., Vappou, J., Breton, E., Boehler, Q., Barbé, L., Renaud, P., de Mathelin, M. (2016). Interventional MR elastography for MRI-guided percutaneous procedures. *Magn. Reson. Med.*, 75, 1110–1118.

Dresner, M.A., Rose, G.H., Rossman, P.J., Muthupillai, R., Manduca, A., Ehman, R.L. (2001). Magnetic resonance elastography of skeletal muscle. *J. Magn. Reson. Imaging*, 13(2), 269–276.

Elgeti, T., Rump, J., Hamhaber, U., Papazoglou, S., Hamm, B., Braun, J., Sack, I. (2008). Cardiac magnetic resonance elastography: Initial results. *Investigative Radiology*, 43(11), 762–772.

Elsheikh, M., Arani, A., Perry, A., Boeve, B.F., Meyer, F.B., Savica, R., Ehman, R.L., Huston III, J. (2017). MR elastography demonstrates unique regional brain stiffness patterns in dementias. *AJR Am. J. Roentgenol.*, 209(2), 403–408.

Garteiser, P., Sahebjavaher, R.S., Ter Beek, L.C., Salcudean, S., Vilgrain, V., Van Beers, B.E., Sinkus, R. (2013). Rapid acquisition of multifrequency, multislice and multi-directional MR elastography data with a fractionally encoded gradient echo sequence. *NMR Biomed.*, 26(10), 1326–1335.

Glaser, K.J., Felmlee, J.P., Manduca, A., Ehman, R.L. (2003). Shear stiffness estimation using intravoxel phase dispersion in magnetic resonance elastography. *Magn. Reson. Med.*, 50, 1256–1265.

Guo, J., Posnansky, O., Hirsch, S., Scheel, M., Taupitz, M., Braun, J., Sack, I. (2012). Fractal network dimension and viscoelastic powerlaw behavior II: An experimental study of structure-mimicking phantoms by magnetic resonance elastography. *Phys. Med. Biol.*, 57(12), 4041–4053.

Kearney, S.P., Majumdar, S., Royston, T., Klatt, D. (2017). Simultaneous 3D MR elastography of the in vivo mouse brain. *Phys. Med. Biol.*, 62(19), 7682–7693.

Khaneja, N., Reiss, T., Kehlet, C., Schulte-Herbrüggen, T., Glaser, S.J. (2005). Optimal control of coupled spin dynamics: Design of NMR pulse sequences by gradient ascent algorithms. *J. Magn. Reson.*, 172(2), 296–305.

Klatt, D., Yasar, T.K., Royston, T.J., Magin, R.L. (2013). Sample interval modulation for the simultaneous acquisition of displacement vector data in magnetic resonance elastography: Theory and application. *Phys. Med. Biol.*, 58(24), 8663–8675.

Knutsson, H., Westin, C.F., Granlund, G. (1994). Local multiscale frequency and bandwidth estimation. *Proceedings ICIP-94*, 1, 36–40.

Lewa, C.J. (1991). Magnetic resonance imaging in the presence of mechanical waves. *Spectroscopy Letters*, 24(1), 55–67.

Manduca, A., Lake, D.S., Kruse, S.A., Ehman, R.L. (2003). Spatio-temporal directional filtering for improved inversion of MR elastography images. *Med. Image Anal.*, 7(4), 465–473.

Mariani, A., Kwiecinski, W., Pernot, M., Balvay, D., Tanter, M., Clement, O., Cuenod, C.A., Zinzindohoue, F. (2014). Real time shear waves elastography monitoring of the rmal ablation: In vivo evaluation in pig livers. *J. Surg. Res.*, 188(1), 37–43.

Murphy, M.C., Huston III, J., Jack Jr., C.R. Glaser, K.J., Manduca, A., Felmlee, J.P., Ehman, R.L. (2011). Decreased brain stiffness in Alzheimer's disease determined by magnetic resonance elastography. *J. Magn. Reson. Imaging*, 34, 494–498.

Muthupillai, R., Lomas, D.J., Rossman, P.J., Greenleaf, J.F., Manduca, A., Ehman, R.L. (1995). Magnetic resonance elastography by direct visualization of propagating acoustic strain waves. *Science*, 269(5232), 1854–1857.

Perriñez, P.R., Kennedy, F.E., Van Houten, E.E.W., Weaver, J.B., Paulsen, K.D. (2010). Magnetic resonance poroelastography: An algorithm for estimating the mechanical properties of fluid-saturated soft tissues. *IEEE Transactions on Medical Imaging*, 29(3), 746–755.

Plewes, D.B., Bishop, J., Samani, A., Sciarretta, J. (2000). Visualization and quantification of breast cancer biomechanical properties with magnetic resonance elastography. *Phys. Med. Biol.*, 45(6), 1591–1610.

Pontryagin, L.S., Boltyanskii, V.G., Gamkrelidze, R.V., Mishechenko, E.F. (1963). The mathematical theory of optimal processes. *Journal of Applied Mathematics and Mechanics*, 43(10/11), 514–515.

Ronot, M., Lambert, S., Elkrief, L., Doblas, S., Rautou, P.E., Castera, L., Vilgrain, V., Sinkus, R., Van Beers, B.E., Garteiser, P. (2014). Assessment of portal hypertension and high-risk oesophageal varices with liver and spleen three-dimensional multifrequency MR elastography in liver cirrhosis. *Eur. Radiol.*, 24(6), 1394–1402.

Runge, J.H., Hoelzl, S.H., Sudakova, J., Dokumaci, A.S., Nelissen, J.L., Guenthner, C., Lee, J., Troelstra, M., Fovargue, D., Stoker, J. et al. (2019). A novel magnetic resonance elastography transducer concept based on a rotational eccentric mass: Preliminary experiences with the gravitational transducer. *Phys. Med. Biol.*, 64(4), 045007.

Sack, I., Beierbach, B., Hamhaber, U., Klatt, D., Braun, J. (2008). Non-invasive measurement of brain viscoelasticity using magnetic resonance elastography. *NMR Biomed.*, 21, 265–271.

Sango Solanas, P., Tse Ve Koon, K., Van Reeth, E., Ratiney, H., Millioz, F., Caussy, C., Beuf, O. (2022). Short echo time dual-frequency MR elastography with optimal control RF pulses. *Scientific Reports*, 12, 1406.

Sinkus, R., Tanter, M., Xydeas, T., Catheline, S., Bercoff, J., Fink, M. (2005). Viscoelastic shear properties of in vivo breast lesions measured by MR elastography. *Magn. Reson. Imaging.*, 23(2), 159–165.

Souchon, R., Salomir, R., Beuf, O., Milot, L., Grenier, D., Lyonnet, D., Chapelon, J.Y., Rouvière, O. (2008). Transient MR elastography (t-MRE) using ultrasound radiation force: Theory, safety, and initial experiments in vitro. *Magn. Reson. Med.*, 60(4), 871–881.

Streitberger, K.J., Sack, I., Kretting, D., Pfüller, C., Braun, J., Paul, F., Wuerfel, J. (2012). Brain viscoelasticity alteration in chronic-progressive multiple sclerosis. *PLoS One*, 7(1), e29888.

Streitberger, K.J., Reiss-Zimmermann, M., Freimann, F.B., Bayerl, S., Guo, J., Artl, F., Wuerfel, J., Braun, J., Hoffmann, K.T., Sack, I. (2014). High-resolution mechanical imaging of glioblastoma by multifrequency magnetic resonance elastography. *PLoS One*, 9(10), e110588.

Testu, J., McGarry, M.D.J., Dittmann, F., Weaver, J.B., Paulsen, K.D., Sack, I., Van Houten, E.E.W. (2017). Viscoelastic power law parameters of in vivo human brain estimated by MR elastography. *J. Mech. Behav. Biomed. Mater.*, 74, 333–341.

Tse, Z.T.H., Janssen, H., Hamed, A., Ristic, M., Young, I., Lamperth, M. (2009). Magnetic resonance elastography hardware design: A survey. *Proc. Inst. Mech. Eng. H.*, 223(4), 497–514.

Tzschätzsch, H., Guo, J., Dittmann, F., Hirsch, S., Barnhill, E., Jöhrens, K., Braun, J., Sack, I. (2016). Tomoelastography by multifrequency wave number recovery from time-harmonic propagating shear waves. *Med. Image. Anal.*, 30, 1–10.

Van Houten, E.E.W., Paulsen, K.D., Miga, M.I., Kennedy, F.E., Weaver, J.B. (1999). An overlapping subzone technique for MR-based elastic property reconstruction. *Magn. Reson. Med.*, 42(4), 779–786.

Van Reeth, E., Lefebvre, P.M., Ratiney, H., Lambert, S.A., Tesch, M., Brusseau, E., Grenier, D., Beuf, O., Glaser, S.J., Sugny, D. et al. (2018). Constant gradient elastography with optimal control RF pulses. *J. Magn. Reson.*, 294, 153–161.

Vappou, J., Breton, E., Choquet, P., Willinger, R., Constantinesco, A. (2008). Assessment of in vivo and post-mortem mechanical behavior of brain tissue using magnetic resonance elastography. *J. Biomech.*, 41(14), 2954–2959.

Vappou, J., Bour, P., Marquet, F., Ozenne, V., Quesson, B. (2018). MR-ARFI-based method for the quantitative measurement of tissue elasticity: Application for monitoring HIFU therapy. *Phys. Med. Biol.*, 63(9), 095018.

Venkatesh, S.K., Yin, M., Ehman, R.L. (2013). Magnetic resonance elastography of liver: Technique, analysis and clinical applications. *J. Magn. Reson. Imaging*, 37(3), 544–555.

Weaver, J.B., Pattison, A.J., McGarry, M.D., Perreard, I.M., Swienckowski, J.G., Eskey, C.J., Lollis, S.S., Paulsen, K.D. (2012). Brain mechanical property measurement using MRE with intrinsic activation. *Phys. Med. Biol.*, 57(22), 7275–7287.

Wuerfel, J., Paul, F., Beierbach, B., Hamhaber, U., Klatt, D., Papazoglou, S., Zipp, F., Martus, P., Braun, J., Sack, I. (2010). MR-elastography reveals degradation of tissue integrity in multiple sclerosis. *NeuroImage*, 49(3), 2520–2525.

Yin, Z., Magin, R.L., Klatt, D. (2014). Simultaneous MR elastography and diffusion acquisitions: Diffusion-MRE (dMRE). *Magn. Reson. Med.*, 71, 1682–1688.

Yin, M., Glaser, K.J., Manduca, A., Mounajjed, T., Malhi, H., Simonetto, D.A., Wang, R., Yang, L., Mao, S.A., Glorioso, J.M. et al. (2017a). Distinguishing between hepatic inflammation and fibrosis with MR elastography. *Radiology*, 284(3), 694–705.

Yin, Z., Kearney, S.P., Magin, R.L., Klatt, D. (2017b). Concurrent 3D acquisition of diffusion tensor imaging and magnetic resonance elastography displacement data (DTI-MRE): Theory and in vivo application. *Magn. Reson. Med.*, 77, 273–284.

Yin, Z., Hughes, J.D., Glaser, K.J., Manduca, A., Van Gompel, J., Link, M.J., Romano, A., Ehman, R.L., Huston III, J. (2017c). Slip interface imaging based on MR-elastography preoperatively predicts meningioma–brain adhesion. *J. Magn. Reson. Imaging*, 46, 1007–1016.

8

Imaging of Dipolar Interactions in Biological Tissues: ihMT and UTE

Guillaume DUHAMEL[1,2], Olivier GIRARD[1,2], Paulo LOUREIRO DE SOUSA[3] and Lucas SOUSTELLE[1,2]

[1] *CRMBM, CNRS, Université Aix-Marseille, France*

[2] *CEMEREM, AP-HM, Hôpital de la Timone, Marseille, France*

[3] *ICUBE, CNRS, Université de Strasbourg, France*

8.1. Introduction

Magnetic dipolar interaction is ubiquitous in MRI. The hydrogen nuclei (commonly called protons or simply spins, and are the focus of this chapter) have a quantum spin number equal to ½, which corresponds to an energy diagram with two distinct levels for a model of isolated spins in the presence of an external magnetic field B_0. The Larmor frequency (i.e. the NMR resonance frequency, see Chapter 1) is determined by the difference between these two energy levels and is directly proportional to the value of the local magnetic field "seen" by the spins. At a microscopic scale, the spins behave like small magnets and create a characteristic magnetic field that affects their close neighbors (this is called magnetic dipolar coupling). This local magnetic field is superposed to the external magnetic field B_0, with a consequent local modification of resonant frequency for close neighbors. This mechanism is the cause of the resonance line broadening (spectral, i.e. frequential, representation, of the NMR signal of the spins (see Chapter 9)) of the protons in macromolecules with restricted motion. This broadening is related to dipolar coupling and corresponds to a very rapid decay of the signal in the time domain with

The Challenges of MRI,
coordinated by Hélène RATINEY and Olivier BEUF.

corresponding ultrashort transverse relaxation times T_2 of the order of tens of microseconds (μs), in contrast to free-water protons which have a T_2 of the order of tens of milliseconds (ms).

In conventional MRI, reducing the echo time to durations shorter than a millisecond is generally not possible due to the presence of the magnetic field gradients required for the spatial encoding of the image (see Chapters 1 and 3). Macromolecules with restricted motion are thus invisible as their MRI signal decays too quickly to provide enough signal at the moment of the echo, contrarily to free water, which is easily detected via MRI. A typical example of macromolecules with these properties can be found in the myelin sheath of the central nervous system (Figure 8.1). This biological structure of primordial importance for brain functioning originates from the membrane of the oligodendrocytes that surround the axons in a very compact way. It carries out the task of electrical isolation of the axons and ensures good functioning of the nervous action potential. Contrary to other biological membranes, where lipids usually represent around 40% of the mass, myelin is very rich in lipids (cholesterol (40%), phospholipids (40%), and glycolipids (20%)) that represent ~75% of its mass. From the structural point of view, the compact wrapping of the membrane results in a multilayer organization of lipid bilayers in which the protons of the methylene groups (-CH_2) of the long carbonate chains are spatially constrained and strongly restricted in their motion (Morell 2013), and thus they are characterized by extremely short T_2 values.

Since it is impossible to directly detect the signal of protons in macromolecules with ultrashort T_2 using conventional MRI, novel techniques, that are the subject of this chapter, have been proposed. They can be classified into two categories: (1) magnetization transfer (MT) techniques and, in particular, inhomogeneous magnetization transfer (ihMT), which exploit the phenomena of exchanges between the populations of protons in macromolecules and the protons in free water in order to detect the presence of the former measuring the signal from the latter; (2) ultrashort echo time (UTE) techniques for which the spatial encoding of the image has been redesigned to reach sufficiently short echo times and thus to detect protons with T_2 values shorter than a millisecond.

The first part of this chapter presents the basics of the mechanisms leading to the dipolar broadening of resonance lines in MRI and helps us to understand the difference between the long relaxation times of protons in very mobile molecules (free water) and the very short ones of protons in macromolecules with restricted motion (usually called semi-solid) such as the lipid membranes that form myelin. The second part of the chapter describes the details of the ihMT and UTE techniques for acquiring images of biological tissues with ultrashort T_2 values, with an emphasis on myelin imaging. Finally, some perspectives and conclusions will be presented.

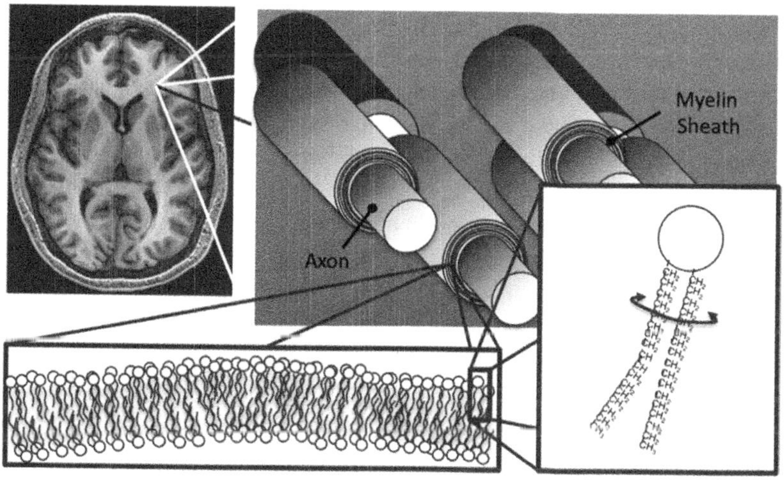

Figure 8.1. *Schematic representation of the myelin sheath formed by a very compact wrapping of lipid bilayers (a hydrophilic head and a long hydrophobic carbonate chain (-CH2)) around the axons. For a color version of this figure, see www.iste.co.uk/ ratiney-beuf/challenges.zip*

8.2. Origins of ultrashort T_2

8.2.1. *Dipolar coupling in NMR*

The magnetic dipolar interaction is the main cause of resonance line broadening in proton NMR (Slichter 1990; Levitt 2008). A classical representation (valid for ½ spins in most situations) consists of considering each hydrogen nucleus as a small magnet (or magnetic dipole containing a north pole and a south pole) that generates a magnetic field in its close vicinity, similar to the lines of the Earth's magnetic field that make a loop to connect the two poles (Figure 8.2). The dipolar interaction is defined as the interaction of these local magnetic fields induced by two neighboring spins, that is, between two magnetic dipoles. By definition, this interaction is mutual: it affects both nuclei and propagates in space without requiring direct physical contact between the two. In practice, for high values of static magnetic field B_0 (of the order of 1 T, i.e. more than 10,000 times the value of the Earth's magnetic field, about 50 μT), only the longitudinal component (i.e. the one aligned with B_0) of these local dipolar fields is of interest, due to the very rapid precession of the spins around the B_0 field that lead to an average zero value for the transverse components of the local dipolar magnetic fields. This is a secular approximation that is commonly used in NMR.

A rigorous treatment of the dipolar interaction in NMR is based on the quantum mechanical formalism of the spin's Hamiltonian, which represents the energy of the interactions (e.g. with an external B_0 field, between the spins, etc.) that occur in the considered spin system. This formalism is often quite complex to comprehend[1], and the treatment differs depending on whether the considered nuclei are of the same kind (homonuclear case) or different kinds (heteronuclear case). The main difference stems from the existence of an additional term in the dipolar Hamiltonian for the homonuclear case, corresponding to an iso-energetic exchange of magnetization between the coupled spins, that is, this exchange does not require any energy contribution from the environment (commonly called the "lattice"). This is typically the case of *flip-flop*, a term used to designate the transition of a spin from its *up* state to its *down* state simultaneously to the opposite transition of the neighbor spin from its *down* state to its *up* state. In the homonuclear case, this double transition is iso-energetic (it does not cost anything from an energy point of view, which is not the case of heteronuclear spins). Therefore, it enables efficient MT between the spins coupled via dipolar interaction and it is, hence, the root of spin diffusion (which is more efficient the stronger the magnetic coupling) that enables the exchange of magnetization within a sample without any physical or chemical exchange of matter. This is an important phenomenon of MT in macromolecules with restricted motion (that present residual nonzero dipolar coupling (see section 8.3)), such as the lipid chains contained in biological membranes (van Zijl et al. 2003; Chen et al. 2006; Malyarenko et al. 2014). In the case of two magnetically coupled ^{1}H protons that we consider here, the dipolar Hamiltonian is directly proportional to the secular dipolar coupling D_{sec} given by:

$$D_{sec} = -\frac{\mu_0}{4\pi}\frac{\gamma_H{}^2\hbar}{r^3}\frac{(3\cos^2\theta - 1)}{2} \qquad [8.1]$$

where μ_0 is the magnetic permeability of vacuum, γ_H is the gyromagnetic ratio of the proton, $\hbar$ is the reduced Planck's constant, r is the distance between the two protons, and θ is the angle obtained by the vector that connects the two spins and the static magnetic field B_0. D_{sec} is expressed in radians per second.

It can be noted that the dipolar coupling strength decreases as a function of the inverse of the distance between the two nuclei to the power of three, and varies with the orientation of the internuclear vector with respect to the external magnetic field.

1 The interested reader is invited to read the excellent textbook by Levitt (2008), in particular section 9.3.

At the "magic angle" $\theta \cong 54.74°$ (value of θ for which $3\cos^2\theta = 1$), the effect of the dipolar coupling is zero, although the nuclei are magnetically coupled.

To give an order of magnitude, let us consider two protons located at 0.2 nm from one another (order of magnitude of the distance between the two protons of a water molecule, for example) and aligned with the magnetic field B_0 ($\theta = 0°$, such that $(3\cos^2\theta - 1)/2 = 1$). In such a case, the secular dipolar coupling is of the order of 15 kHz (expressed here in Hz for direct comparison with the Larmor frequency, of the order of 64 MHz for a field of 1.5 T).

8.2.2. *Dipolar resonance line broadening*

In a heterogeneous sample rich in protons, as is the case of biological tissues, there is a multitude of molecules and possible dipolar couplings between the different protons (Calucci et al. 2009).

The latter can take place between protons of the same molecule (intramolecular) or between two different molecules (intermolecular). The intramolecular couplings are generally stronger due to the rapid decay of the dipolar coupling with the distance.

First, let us consider the simplified case of purely static nuclei (the spins are motionless). A dipolar coupling constant could be calculated for all pairs of hydrogen nuclei and, hence, the local magnetic field perceived by each proton could be obtained. Due to the multitude of interaction distances and possible orientations within the nuclei pairs, a quasi-continuum of dipolar coupling values is expected, with an almost continuous distribution of the resonance frequency values that are intrinsic to each proton in the medium. The corresponding NMR line could then be calculated simply by integrating (i.e. summing up) the spectra of all of the protons contributing to the NMR signal.

Although this mental exercise is almost impossible to perform in practice because of the too-high number of protons and couplings, intuitively, we can understand that the width of the obtained line for such a sample (a static one, as a reminder) would be of the order of magnitude of the strongest dipolar coupling values, that is, tens of kHz. This phenomenon is called the dipolar broadening of the resonance lines. However, the spins are not static, but in motion because of the thermal oscillations in the medium, and these motions will also affect the line width.

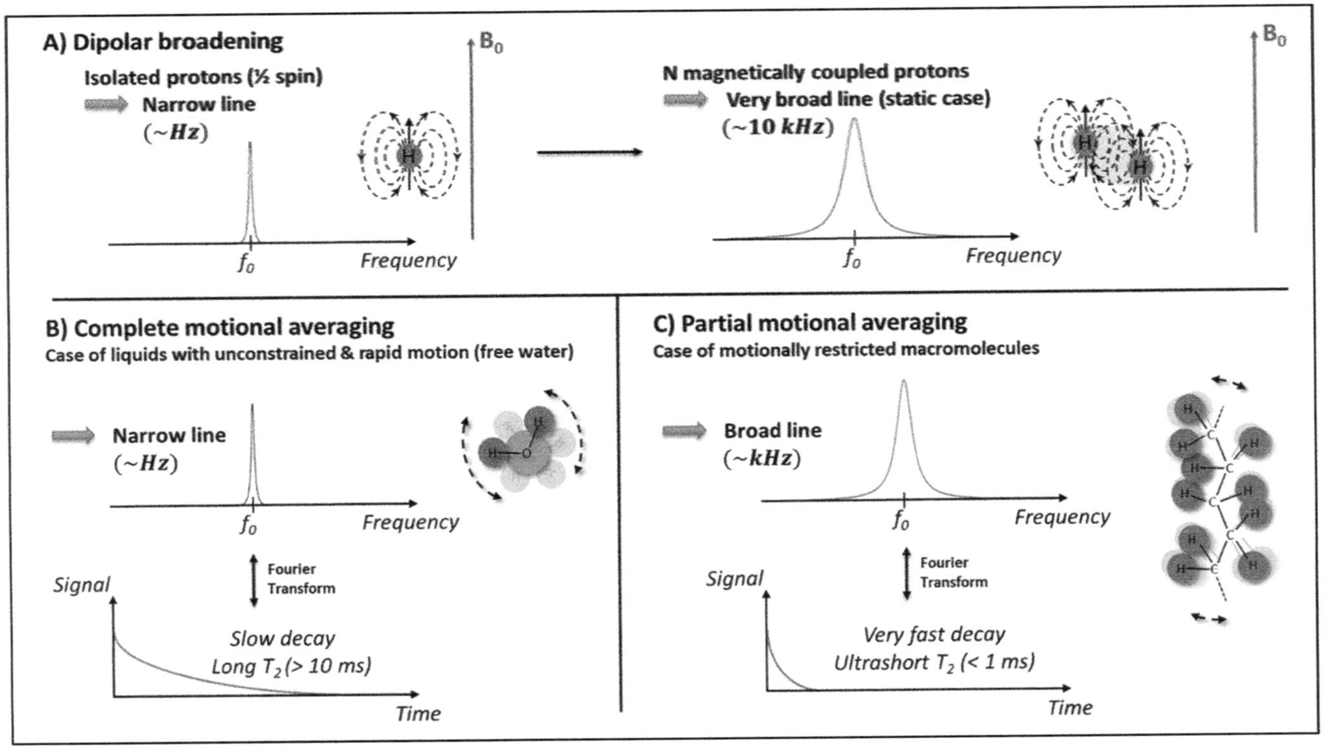

Figure 8.2. *Illustration of the concepts of dipolar broadening resonance line (a) and complete (b) and partial (c) motional averaging. For a color version of this figure, see www.iste.co.uk/ratiney-beuf/challenges.zip*

8.2.3. *Motional averaging*

When the spins are in motion, they do not experience the same value of magnetic field induced by their close neighbors over time, and they are sensitive to its average value over time. Different types of molecular motion can be distinguished: the motion that occurs internally to each molecule, the translational diffusion of the molecules, or the rotation of the molecules around themselves when they are free (see Levitt 2008; see also in particular section 8.6). These motions may be rapid or slow depending on the considered medium (e.g. the viscosity of a fluid changes the speed of the molecules' displacement or rotation around themselves). From a formal point of view, a correlation time (τ_c) can be associated with each type of movement to quantify the time limit when the dipolar Hamiltonian is no longer correlated with its initial value since it has significantly evolved over time due to the motion. The fastest motion is the determining factor of the motional averaging in dipolar interactions. The more the motion is rapid, the shorter the associated correlation time and the stronger the averaging effects.

In the case of free water (or isotropic liquid[2]), the correlation time of translational diffusion and molecular rotations is of the order of 10^{-12} s (Calucci et al. 2009). All of the molecular orientations have the same probability over time, hence the average dipolar Hamiltonian (that describes the average local dipolar field) is zero because the integral of the function $(3\cos^2\theta - 1)$ for all of the possible orientations equals 0. Therefore, although a strong dipolar coupling between the two water protons exists in the static case, it does not have any effect on the observed resonance frequency for each proton in the case of free water and the resonance line is very thin, typically of the order of a few Hz. The line width is then representative of the pure transverse relaxation phenomena related to the fluctuations of the surrounding dipolar fields (T_2 relaxation) or the non-uniformity of the B_0 field, which can be related to an imperfect design of the MRI magnet or magnetic susceptibility effects (T_2* relaxation contributions).

In the case of macromolecules with constrained motion (e.g. myelin lipid chains), several couplings exist between protons but, in this case, the restricted molecular mobility hinders some of the possible orientations. The value of the average dipolar field perceived by the spins corresponds in such a case to the average of the dipolar field over all possible orientations of the molecule. In this

---

2 In some conditions, although the liquid is very mobile, its motion is restricted such that the molecular orientations do not all have the same probability; this is, for example, the case of liquid crystals. Such liquids are called anisotropic liquids.

case, the term residual dipolar coupling (RDC) is employed to describe the value of the dipolar coupling that remains after the time averaging due to motion. The RDC is weaker than the coupling obtained in the static case. It is relatively weak in the case of anisotropic liquids but can be strong (of the order of kHz) for non-mobile macromolecules or semi-solids that are present[3] in biological tissues. In such cases, the line width is a combination of the transverse relaxation phenomena related to the fluctuations of the local dipolar fields and dipolar broadening effects induced by the residual component of the dipolar interaction. Often, a unique value of T_2 (inversely proportional to the line width) is used, typically equal to a few tens of microseconds for semi-solid macromolecules in biological tissues.

8.3. Imaging of the inhomogeneous magnetization transfer

The RDC observed in such motion-restricted macromolecules is the basis of the dipolar order, that is, polarization of coupled spins in the local dipolar field produced by their close neighbors. This dipolar order is particularly relevant for ihMT imaging as we will see in this chapter.

8.3.1. *Dipolar order and radiofrequency saturation*

Quite often, a simplified biophysical model composed of two separate compartments is used in MRI to describe biological tissues. The first compartment describes the magnetization of liquid protons (i.e. mobile protons) and the second represents the magnetization of the so-called semi-solid protons (i.e. protons with restricted motion, such as those in the macromolecules composing the myelin). These two compartments are supposed to exchange energy since there are physiochemical phenomena, such as chemical exchange of protons or cross-relaxation, enabling magnetization to be transferred from one compartment to another.

While the liquid compartment can be described by the so-called Zeeman magnetization (the classical concept of macroscopic nuclear magnetization in NMR), the semi-solid compartment (that differs from the other due to the existence of a nonzero RDC) requires considering two degrees of freedom for describing the

3 It should be noted that the notion of semi-solid macromolecules is intrinsically related to their degree of mobility and is not related to their size expressed in units of atomic mass. For instance, solute proteins are highly mobile, while the lipids that compose the myelin are very restricted in their motion.

distribution of energy levels populations of the corresponding system of spins. In this way, in addition to the Zeeman magnetization that corresponds to the polarization of the spins in the external magnetic field B_0, another type of magnetization coexists, called the dipolar order, which corresponds to the polarization of the spins in the local dipolar fields created by their neighbors.

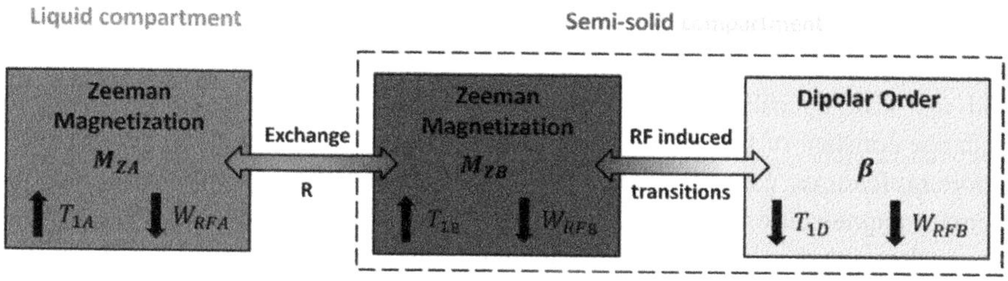

Figure 8.3. *Biophysical model of biological tissue subjected to an RF saturation pulse. For a color version of this figure, see www.iste.co.uk/ratiney-beuf/challenges.zip*

The effects of an MRI scan during which a saturation radiofrequency (RF) pulse is applied to the biological tissue can be modeled using the Bloch equations[4] modified to take into account the MT (Henkelman et al. 1993) and the theory of RF saturation in solids, initially developed by Provotorov (1962) and later reinterpreted and made widely popular by Goldman (1970). This theory considers the dipolar order (Figure 8.3) and describes the coupling of the magnetization's degrees of freedom of the semi-solid protons compartment, the Zeeman magnetization (M_Z^B), and the dipolar order (β) under the effect of RF saturation off-resonance at a frequency Δ (the term single frequency RF saturation is employed in this case). Thus, a system of coupled differential equations [8.2] (equations of Bloch–Provotorov) describing the evolution of the magnetizations M_Z^A, M_Z^B and β is obtained:

$$\begin{cases} \frac{dM_Z^A}{dt} = \frac{1}{T_{1A}}(M_0^A - M_Z^A) - R_{rfA}M_Z^A + R(M_0^A M_Z^B - M_0^B M_Z^A) \\ \frac{dM_Z^B}{dt} = \frac{1}{T_{1B}}(M_0^B - M_Z^B) - R_{rfB}M_Z^B + 2\pi\Delta R_{rfB}\beta + R(M_0^B M_Z^A - M_0^A M_Z^B) \\ \frac{d\beta}{dt} = -\frac{1}{T_{1D}}\beta - \left(\frac{2\pi\Delta}{D}\right)^2 R_{rfB}\beta + \frac{2\pi\Delta}{D^2} R_{rfB} M_Z^B \end{cases} \quad [8.2]$$

4 Bloch equations are valid for liquid protons and correspond to a Lorentzian shape of the resonance line in the frequency domain, which corresponds to an exponential decay of the transverse magnetization in time.

T_{1A}, T_{1B} and T_{1D} correspond to the longitudinal relaxation constant of the Zeeman magnetization of the liquid and semi-solid compartments and of the dipolar order, respectively. The terms $R_{rfA,B} = \pi\omega_1{}^2 g_{A,B}(2\pi\Delta)$ correspond to the rate of RF saturation of the liquid and semi-solid compartments induced by an RF pulse of intensity ω_1 (expressed in rad/s[5]) and of a frequency offset Δ, where g_A and g_B correspond to the normalized absorption lines associated with the liquid (Lorentzian line shape) and semi-solid compartment (usually assumed to have a super-Lorentzian shape) (Morrison et al. 1995). D corresponds to the local dipolar field that can be calculated using the second moment of g_B. Finally, R is the exchange constant of the MT between the liquid and semi-solid compartments. Two important features can be observed from the system of equations [8.2]: (i) the Zeeman magnetization of the semi-solid compartment ($M_Z{}^B$) and the dipolar order (β) are decoupled in the absence of RF saturation ($R_{rfB} = 0$) or when the pulse is played on resonance ($\Delta = 0$); (ii) the RF saturation acts on $M_Z{}^B$ in two opposed ways, promoting its attenuation ($-R_{rfB}M_Z{}^B$ term) as well as its recovery by means of the inflow from dipolar order ($+2\pi\Delta R_{rfB}\beta$ term). Besides, if the system of spins is exposed to saturation with a total RF power $\omega_1{}^2$ that is simultaneously split into two symmetric saturation frequencies $+\Delta$ and $-\Delta$ (symmetric dual RF saturation) then, using the full expression of R_{rfB} at the frequencies $+\Delta$ and $-\Delta$, the Provotorov equations can be rewritten as:

$$\begin{cases} \frac{dM_Z^B}{dt} = \frac{1}{T_{1B}}(M_0^B - M_Z^B) - \left\{\pi\frac{\omega_1^2}{2}g_B(2\pi\Delta) + \pi\frac{\omega_1^2}{2}g_B(-2\pi\Delta)\right\}M_Z^B + \\ \quad 2\pi\left\{\Delta\frac{\omega_1^2}{2}g_B(2\pi\Delta) - \Delta\frac{\omega_1^2}{2}g_B(-2\pi\Delta)\right\}\beta + R(M_0^B M_Z^A - M_0^A M_Z^B) \\ \frac{d\beta}{dt} = -\frac{1}{T_{1D}}\beta - \left(\frac{2\pi}{D}\right)^2\left\{\Delta^2\pi\frac{\omega_1^2}{2}g_B(2\pi\Delta) + (-\Delta)^2\pi\frac{\omega_1^2}{2}g_B(-2\pi\Delta)\right\}\beta + \\ \quad \frac{2\pi}{D^2}\left\{\Delta\pi\frac{\omega_1^2}{2}g_B(2\pi\Delta) - \Delta\pi\frac{\omega_1^2}{2}g_B(-2\pi\Delta)\right\}M_Z^B \end{cases} \quad [8.3]$$

The symmetry hypothesis for the line shape of the semi-solid pool[6] ($g_B(2\pi\Delta) = g_B(-2\pi\Delta)$) allows the system of equations [8.3] to be simplified such that the

5 In NMR, the intensities of the magnetic field are usually expressed in Hz or rad/s following the Larmor relationship that associates the value of the magnetic field with the frequency of precession around this field (see Chapter 1).

6 We are reminded that, by definition, the dipolar coupling induces a symmetric broadening of the resonance lines; however, the corresponding line can be slightly shifted with respect to the free water line due to the chemical shift (see Chapter 9), which can introduce a small asymmetry with respect to the centered frequencies of free water (Prevost et al. 2016).

Bloch-Provotorov equations describing the evolution of the system of spins subjected to symmetric dual RF saturation are reduced to:

$$\begin{cases} \frac{dM_Z^A}{dt} = \frac{1}{T_{1A}}(M_0^A - M_Z^A) - R_{rfA}M_Z^A + R(M_0^A M_Z^B - M_0^B M_Z^A) \\ \frac{dM_Z^B}{dt} = \frac{1}{T_{1B}}(M_0^B - M_Z^B) - R_{rfB}M_Z^B + R(M_0^B M_Z^A - M_0^A M_Z^B) \\ \qquad \frac{d\beta}{dt} = -\frac{1}{T_{1D}}\beta - \left(\frac{2\pi\Delta}{D}\right)^2 R_{rfB}\beta \end{cases} \quad [8.4]$$

Remarkably, the dipolar order is decoupled from the Zeeman magnetization of the macromolecular compartment: the dual RF saturation does not act in opposite ways anymore and the attenuation of $M_Z{}^B$ is greater than in the case of *simple* frequency RF saturation.

An analytical solution[7] of the equation systems [8.2] and [8.4] can be obtained for a stationary state (i.e. time derivatives equal to zero) for the magnetization of the liquid compartment in the case of *single* ($M_Z{}^{A+}$) and *dual* ($M_Z{}^{A+/-}$) frequency RF saturation. Since the dipolar order effects are present in $M_Z{}^{A+}$ and canceled out in $M_Z{}^{A+/-}$, the difference between $M_Z{}^{A+}$ and $M_Z{}^{A+/-}$ mainly reflects the contribution of the dipolar order to MT effects.

8.3.2. *Dipolar order and inhomogeneous magnetization transfer*

Experimentally, assessing the dipolar order ($M_Z{}^{A+} - M_Z{}^{A+/-}$) is done via ihMT imaging (Varma et al. 2015a, 2015b). The application of single frequency saturation generates an image MT^+ representing $M_Z{}^{A+}$ and the application of dual saturation leads to an image $MT^{+/-}$ corresponding to $M_Z{}^{A+/-}$ (Figure 8.4). The inhomogeneous magnetization transfer image ihMT and ratio ihMTR are then defined as:

$$ihMT = MT^+ - MT^{+/-}$$

$$ihMTR = \frac{ihMT}{M_0}$$

where M_0 corresponds to a reference image acquired without RF saturation, representing the magnetization of the liquid compartment $M_0{}^A$.

In practice, the MT^+ image is obtained via the application of a saturation block, typically a pulse train of off-resonance RF saturations (frequency $+\Delta$, power $\omega_1{}^2$)

7 We recommend reading Varma et al. (2015b) for complete analytical formulations.

applied before the image readout block (on-resonance RF pulse followed by an image acquisition pattern such as GRE or SE)[8]. For the $MT^{+/-}$ image, dual saturation can be obtained via the same kind of RF pulses applied on resonance and with their amplitude modulated by a sinusoidal function ($\sqrt{2}sin(2\pi\Delta\tau)$). The sinusoidal function modulation excites the two frequency bands centered at $+\Delta$ and $-\Delta$ simultaneously. The $\sqrt{2}$ factor is introduced in the amplitude modulation to maintain the same total power applied at $+\Delta$ and $-\Delta$ as the power applied at $+\Delta$ in the single frequency saturation case (Figure 8.5).

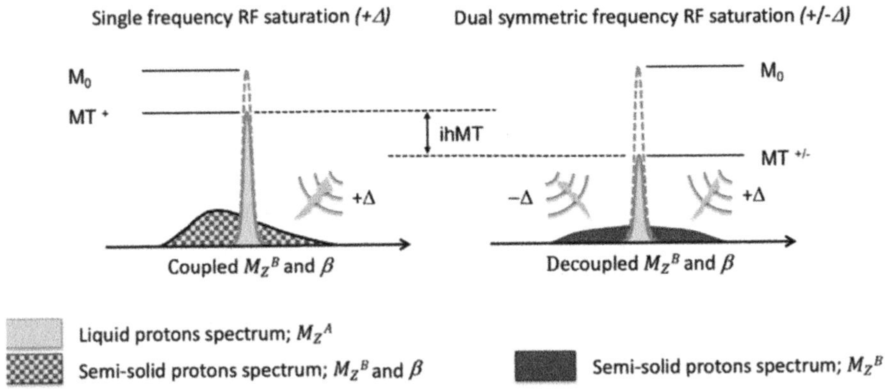

Figure 8.4. *Schematic illustration of inhomogeneous magnetization transfer. For a color version of this figure, see www.iste.co.uk/ratiney-beuf/challenges.zip*

COMMENT ON FIGURE 8.4.– *The application of single frequency off-resonance RF saturation attenuates the Zeeman magnetization of the semi-solid compartment. The attenuation is however counterbalanced by the influx of the coupled dipolar order. The magnetization transfer between the semi-solid compartment and the liquid compartment results in a decrease in the magnetization of the liquid compartment. This decrease is represented in the* MT^{+} *image. The application of dual saturation decouples the dipolar order and the Zeeman magnetization of the semi-solid compartment causing a greater attenuation of the latter. Consequently, the exchange of spins between the semi-solid compartment and the liquid one results in a greater reduction of the liquid compartment's magnetization. This translates into an* $MT^{+/-}$

8 It is also common to acquire a single frequency acquisition MT^{-} with an opposite offset (frequency $-\Delta$), and to define $ihMT = MT^{+} + MT^{-} - 2MT^{+/-}$. Conceptually, the discussion remains the same; this double difference simply reduces the asymmetry effects of dual saturation (Prevost et al. 2016).

image having a lower intensity than the MT^+ image. The ihMT image corresponds to the difference between MT^+ and $MT^{+/-}$ images.

Representative examples of ihMT images obtained in humans at 1.5 T and in small animals at 7 T are shown in Figure 8.6. The contrast of ihMT images clearly shows the white matter structures made up of myelinated axon fibers (e.g. corpus callosum, internal capsules, optic nerves) as hyperintense and the gray matter (neurons) as hypointense.

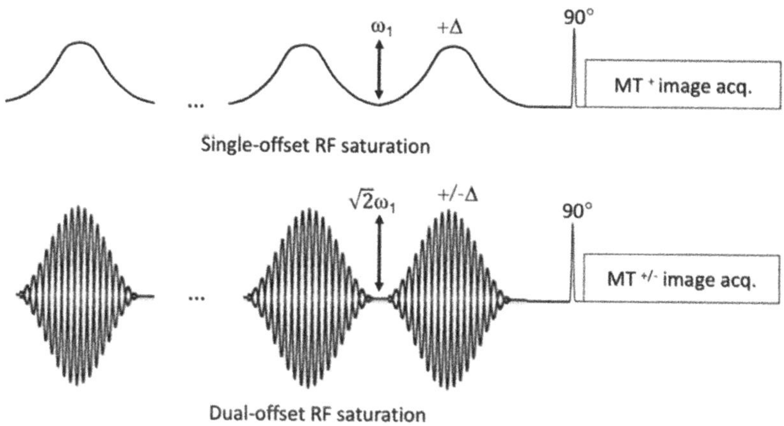

Figure 8.5. *Schematic illustration of an inhomogeneous magnetization transfer MRI sequence*

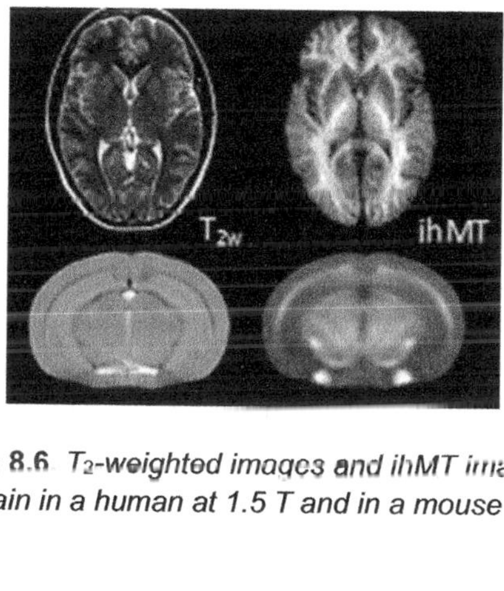

Figure 8.6 *T_2-weighted images and ihMT images of the brain in a human at 1.5 T and in a mouse at 7 T*

8.3.3. *Specificity of the ihMT signal and relaxation of the dipolar order*

The ihMT signal represents the dipolar order and is thus intrinsically sensitive to its longitudinal relaxation characterized by the time constant T_{1D}. This value varies with the composition and structure of the tissues. Although the evaluation of T_{1D} values in biological tissues is still an exploratory research topic, some orders of magnitude can be given here. Lamellar liquid crystals, as well as myelinated tissues (with an analogous structure to lamellar liquid crystals and in terms of molecular dynamics), have relatively long dipolar relaxation times, of the order of tens of milliseconds. No other biological tissue is known to have such long T_{1D} values and several structured tissues with a nonzero RDC, such as muscles, cartilages or tendons, have T_{1D} values of the order of or lower than a millisecond. Hence, weighting the ihMT signal towards some specific T_{1D} value ranges can provide images with more or less contrast and specificity for certain tissues, and in particular to the myelin in the case of the central nervous system.

The T_{1D} weighting of the ihMT signal is modulated by adjusting the saturation parameters (power and repetition times of the saturation pulses) of the MT^{+} and $MT^{+/-}$ images. The power of the RF saturation pulses (ω_1^2) used for acquiring the MT^{+} image defines the range of dipolar order that contributes to the MT^{+} image according to the empirical law (Manning et al. 2016) $R_{rfB}.T_{1D} > 0.01$. In other words, the power required to detect the dipolar order contributing to the ihMT image is greater for shorter T_{1D} relaxation constants. For the $MT^{+/-}$ image, the application of on-resonance RF pulses, modulated by a sinusoidal function (Figure 8.7(a)) leads to simultaneous saturation at $+\Delta$ and $-\Delta$ frequencies, independently of the T_{1D} value. The resulting ihMT image is thus sensitive to all of the T_{1D} components observed in the MT^{+} image. The application of a train of off-resonance RF saturation pulses whose frequency alternates between $+\Delta$ and $-\Delta$ every Δt is another way of performing dual saturation (Figures 8.7(b) and (c)). In this approach, dual saturation is sequential and effective only at the end of a dual-frequency pulse cycle $(+\Delta, -\Delta)$, that is, after a time $2\Delta t$. The degree of freedom provided by this time variable enables the selection of a range of T_{1D} components contributing to the ihMT signal. In fact, if $\Delta t << T_{1D}$ (Figure 8.7(b)), the dipolar order created by the pulses at the frequency $+\Delta$ does not relax during Δt and is, as a consequence, entirely compensated by the pulses at the opposite frequency $-\Delta$. The dual saturation is effective, and the dipolar order associated with $T_{1D} >> \Delta t$ contributes to the ihMT signal in its entirety. On the other hand, if $\Delta t > T_{1D}$ (Figure 8.7(c)), the dipolar order created by the pulses at the offset frequency $+\Delta$ will relax during Δt and will only be partially compensated (or even uncompensated if $\Delta t >> T_{1D}$). The dual saturation is then only partially effective (or even completely ineffective), and the dipolar order gives only a partial contribution (or no at all) to the ihMT signal.

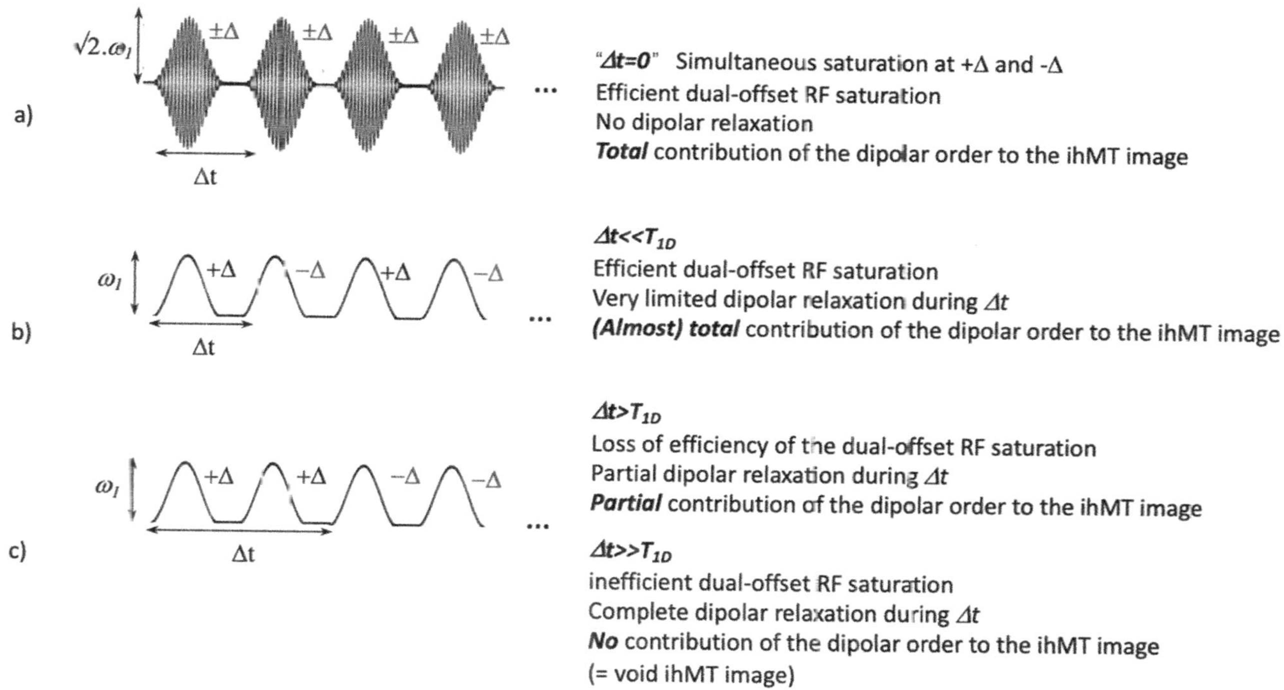

Figure 8.7. *Dual saturation: (a) simultaneous, performed with a sinus modulation of the RF pulses; (b and c) sequential, performed via RF pulses whose frequency is alternated every Δt. For a color version of this figure, see www.iste.co.uk/ratiney-beuf/challenges.zip*

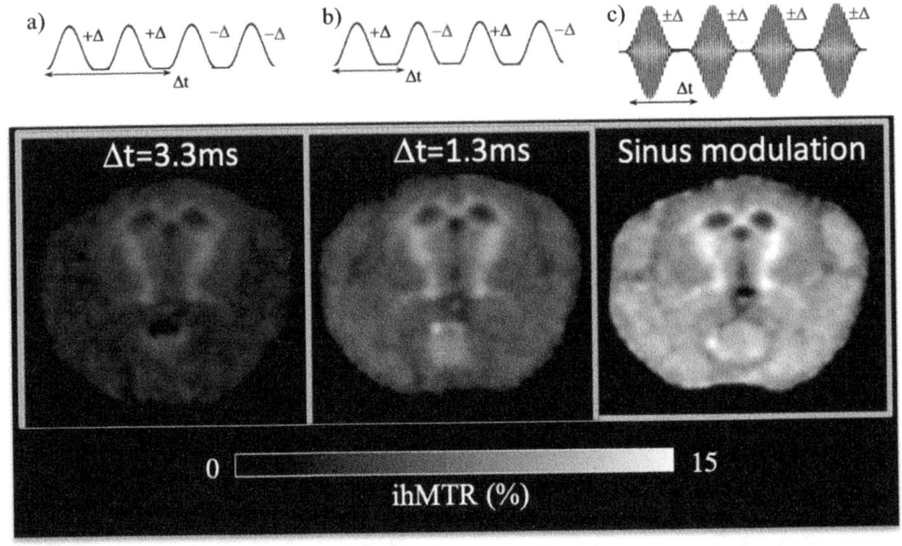

Figure 8.8. *ihMTR images of a mouse brain for different dual saturation patterns: application of RF pulses whose frequency is alternated every Δt = 3.3 ms (a); Δt = 1.3 ms (b); simultaneous dual saturation obtained via modulation of RF pulses by a sinusoidal function (c). For a color version of this figure, see www.iste.co.uk/ratiney-beuf/challenges.zip*

In conclusion, dual RF saturation performed by alternating RF pulses with a opposite frequency offset every Δt attenuates or removes the contribution to the ihMT signal of the T_{1D} components for which $T_{1D} < \Delta t$, that is, of short-T_{1D} components, and the signal is intrinsically weighted toward longer T_{1D} values.

This approach, called T_{1D}-filtering (Prevost et al. 2017), is used to modulate the contrast of ihMT images (Figure 8.8).

As previously mentioned, it is possible not to filter short T_{1D} components by performing simultaneous dual saturation and thus to reveal the ihMT signal in all of the structures where the dipolar order is characterized by T_{1D} values that satisfy $R_{rfB}.T_{1D} > 0.01$. Thus, such an ihMTR image shows a high signal in the structures with a long T_{1D} (e.g. white matter $T_{1D} \approx 6$ ms) but also a visible signal in structures with a short T_{1D} (muscle $T_{1D} \approx 1$ ms) (Prevost et al. 2017). On the opposite hand, using pulses with alternated frequencies for dual saturation attenuates or even removes (filters) the ihMT signal of components with a short T_{1D} by modulating the value of Δt. The T_{1D} filtering mechanism leads to a global reduction in the intensity of the ihMT signal, but also leads to an important increase in the contrast of the ihMTR image favoring structures with long T_{1D}. Therefore, ihMTR images with T_{1D} filtering provide a very clear apparent specificity for myelinated structures (Figure 8.8).

8.3.4. *Specificity of the ihMT signal to myelin*

The molecular origin of the dipolar order characterized by long T_{1D} values in myelinated structures has not yet been determined. Nevertheless, validation of the sensitivity and specificity of the ihMT technique for myelin imaging has been performed experimentally in comparison to another reference myelin imaging method, fluorescence microscopy (Duhamel et al. 2019). The experiments have been performed on a model of transgenic mice (PLP-GFP) where GFP (green fluorescent protein) is co-expressed with one of the major proteins constituting myelin, the PLP (proteolipid protein) (Figure 8.9).

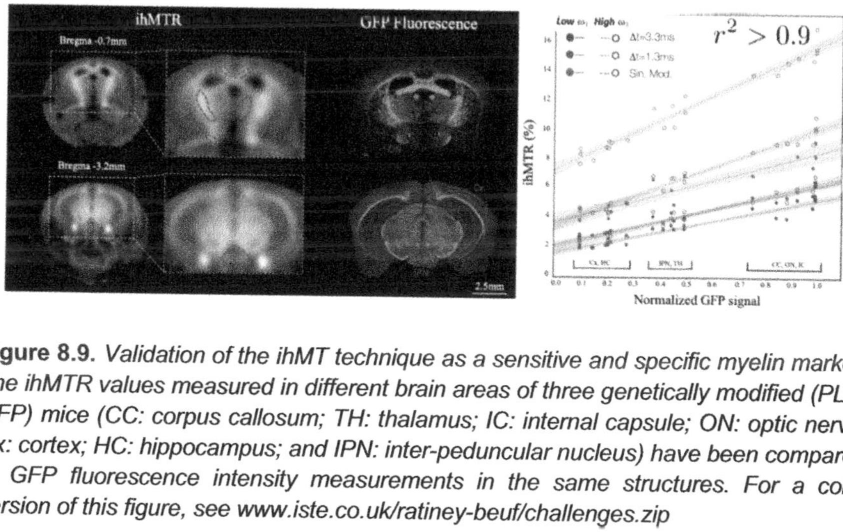

Figure 8.9. *Validation of the ihMT technique as a sensitive and specific myelin marker. The ihMTR values measured in different brain areas of three genetically modified (PLP-GFP) mice (CC: corpus callosum; TH: thalamus; IC: internal capsule; ON: optic nerve; Cx: cortex; HC: hippocampus; and IPN: inter-peduncular nucleus) have been compared to GFP fluorescence intensity measurements in the same structures. For a color version of this figure, see www.iste.co.uk/ratiney-beuf/challenges.zip*

The excellent correlation between the GFP signal and the ihMT signal for all employed dual saturation schemes and intensities validates the sensitivity of the ihMT technique to myelin content. Moreover, the very low intercept values[9] of the correlation lines obtained for the configurations with $\Delta t \geq 1.3$ ms validate the strong specificity of the ihMT technique with short T_{1D} filtering for myelin.

9 Actually, the intercept corresponds to the ihMT signal measured when the reference technique has confirmed the absence of myelin, and this is therefore a part of the ihMT signal that is not specific to myelin.

8.3.5. *Research outlook*

The ihMT technique is a mature method for acquiring images of myelin via MRI both in humans and animal models. It has been investigated in clinical studies on patients with multiple sclerosis, a demyelinating disease of the central nervous system (e.g. van Obberghen et al. 2018). However, many research directions still need to be explored to better understand the contrast mechanisms associated with pathological tissues and the underlying physicochemical phenomena, and make the link with the physiopathology of diseases that affect myelin integrity.

More fundamentally, it has been shown that the ihMT signal of lipid membranes contain several components associated with distinct T_{1D} values. Research on the attribution of these signal components to specific molecular species is ongoing and performed both on synthetic membrane models and myelin. In addition, the features of molecular dynamics, such as the type and amplitude of specific motions of chemical groups within the molecules that could explain the orders of magnitude of the observed T_{1D} values, are other research topics of great interest for better understanding the causes of the ihMT signal variations in a pathological context.

Finally, the derivation of a biophysical model that would be both sufficiently simple for a reliable quantitative estimation of tissue parameters via MRI and sufficiently comprehensive for faithfully describing the degrees of freedom causing the variations in signal and contrast observed in the ihMT images is an important research topic for providing quantitative parameters and potential biomarkers of the central nervous system pathologies.

For more in-depth material, the interested reader can find complementary information in the following references regarding the different topics:

– Physics underlying the ihMT technique: effects of RF features on the ihMT signal (Girard et al. 2015; Mchinda et al. 2017; Varma et al. 2018); measurement of the dipolar relaxation constant T_{1D} (Varma et al. 2017); observation of the existence of several dipolar compartments in the central nervous system (Carvalho et al. 2020).

– Optimized implementation of an ihMT sequence for preclinical and clinical in vivo scans (Mchinda et al. 2017; Duhamel et al. 2019; Varma et al. 2020).

– First applications in clinics and neuroscience research (Taso et al. 2016; Rasoanandrianina et al. 2017; van Obberghen et al. 2018; Munsch et al. 2020; Rasoanandrianina et al. 2020).

8.4. Ultrashort echo time imaging

8.4.1. *Definition of T_2 ranges*

As we have seen in section 8.2, the incomplete averaging of dipolar interactions due to the restricted motion of macromolecules implies a shortening of the transverse relaxation time T_2 in biological tissues. Since the NMR signal is composed of the contribution of water and non-water protons, the biological tissues are characterized by several ranges of T_2, arbitrarily defined as "long", "short" and "ultrashort" depending on their interval of values (Table 8.1); examples of T_2 measured in tissues are given in Table 8.2.

Long T_2	>10 ms
Short T_2	1–10 ms
Ultrashort T_2	0.1–1 ms

Table 8.1. *Classification of the transverse relaxation constant T_2*

Structure	$T_2 \approx T_2^*$
Myelin	0.15–0.3 ms
Cortical bone	0.39 ms
Cartilage	0.5 ms
Patella	0.3 ms
Tendon	0.78–15 ms

Table 8.2. *Examples of T_2 values estimated in different biological tissues*

In the remainder of this chapter, we shall not distinguish between T_2 and T_2^* values of the shortest components, following the assumption that the dipolar resonance line broadening is the dominant contribution to the transverse relaxation, that is, that the effects of magnetic susceptibility (that contribute to T_2^* and not to T_2 (see Chapter 10)) do not cause significative dephasing of the MRI signal when the T_2 is of the order of tens of μs. In other words, these susceptibility effects do not have enough time to affect the shortening of T_2 in ultrashort components.

8.4.2. *Distribution of short T_2 values in cerebral tissue*

Two NMR studies suggest a selectivity of the signal with ultrashort T_2 in brain tissue to the presence and content of myelin (Horch et al. 2011; Wilhelm et al. 2012). These studies investigated, respectively, the distribution of short T_2 components in myelinated tissues and the correlations between the amount of myelin and its spectral NMR content. Horch et al. (2011) have shown that the main origin of the ultrashort T_2 signal in the white matter was related to the pool of protons of chemical methylene groups (-CH2), by performing an analysis via in vitro T_2 relaxometry on representative myelin samples, with and without substitution of mobile ^{1}H protons (i.e. exchangeable, nonmethylene protons) by deuterium atoms. In an NMR spectrometry study conducted by Wilhelm et al. (2012), the protonic spectral content was adjusted by a sum of superlorentzian functions and, consequently, confirmed the prevalence of methylene protons contribution to the signal in a purified myelin bovine sample.

8.4.3. *What are the technical challenges for detecting signals with ultrashort T_2?*

8.4.3.1. *Ultrashort echo times and capabilities of the imaging system*

The lower range of echo times (TE) achievable in clinical and preclinical scanners for a conventional Cartesian acquisition of an image is of the order of 10 ms in spin echo sequences and between 1 and 2 ms in gradient echo sequences. As a result, the signal of ultrashort T_2 components decreases significantly between its creation (excitation via an RF pulse) and its detection (sampling of the signal at the time of the echo), intrinsically reducing the available signal of the component of interest. In gradient echo sequences, the echo time can be decreased below a millisecond, but the minimum value is constrained by the capabilities of the gradients system with respect to the geometric parameters (e.g. the field of view size and the acquisition matrix), and most often is greater than 0.5 ms.

Acquiring images of the components of interest requires the considerable shortening of TE, while allowing for spatial encoding of the signal. For this purpose, different types of sequences have been developed to obtain a minimum TE of the order of tens of microseconds, depending on the characteristic time of the imaging systems for the excitation of the spins (RF pulse) and the reception of the signal (sampling of the signal). For example, on recent preclinical systems, this transition time is of the order of 6 μs. Adaptation efforts have been done by some manufacturers of clinical scanners on their systems, enabling transition times of the order of 1–8 μs (Du et al. 2013; Brunner et al. 2015; Froidevaux et al. 2017, 2021).

8.4.3.2. *Types of UTE sequences*

The favored strategy for filling the k-space with the minimum echo time consists of a centric-out radial encoding, that is, a k-space line is acquired along a trajectory starting from the center (encoding of null spatial frequencies) toward the periphery. Besides, this encoding pattern does not require echo generation to acquire the signal and enables the measurement very shortly after the excitation, similar to an FID as typically measured in MR spectroscopy.

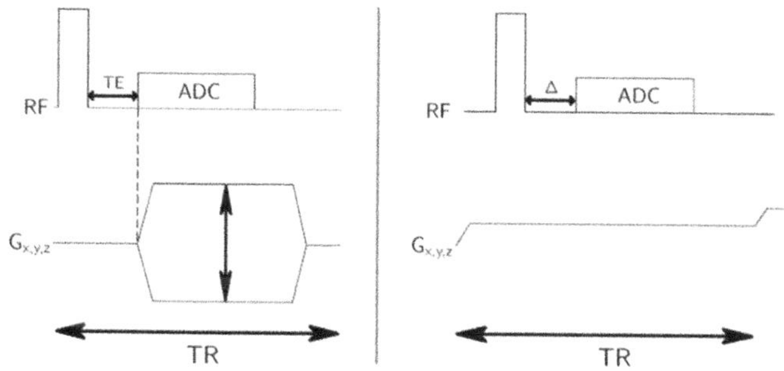

Figure 8.10. *Typical patterns of UTE and ZTE sequences*

Two different types of sequences implementing such kind of encoding can be distinguished: UTE and ZTE (zero time-to-echo) sequences. In a UTE sequence, the signal is sampled after a minimum delay (TE) following the RF excitation and, with a simultaneous application of the encoding gradients. On the other hand, in a ZTE sequence, the encoding gradients are already set at their nominal amplitude when the RF pulse is run (Figure 8.10). Two undesired aspects of ZTE sequences should be highlighted: (i) during the transition time (Δ), the magnetization is slightly dephased by the application of the spatial encoding gradients; and (ii) the presence of gradients during the RF pulse implies an undesired spatial selectivity that varies depending on the relative amplitudes of these gradients and the features of the RF pulse. The first aspect is tackled by filling the missing points at the center of the k-space via an independent acquisition (e.g. using single point imaging) (Madio et al. 1995; Wu et al. 2003; Grodzky et al. 2012) or via interpolation (Weiger et al. 2011), and the second one is addressed by using sufficiently short RF pulses (of the order of tens of microseconds).

8.4.3.3. *Relaxation during the excitation*

The relaxation during the RF pulse is mostly negligible in conventional imaging of water protons, but it cannot be neglected in the context of the excitation of protons having a T_2 of the order or shorter than the pulse duration. This phenomenon translates into a decrease in the efficiency of the magnetization tipping, affecting the signal of the species of interest (Figure 8.11). A solution to this problem consists of using sufficiently short RF pulses, which however hinders the possibility of applying large flip angles due to hardware limitations (e.g. maximum B_1 amplitude, temporal resolution of the RF amplifier for non-rectangular pulses), or phase-modulated pulses (Li et al. 2017).

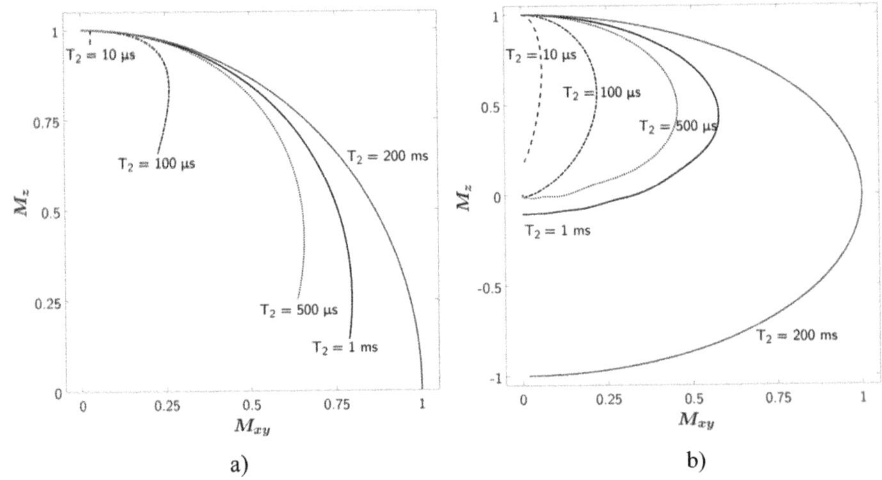

Figure 8.11. *Time evolution of the longitudinal and transverse magnetizations according to a simulation of the Bloch equations during (a) rectangular excitation with a 90° flip angle and a duration τ_{RF}= 500 µs, and (b) adiabatic inversion with a first order hyperbolic secant, on-resonance, and for different T_2 species. For a color version of this figure, see www.iste.co.uk/ratiney-beuf/challenges.zip*

8.4.3.4. *Relaxation during the detection*

The relaxation during the signal encoding (with a duration of the order of the T_2 of the species of interest) also affects the reconstructed image. It manifests as a blurring effect that can be studied using the concept of the point-spread function depending on the type of encoding and the duration of the signal readout. Rahmer et al. (2006) have evaluated this effect for a radial type of k-space encoding (Figure 8.12), showing that a trade-off between the SNR of the species of interest, the readout duration and the blurring amount has to be considered.

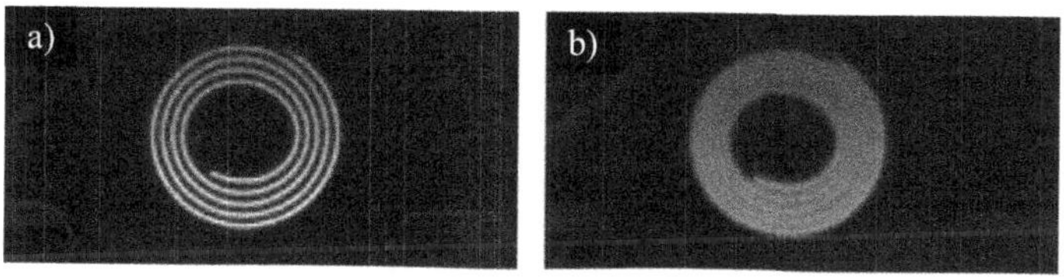

Figure 8.12. *Imaging scan using UTE 3D (voxel size: 0.83 mm isotropic) of adhesive tape roll ($T_2 \approx 660$ μs) for different signal readout durations (T_{read}) (a: $T_{read} = 450$ μs; b: $T_{read} = 1430$ μs). Image modified from Rahmer et al. (2006) with the author's permission*

8.4.3.5. *Trajectories and reconstruction*

The "non-Cartesian" trajectories for filling the k-space that perform a centric-out acquisition are numerous: radial "Kooshball" (Boada et al. 1997; Riemer et al. 2014), radial cone (Gurney et al. 2006), spiral (Cha et al. 2018), hybrid radial cone (Johnson et al. 2017), etc. All of these strategies have advantages and disadvantages (e.g. versatility regarding k-space filling criteria and point-spread function features).

By definition, the k-space coefficients are not located exactly on a Cartesian grid, which is a condition for applying a fast Fourier transform (FFT) for image reconstruction. Most often, re-gridding over a Cartesian grid is performed as an intermediate step, consisting of interpolations using a predefined kernel to compensate for the local information densities; general consensus agrees on a Kaiser–Bessel window (Jackson et al. 1991).

8.4.3.6. *Background signal contamination*

The coils required for the excitation and the reception of the NMR signal are most often enclosed in some support structure made of plastic polymers containing ^{1}H protons. These materials have T_2 values of the order of 10–100 μs and, as a consequence, their signal is absent in conventional Cartesian MRI sequences. On the other hand, UTE acquisitions can be sensitive to these materials (Weiger et al. 2011, 2012; Dreher et al. 2015) (Figure 8.13), although the components are located outside the nominal field of view, contamination of the image occurs due to the phenomenon of spatial folding of information (see Chapter 3).

Different methods can be considered to reduce this effect such as selectively saturating the undesired parts (Dreher et al. 2015), using binomial pulse preparation (Weiger et al. 2012) which does however reduce SNR, or using coil supports made of Teflon (devoid of ^{1}H protons).

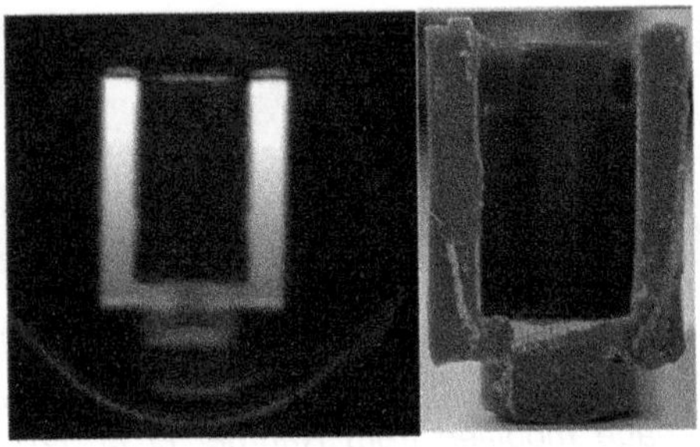

a) b)

Figure 8.13. *Image acquired with a UTE 2D sequence (a) of a plastic ABS polymer piece (b). For a color version of this figure, see www.iste.co.uk/ratiney-beuf/challenges.zip*

8.4.4. *What are the challenges for the characterization of signals with ultrashort T_2 in the cerebral tissue?*

In tissues that include a mixture of components with ultrashort and long T_2, observing the ultrashort components directly can be difficult due to the dominant amount of protons with long T_2: white matter and gray matter contain 72% and 82% of water, respectively (Knaap et al. 2005), and it is worth using some strategy to suppress these undesired components.

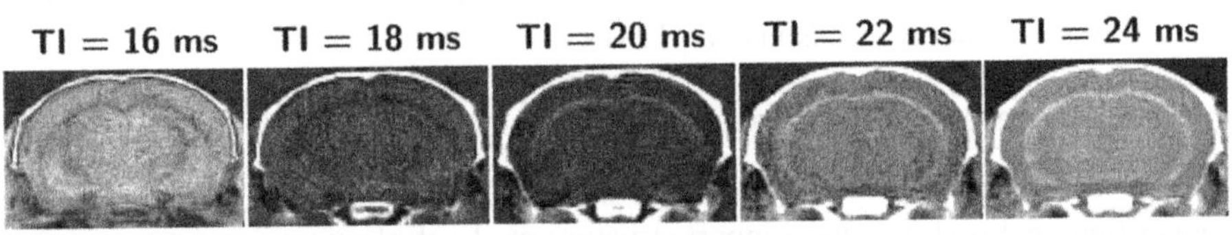

Figure 8.14. *IR-UTE 3D ex vivo images in a mouse brain, where the contrast between the long and ultrashort components changes depending on the inversion time*

8.4.4.1. *Inversion-recovery*

The suppression of the water signal via an inversion pulse followed by a delay (IR: inversion-recovery) is a widely used MRI method for generating contrast between structures with different T_1 values. As has been previously introduced in Figure 8.11, the effect of an RF pulse on the transverse magnetization depends on the T_2 value, the duration of the pulse, and its amplitude. Based on these two effects (excitation followed by longitudinal relaxation), the duration of an RF pulse and the inversion time (TI) can be optimized such that the signal of components with a long

T_2 is significantly suppressed, while the components with ultrashort T_2 are only partially saturated (Figure 8.14).

8.4.4.2. *Echo subtraction*

Based on the ranges of components with ultrashort T_2 ($T_{2S} < 1$ ms) and long T_2 ($T_{2L} >> 10$ ms), the suppression of the long component is also possible via the subtraction between the signal acquired at short TE (TE_S) and the signal acquired at long TE (TE_L). The suppression is based on the hypothesis of negligible relaxation of the long component ($\exp(-TE_L/T_{2L}) \approx \exp(-TE_S/T_{2L})$), while the ultrashort component has completely decayed at TE_L ($\exp(-TE_L/T_{2S}) \approx 0$), leading to a contrast between the components of interest.

This method is often used in combination with the inversion-recovery UTE method: when some tissue is targeted for suppression (e.g. white matter), tissues with a longer T_1 (e.g. gray matter) will be only partially suppressed. Echo subtraction removes the residual signal to provide selective contrast of the targeted tissue (Figure 8.15) (Jang et al. 2021). The price for this suppression is a decrease in SNR by a factor of $\sqrt{2}$ due to the subtraction operation.

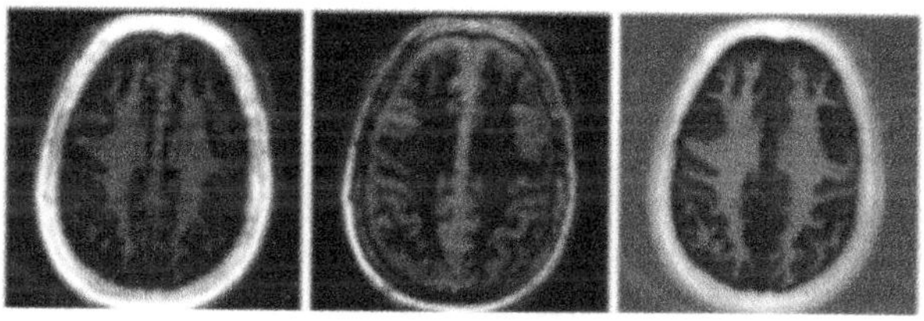

a) b) c)

Figure 8.15. *Images of a human brain with an IR-UTE sequence at TE = 8 μs (a) and TE = 2.3 ms (b), and the subtraction of the two images (c) for suppressing the residual signal of the gray matter and to yield a selective contrast of the white matter. Image modified from Jang (2021) with the author's permission*

8.4.4.3. *Diffusion-weighted suppression*

A recent method for suppressing components with long T_2 consists of exploiting their diffusion behavior (Soustelle et al. 2018). In a sequence with a short TR in comparison to T_1 and T_2, the transverse and longitudinal magnetizations of this component can be weighted by the diffusion effect by means of strong gradients (with a moment greater than 100 mT/m.ms, similar to the gradients commonly used in diffusion imaging; see Chapter 4). With appropriate sequence parameters, it is possible to produce a transverse magnetization equal to zero following the RF excitation of the UTE readout block (Diff-UTE). Compared to inversion-recovery techniques, this method has been shown to be superior in terms of SNR per unit time of the components with ultrashort T_2, while providing white matter contrast with respect to gray matter (Figure 8.16).

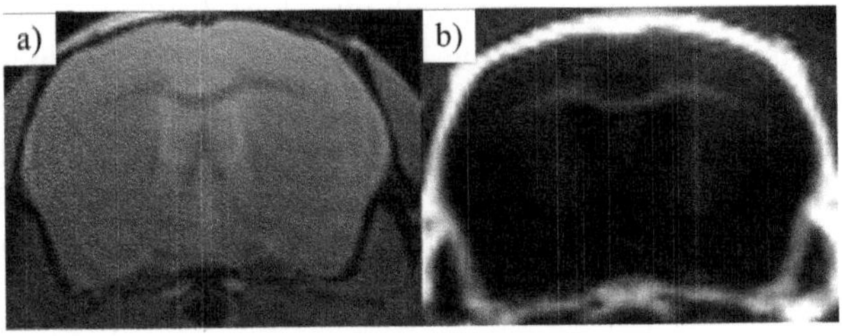

Figure 8.16. *Axial slices with T_2 weighting (a) and with an optimized Diff-UTE sequence (b) of an ex vivo mouse brain. The hypersignal surrounding the brain corresponds to the head skull*

8.4.5. *Applications: myelin imaging*

8.4.5.1. *Contrast and selectivity of ultrashort-T_2 signals in white matter*

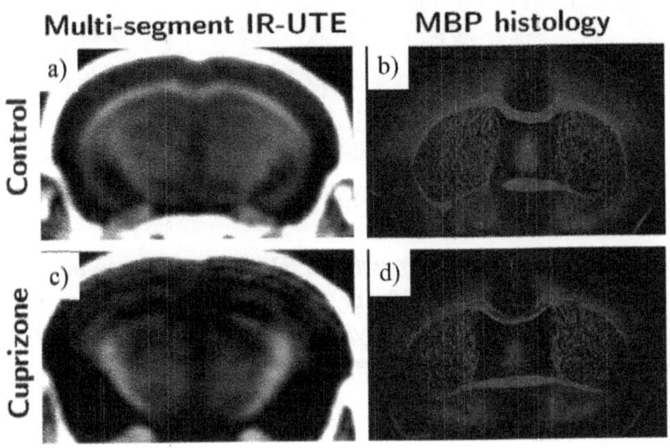

Figure 8.17. *Representative IR-UTE images (a, c) and histological MBP-marked images (b, d) of the brain of a healthy mouse (a, b) and a demyelinated mouse fed with the cuprizone copper chelator (c, d). For a color version of this figure, see www.iste.co.uk/ratiney-beuf/challenges.zip*

The specific detection of components with ultrashort T_2 of the white matter, mainly ascribed to myelin, is most often performed via IR-UTE sequences in combination, if necessary, with the echo subtraction method to guarantee the selectivity of the signal to ultrashort-T_2 components. An example of contrast generated by an IR-UTE sequence in a control mouse brain and a demyelinated mouse brain (cuprizone model) is given in Figure 8.17. This study shows a joint variation of the UTE signal with a specific alteration of the white matter confirmed via histology (immunofluorescence of the basic myelin protein (MBP)). The selectivity of the IR-UTE signal to myelin has also been shown in focal lesions of multiple sclerosis (Ma et al. 2020; Jang et al. 2021). A study performed on a cohort of ex vivo healthy and demyelinated mice using a Diff-UTE sequence has established a significant correlation ($\rho = 0.81$) between the UTE signal and histology (Soustelle et al. 2019).

8.4.5.2. *Extraction of T_1 and T_2 values of ultrashort components*

The characterization of ultrashort-T_2 signal components is of interest for establishing myelin-specific biomarkers. The T_2 quantification of these species has been usually addressed using mono- and multi-exponential models on data acquired at different echo times, leading to T_2 estimations ranging from about 150 μs in mice (Figure 8.18) to 300 μs in humans, with shortened values in the white matter of patients with multiple sclerosis ($T_2 \approx 216$ μs) (Sheth et al. 2016).

The T_1 quantification of species with ultrashort T_2 is less frequently investigated due to technical difficulties (e.g. the suppression of the component with long T_2 has to be ensured) and acquisition time, with first estimations in the white matter of a human brain yielding values of approximately 350 ms (Du et al. 2014).

A promising metric for the characterization of myelinated tissues that combines the estimations of T_1 and T_2 consists of estimating the density of macromolecular protons. The general equation of the ultrashort-T_2 signal in a voxel is expressed as:

$$S = \rho \times RG \times M_z e^{-TE/T_2} \qquad [8.5]$$

where M_z and ρ are, respectively, the longitudinal magnetization (depending on T_1 and sequence parameters) and the proton density of the species of interest, and RG is a factor related to the gain and sensitivity of the reception system of the scanner. Then, from an external reference (ref) with known ρ, T_2, and T_1, the density of macromolecular protons (ρ_m) can be quantified from the ratio of the equations of the respective signals as:

$$\rho_m - \rho_{ref} \frac{S_m M_{z,ref} e^{-TE/T2,ref}}{S_{ref} M_{z,m} e^{-TE/T2,m}} \qquad [8.6]$$

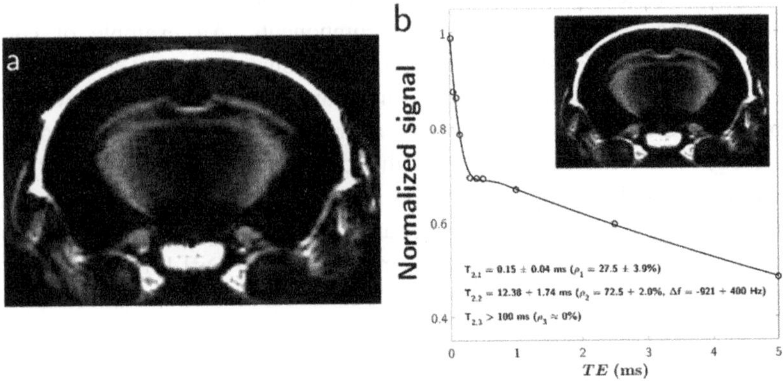

Figure 8.18. *Image of a healthy mouse brain using an IR-UTE 2D sequence (a) and example of T_2 quantification in the corpus callosum using a multi-exponential model (b). For a color version of this figure, see www.iste.co.uk/ratiney-beuf/challenges.zip*

Preliminary estimations of proton densities for the ultrashort-T_2 component are of about 8 mol/L in the white matter of healthy volunteers, and respectively 7.2 mol/L and 3.8 mol/L in normal white matter and in the lesions of multiple sclerosis patients (Ma et al. 2020).

8.5. Conclusion

Conventional MRI commonly used in clinical practice mainly focuses on the measurement of water protons, whose NMR signal decays sufficiently slowly to be easily detected (relatively long T_2). In parallel, advanced MRI techniques have emerged in recent years for directly (UTE) or indirectly imaging ((inhomogeneous) MT) tissues associated with ultrashort T_2 values resulting from strong RDCs in the semi-solid macromolecular matrix. These two research fields are very active today and, although several challenges remain unsolved, some applications, in particular myelin imaging, are possible nowadays in clinical practice. Today, MRI is a very versatile technique thanks to its sensitivity to multiple contrast phenomena allowing for proven clinical usage for several pathologies. In the future, more specific approaches could enable more accurate information to be extracted from the measurements and thus more precise tissue characterization, somewhat similar to a quantitative histology technique that could be applicable in vivo. Ultrashort echo time imaging and MT imaging are very promising techniques for reaching this goal.

8.6. References

ihMT

Calucci, L. and Forte, C. (2019). Proton longitudinal relaxation coupling in dynamically heterogeneous soft systems. *Prog. Nucl. Magn. Reson. Spectrosc.*, 55, 296–323.

Carvalho, V.N.D., Hertanu, A., Grélard, A., Mchinda, S., Soustelle, L., Loquet, A., Dufourc, E.J., Varma, G., Alsop, D.C., Thureau, P. et al. (2020). MRI assessment of multiple dipolar relaxation time (T_{1D}) components in biological tissues interpreted with a generalized inhomogeneous magnetization transfer (ihMT) model. *J. Magn. Reson.*, 311, 106668.

Chen, J.H., Sambol, E.B., Decarolis, P., O'Connor, R., Geha, R.C., Wu, Y.V., Singer, S. (2006). High-resolution MAS NMR spectroscopy detection of the spin magnetization exchange by cross-relaxation and chemical exchange in intact cell lines and human tissue specimens. *Magn. Reson. Med.*, 55, 1246–1256.

Duhamel, G., Prevost, V.H., Cayre, M., Hertanu, A., Mchinda, S., Carvalho, V.N.D., Varma, G., Durbec, P., Alsop, D.C., Girard, O.M. (2019). Validating the sensitivity of inhomogeneous magnetization transfer (ihMT) MRI to myelin with fluorescence microscopy. *NeuroImage*, 199, 289–303.

Girard, O.M., Prevost, V.H., Varma, G., Cozzone, P.J., Alsop, D.C., Duhamel, G. (2015). Magnetization transfer from inhomogeneously broadened lines (ihMT): Experimental optimization of saturation parameters for human brain imaging at 1.5 Tesla. *Magn. Reson. Med.*, 73, 2111–2121.

Goldman, M. (1970). *Spin Temperature and Nuclear Magnetic Resonance in Solids*. Oxford University Press, Oxford.

Henkelman, R.M., Huang, X., Xiang, Q.S, Stanisz, G.J., Swanson, S.D., Bronskill, M.J. (1993). Quantitative interpretation of magnetization transfer. *Magn. Reson. Med.*, 29, 759–766.

Levitt, M.H. (2008). *Spin Dynamics: Basics of Nuclear Magnetic Resonance*. Wiley, New York.

Malyarenko, D.I., Zimmermann, E.M., Adler, J., Swanson, S.D. (2014). Magnetization transfer in lamellar liquid crystals. *Magn. Reson. Med.*, 72, 1427–1434.

Manning, A.P., Chang, K.L., MacKay, A.L., Michal, C.A. (2016). The physical mechanism of "inhomogeneous" magnetization transfer MRI. *J. Magn. Reson.*, 274, 125–136.

Mchinda, S., Varma, G., Prevost, V.H., Le Troter, A., Rapacchi, S., Guye, M., Pelletier, J., Ranjeva, J.-P., Alsop, D.C., Duhamel, G., Girard, O.M. (2017). Whole brain inhomogeneous magnetization transfer (ihMT) imaging: Sensitivity enhancement within a steady state gradient echo sequence. *Magn. Reson. Med.*, 79, 2607–2619.

Morell, P. (2013). *Myelin*. Springer, Berlin.

Morrison, C. and Mark Henkelman, R. (1995). A model for magnetization transfer in tissues. *Magn. Reson. Med.*, 33, 475–482.

Munsch, F., Varma, G., Taso, M., Girard, O., Guidon, A., Duhamel, G., Alsop, D.C. (2021). Characterization of the cortical myeloarchitecture with inhomogeneous magnetization transfer imaging (ihMT). *NeuroImage*, 225, 117442.

Prevost, V.H., Girard, O.M., Varma, G., Alsop, D.C., Duhamel, G. (2016). Minimizing the effects of magnetization transfer asymmetry on inhomogeneous magnetization transfer (ihMT) at ultra-high magnetic field (11.75 T). *Magn. Reson. Mater. Phys. Biol. Med.*, 29, 699–709.

Prevost, V.H., Girard, O.M., Mchinda, S., Varma, G., Alsop, D.C., Duhamel, G. (2017). Optimization of inhomogeneous magnetization transfer (ihMT) MRI contrast for preclinical studies using dipolar relaxation time (T_{1D}) filtering. *NMR Biomed.*, 30(6), e3706.

Provotorov, B. (1962). Magnetic resonance saturation in crystals. *Zh. Eksp. Teor. Fiz.*, 14, 1126–1131.

Rasoanandrianina, H., Grapperon, A.M., Taso, M., Girard, O.M., Duhamel, G., Guye, M., Ranjeva, J.-P., Attarian, S., Verschueren, A., Callot, V. (2017). Region-specific impairment of the cervical spinal cord (SC) in amyotrophic lateral sclerosis: A preliminary study using SC templates and quantitative MRI (diffusion tensor imaging/inhomogeneous magnetization transfer). *NMR Biomed.*, 30(12), e3801.

Rasoanandrianina, H., Demortière, S., Trabelsi, A., Ranjeva, J.-P., Girard, O., Duhamel, G., Guye, M., Pelletier, J., Audoin, B., Callot, V. (2020). Sensitivity of the inhomogeneous magnetization transfer imaging technique to spinal cord damage in multiple sclerosis. *Am. J. Neuroradiol.*, 41, 929–937.

Slichter, C.P. (1990). *Principles of Magnetic Resonance*. Springer, Berlin.

Taso, M., Girard, O.M., Duhamel, G., Le Troter, A., Feiweier, T., Guye, M., Ranjeva, J.-P., Callot, V. (2016). Tract-specific and age-related variations of the spinal cord microstructure: A multi-parametric MRI study using diffusion tensor imaging (DTI) and inhomogeneous magnetization transfer (ihMT): Spinal cord microstructure assessment using DTI and ihMT. *NMR Biomed.*, 29(6), 817–832.

Van Obberghen, E., Mchinda, S., Le Troter, A., Prevost, V.H., Viout, P., Guye, M., Varma, G., Alsop, D.C., Ranjeva, J.-P., Pelletier, J. et al. (2018). Evaluation of the sensitivity of inhomogeneous magnetization transfer (ihMT) MRI for multiple sclerosis. *AJNR Am. J. Neuroradiol.*, 39, 634–641.

Van Zijl, P.C.M., Zhou, J., Mori, N., Payen, J.F., Wilson, D., Mori, S. (2003). Mechanism of magnetization transfer during on-resonance water saturation. A new approach to detect mobile proteins, peptides, and lipids. *Magn. Reson. Med.*, 49, 440–449.

Varma, G., Duhamel, G., de Bazelaire, C., Alsop, D.C. (2015a). Magnetization transfer from inhomogeneously broadened lines: A potential marker for myelin. *Magn. Reson. Med.*, 73, 614–622.

Varma, G., Girard, O.M., Prevost, V.H., Grant, A.K., Duhamel, G.D., Alsop, D.C. (2015b). Interpretation of magnetization transfer from inhomogeneously broadened lines (ihMT) in tissues as a dipolar order effect within motion restricted molecules. *J. Magn. Reson.*, 260, 67–76.

Varma, G., Girard, O.M., Prevost, V.H., Grant, A.K., Duhamel, G.D., Alsop, D.C. (2017). In vivo measurement of a new source of contrast, the dipolar relaxation time, T_{1D}, using a modified inhomogeneous magnetization transfer (ihMT) sequence. *Magn. Reson. Med.*, 78, 1362–1372.

Varma, G., Girard, O.M., Mchinda, S., Prevost, V.H., Grant, A.K., Duhamel, G.D., Alsop, D.C. (2018). Low duty-cycle pulsed irradiation reduces magnetization transfer and increases the inhomogeneous magnetization transfer effect. *J. Magn. Reson.*, 296, 60–71.

Varma, G., Munsch, F., Burns, B., Duhamel, G., Girard, O.M., Guidon, A., Lebel, R.M., Alsop, D.C. (2020). Three-dimensional inhomogeneous magnetization transfer with rapid gradient-echo (3D ihMTRAGE) imaging. *Magn. Reson. Med.*, 84(6), 2964–2980.

UTE

Boada, F.E., Gillen, J.S., Shen, G.X., Chang, S.Y., Thulborn, K.R. (1997). Fast three dimensional sodium imaging. *Magn. Reson. Med.*, 37, 706–715.

Brunner, D.O., Furrer, L., Weiger, M., Baumberger, W., Schmid, T., Reber, J., Dietrich, B.E., Wilm, B.J., Froidevaux, R., Pruessmann, K.P. (2016). Symmetrically biased T/R switches for NMR and MRI with microsecond dead time. *J. Magn. Reson.*, 263, 147–155.

Cha, M.J., Park, H.J., Paek, M.Y., Stemmer, A., Lee, E.S., Park, S.B., Kim, Y.S. (2018). Free-breathing ultrashort echo time lung magnetic resonance imaging using stack-of-spirals acquisition: A feasibility study in oncology patients. *Magn. Reson. Imaging*, 51, 137–143.

Dreher, W., Bardenhagen, I., Huang, L., Bäumer, M. (2015). On the suppression of background signals originating from NMR hardware components. Application to zero echo time imaging and relaxation time analysis. *Magn. Reson. Imaging*, 34, 264–270.

Du, J., Ma, G., Li, S., Carl, M., Szeverenyi, N.M., VandenBerg, S., Corey-Bloom, J., Bydder, G.M. (2014). Ultrashort echo time (UTE) magnetic resonance imaging of the short T_2 components in white matter of the brain using a clinical 3T scanner. *NeuroImage*, 87, 32–41.

Froidevaux, R., Weiger, M., Brunner, D.O., Dietrich, B.E., Wilm, B.J., Pruessmann, K.P. (2017). Filling the dead-time gap in zero echo time MRI: Principles compared. *Magn. Reson. Med.*, 28, 1–135.

Froidevaux, R., Weiger, M., Rösler, M.B., Brunner, D.O., Pruessmann, K.P. (2021). HYFI: Hybrid filling of the dead-time gap for faster zero echo time imaging. *NMR Biomed.*, 34(6), 1–14.

Grodzki, D.M., Jakob, P.M., Heismann, B. (2012). Ultrashort echo time imaging using pointwise encoding time reduction with radial acquisition (PETRA). *Magn. Reson. Med.*, 67, 510–518.

Gurney, P.T., Hargreaves, B.A., Nishimura, D.G. (2006). Design and analysis of a practical 3D cones trajectory. *Magn. Reson. Med.*, 55, 575–582.

Horch, R.A., Gore, J.C., Does, M.D. (2011). Origins of the ultrashort-T_2 ^{1}H NMR signals in myelinated nerve: A direct measure of myelin content? *Magn. Reson. Med.*, 66, 24–31.

Jackson, J.I., Meyer, C.H., Nishimura, D.G., Macovski, A. (1991). Selection of a convolution function for Fourier inversion using gridding (computerised tomography application). *IEEE Trans. Med. Imaging*, 10, 473–478.

Jang, H., Ma, Y.J., Chang, E.Y., Fazeli, S., Lee, R.R., Lombardi, A.F., Bydder, G.M., Corey-Bloom, J., Du, J. (2021). Inversion recovery ultrashort TE MR imaging of myelin is significantly correlated with disability in patients with multiple sclerosis. *Am. J. Neuroradiol.*, 42(5), 868–874.

Johnson, K.M. (2017). Hybrid radial-cones trajectory for accelerated MRI. *Magn. Reson. Med.*, 77, 1068–1081.

Knaap, M.S. and van der Valk, J. (2005). *Magnetic Resonance of Myelination and Myelin Disorders*. Springer, Berlin.

Li, C., Magland, J.F., Zhao, X., Seifert, A.C., Wehrli, F.W. (2017). Selective in vivo bone imaging with long-T_2 suppressed PETRA MRI. *Magn. Reson. Med.*, 77, 989–997.

Ma, Y., Jang, H., Wei, Z., Cai, Z., Xue, Y., Lee, R.R., Chang, E.Y., Bydder, G.M., Corey-Bloom, J., Du, J. (2020a). Myelin imaging in human brain using a short repetition time adiabatic inversion recovery prepared ultrashort echo time (STAIR-UTE) MRI sequence in multiple sclerosis. *Radiology*, 200425, 297(2), 392–404.

Ma, Y., Searleman, A.C., Jang, H., Fan, S.-J., Wong, J., Xue, Y., Cai, Z., Chang, E.Y., Corey-Bloom, J., Du, J. (2020b). Volumetric imaging of myelin in vivo using 3D inversion recovery-prepared ultrashort echo time cones magnetic resonance imaging. *NMR Biomed.*, 33(10), 1–12.

Madio, D.P. and Lowe, I.J. (1995). Ultra-fast imaging using low flip angles and fids. *Magn. Reson. Med.*, 34, 525–529.

Rahmer, J., Börnert, P., Groen, J., Bos, C. (2006). Three-dimensional radial ultrashort echo-time imaging with T_2 adapted sampling. *Magn. Reson. Med.*, 55, 1075–1082.

Riemer, F., Solanky, B.S., Stehning, C., Clemence, M., Wheeler-Kingshott, C.A.M., Golay, X. (2014). Sodium (23Na) ultra-short echo time imaging in the human brain using a 3D-cones trajectory. *Magn. Reson. Mater. Phys. Biol. Med.*, 27, 35–46.

Sheth, V., Shao, H., Chen, J., VandenBerg, S., Corey-Bloom, J., Bydder, G.M., Du, J. (2016). Magnetic resonance imaging of myelin using ultrashort echo time (UTE) pulse sequence: Phantom, specimen, volunteer and multiple sclerosis patient studies. *NeuroImage*, 136, 37–44.

Soustelle, L., Lamy, J., Rousswater, F., Armspach, J.P., Loureiro de Sousa, P. (2018). Diffusion-based method for long-T_2 suppression in steady state sequence: Validation and application for 3D-UTE imaging. *Magn. Reson. Med.*, 80, 548–559.

Soustelle, L., Antal, M.C., Lamy, J., Rousswater, F., Armspach, J.P., Loureiro de Sousa, P. (2019). Correlations of quantitative MRI metrics with myelin basic protein (MBP) staining in a murine model of demyelination. *NMR Biomed.*, 32, e4116.

Weiger, M. and Pruessmann, K.P. (eds) (2012). MRI with zero echo time. In *Encyclopedia of Magnetic Resonance 1*. John Wiley & Sons, Ltd, New York.

Weiger, M., Pruessmann, K.P., Hennel, F. (2011). MRI with zero echo time: Hard versus sweep pulse excitation. *Magn. Reson. Med.*, 66, 379–389.

Wilhelm, M.J., Ong, H.H., Wehrli, S.L., Li, C., Tsai, P.-H., Hackney, D.B., Wehrli, F.W. (2012). Direct magnetic resonance detection of myelin and prospects for quantitative imaging of myelin density. *Proc. Natl. Acad. Sci.*, 109, 9605–9610.

Wu, Y., Ackerman, J.L., Chesler, D.A., Graham, L., Wang, Y., Glimcher, M.J. (2003). Density of organic matrix of native mineralized bone measured by water- and fat-suppressed proton projection MRI. *Magn. Reson. Med.*, 50, 59–68.

9

In Vivo MR Spectroscopy and Metabolic Imaging

Julien FLAMENT[1], Hélène RATINEY[2] and Fawzi BOUMEZBEUR[3]

[1] *MIRCen, CEA, Fontenay-aux-Roses, France*

[2] *CREATIS, CNRS, Inserm, INSA Lyon, Université Claude Bernard Lyon 1, France*

[3] *NeuroSpin, CEA, Gif-sur-Yvette, France*

9.1. Introduction

NMR spectroscopy (MRS) is a technique used to study the magnetic properties of nuclei with non-zero spin; it was invented concomitantly soon after the second world war by Purcell (1946), Bloch (1946) (Nobel Prize in Physics 1952) and their collaborators based on the work of Rabi (1938) (Nobel Prize in Physics 1944). Very quickly, MRS developed into a method for chemical structure analysis, in particular thanks to the discovery of chemical shift effects in 1950 by Proctor and Yu (1950) and by Dickinson (1950). In the following decades, other important discoveries and inventions have been made for the development of MRS such as pulsed NMR by Ernst (1991 Nobel prize in chemistry) in Zurich (Ernst and Anderson 1966) and Waugh in Boston at MIT (Waugh 1968).

Although MRS is a spectroscopy technique with relatively low sensitivity (compared to other chemical analysis methods exploiting higher energies), it has been rapidly adopted for non-invasive investigations of biological samples, from vegetal ones (Shaw and Elsken 1950) to prepared tissue samples (Odebald and Lindstrom 1954), or cells (Odebald 1956), and gradually for studying intact excised

For a color version of all the figures in this chapter, see www.iste.co.uk/ratiney-beuf/challenges.zip.

The Challenges of MRI,
coordinated by Hélène RATINEY and Olivier BEUF. © ISTE Ltd 2024.

organs (Moon and Richards 1973; Hoult 1974). However, it was not until the invention of MRI by Mansfield and Lauterbur (Nobel Prize in Medicine 2004) that in vivo MRS in intact and functional organs or animals could be performed (Ackerman 1980).

Contrary to MRI, NMR spectroscopy is not (yet) commonly used in clinical routine, partly due to its limited spatial resolution. Nevertheless, it is recognized as a valuable tool for clinical research, in particular for the study of the central nervous system. Indeed, in vivo MRS enables the non-invasive characterization of metabolic changes occurring in many neurological and psychiatric pathologies as well as when monitoring their evolution.

This chapter is dedicated to the presentation of the basics of in vivo NMR spectroscopy and metabolic imaging, in particular via chemical exchange saturation transfer (CEST) and non-proton (X) nuclei MRI, with an overview of specific acquisition and analysis methods.

9.2. In vivo MR spectroscopy

Like MRI, NMR spectroscopy is based on the nuclear magnetic resonance phenomenon. Within a strong magnetic field $\boldsymbol{B_0}$, nuclei with a non-zero spin possess quantized magnetic moments precessing around $\boldsymbol{B_0}$ associated with discrete energy levels. From a macroscopic point of view, a magnetization $\boldsymbol{M_0}$ is observed and can be manipulated by means of radiofrequency (RF) waves applied at the Larmor frequency ($\nu_0 = \gamma B_0/2\pi$). The macroscopic magnetization $\boldsymbol{M_0}$ is calculated from the sum across the sample of all those individual nuclear magnetic moments via the application of Boltzmann's statistics (see section 1.2.1), where T is the temperature and N is the number of spins:

$$M_0 \approx {(\gamma\hbar)^2 N B_0}/{4k_B T}, \text{ for a spin } 1/2 \text{ and for } k_B T \ll h\nu_0 \quad [9.1]$$

As a result, the macroscopic magnetization $\boldsymbol{M_0}$ increases with the intensity of the magnetic field $\boldsymbol{B_0}$ and the number N of spins in the sample and decreases with the temperature (expressed in K). It should be noted that this magnetization and the Larmor frequency depend on the value of the gyromagnetic ratio γ of the considered nucleus (see Table 9.1). Hence, great differences in sensitivity exist between nuclei. The hydrogen nucleus (^1H) or "proton" presents the most favorable sensitivity thanks to its high gyromagnetic ratio and its ubiquity in biochemistry, in particular as water (^1H_2O) in tissues.

	Spin	Gyromagnetic ratio (10^7rad.T^{-1}.s^{-1})	Frequency @ 11.7T (MHz)	Natural abundance (%)	Relative sensitivity	$[\ ]_{in\ vivo}$ (mol/L)
^{1}H	1/2	26.752	498.19	99.98	1.00	80
^{3}He	1/2	-20.380	379.43	1.4 10^{-4}	5.75 10^{-7}	–
^{7}Li	3/2	10.398	193.63	92.58	0.272	~ 10^{-3}
^{13}C	1/2	6.728	125.19	1.11	1.76 10^{-4}	1-20 10^{-3}
^{15}N	1/2	-2.712	50.54	0.37	3.86 10^{-6}	1-20 10^{-3}
^{17}O	5/2	-3.628	67.51	0.04	1.08 10^{-5}	40
^{19}F	1/2	25.181	468.59	100.00	0.834	–
^{23}Na	3/2	7.080	131.74	100.00	9.27 10^{-2}	IC~ 14.10^{-3} EC~ 145.10^{-3}
^{31}P	1/2	10.841	201.71	100.00	6.65 10^{-2}	1-20 10^{-3}
^{35}Cl	3/2	2.626	29.26	75.76	3.58 10^{-3}	IC~ 4.10^{-3} EC~ 100.10^{-3}
^{39}K	3/2	1.250	23.28	93.26	4.75 10^{-4}	EC~ 145.10^{-3} IC~ 4.10^{-3}
^{129}Xe	1/2	-7.452	83.02	26.44	5.71 10^{-3}	–

Table 9.1. *NMR properties of most nuclei-of-interest in biomedical research. IC: intracellular concentration; EC: extracellular concentration*

9.2.1. *Free induction decay signal*

In the most simple NMR experiment, a *radiofrequency pulse* $\boldsymbol{B_1(t)}$ is applied, ideally at the sole Larmor frequency, to excite the spins and tip entirely or partially the macroscopic magnetization $\boldsymbol{M_0}$ into the transverse plane. In practice, the radiofrequency pulse $\boldsymbol{B_1(t)}$ has a finite selectivity in frequency, as defined by its Fourier transform.

The transverse component $\boldsymbol{M_T}$ of the magnetization induces an electromotive force within the receiver coil (see section 2.4). A time-domain signal $S(t)$, called free induction decay (FID), can be recorded, and its frequency-domain representation $\hat{S}(\nu)$, called the NMR spectrum, is obtained after a Fourier transform (Ernst and Anderson 1966):

$$S(t) \propto M_x(t) + iM_y(t) = M_T(0)\, e^{-(i2\pi(\nu_0-\nu)+1/T_2^*)t}, \text{ for a single resonance}$$

$$\hat{S}(\nu) = \int_{-\infty}^{+\infty} S(t)\, e^{-i2\pi\nu t} dt \ = R(\nu) + i\, I(\nu) \qquad [9.2]$$

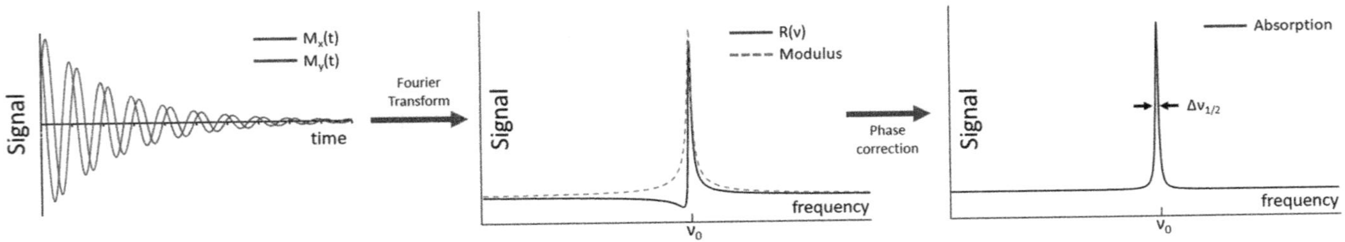

Figure 9.1. *Free induction decay (FID) signal and its spectral representation before and after phase correction*

Typically, a phase-correcting term $\varphi_c = \varphi_0 + 2\pi(\nu_0 - \nu)\varphi_1$ has to be applied with φ_0 and φ_1, denoted as the "zero-" and "first-" order phases, respectively (see section 9.3.1.1), to visualize the absorption spectrum $A(\nu)$:

$$A(\nu) = \frac{M_T(0)\, T_2^* \, e^{-(1/T_2^*)}}{1+\left[2\pi(\nu_0-\nu)T_2^*\right]^2} = R(\nu)\cos\varphi_c + I(\nu)\sin\varphi_c \qquad [9.3]$$

As illustrated in Figure 9.1, for a single resonance, the absorption spectrum corresponds to a Lorentzian distribution centered at the Larmor frequency and with a full width at half maximum (FWHM) $\Delta\nu_{1/2}$ equal to $1/\pi T_2^*$. Otherwise, the modulus $|\hat{S}(\nu)| = \sqrt{R(\nu)^2 + I(\nu)^2}$ can be considered.

9.2.2. Chemical shift and dipolar coupling

If MRS could distinguish only different nuclei, that is, ^1H and ^{13}C, its utility would be very limited. Luckily, the chemical shift phenomenon allows MRS to differentiate between nuclei of the same element depending on their electronic environment.

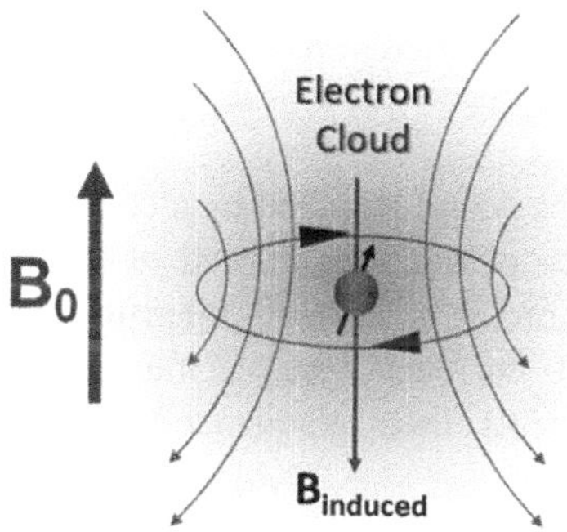

Figure 9.2. *In presence of an external magnetic field B_0, electrons generate an opposing magnetic field around the nucleus leading to a local field $B_{local} = B_0 - B_{induced}$*

9.2.2.1. *Electron shielding and shielding constant*

Every nucleus is affected not only by the static magnetic field $\boldsymbol{B_0}$ but also by an opposing magnetic field $\boldsymbol{B_{induced}}$ (Figure 9.2) induced by the motion of electrons, proportional to $\boldsymbol{B_0}$. Therefore, the nucleus perceives a local field $B_{local} = B_0 - B_{induced} = (1 - \sigma)B_0$ and precesses at a specific frequency $\nu_0 = \frac{\gamma}{2\pi}(1 - \sigma)B_0$.

Although σ is a tensor of the second order, only its trace can be observed if the molecule is in a liquid phase solution. This shielding constant is independent of $\boldsymbol{B_0}$ and is expressed in ppm (parts per million). Experimentally, the chemical shift δ is defined as $\delta = \sigma_{ref} - \sigma$, with σ_{ref} the shielding constant of a reference compound such as tetramethylsilane (TMS). Thus, δ of water is equal to 4.786 ppm at T = 37°C for in vivo ^{1}H MRS.

For a given molecule, one can observe as many different resonance frequencies as there are non-identical electronic environments. Although it does not depend on the intensity of the magnetic field, the electronic environment can vary depending on the employed solvent, its pH and temperature. The range of chemical shifts depends of course on the considered nucleus. For ^{1}H, it extends over less than 10 ppm, while for ^{13}C it covers about 200 ppm.

9.2.2.2. *Spin–spin coupling*

Besides the chemical shift, direct (through space) or indirect (via shared electrons and thus via chemical bonds) dipolar interactions between nuclear spins help distinguish the molecules of interest according to their NMR spectrum. While the first type of interaction has an average value of zero for solutes in liquids, the second type, also called scalar couplings, spin-spin or J-couplings, influences the energy levels associated with the different possible quantum states of the considered spin system.

Thus, for two nuclear spins A and B linked by a covalent bond, one observes, on the one hand, the appearance of doublets instead of single resonances associated with two isolated spins, and, on the other hand, intensity distortions, also referred to as "roof effect" (Figure 9.3). For each possible transition of the spin system AB, table C in Figure 9.3 presents their resonance frequencies and their relative intensities.

The values of the scalar coupling constant J are in the range of 100–200 Hz for ^{1}H-^{13}C, 70–110 Hz for ^{1}H-^{15}N, 30–80 Hz for ^{13}C-^{13}C, and 10–20 Hz for ^{1}H-^{31}P. Coupling constants for n bonds exist as well, indicated as ^{n}J, for example, the two-bond coupling $^{2}J_{HH}$ typically is comprised between –20 and +40 Hz, while $^{2}J_{CH}$ coupling equals approximately half of $^{2}J_{HH}$ for a comparable geometry. For two given nuclei, the values of J are quite stable and mainly vary with the geometry, type and number of bonds.

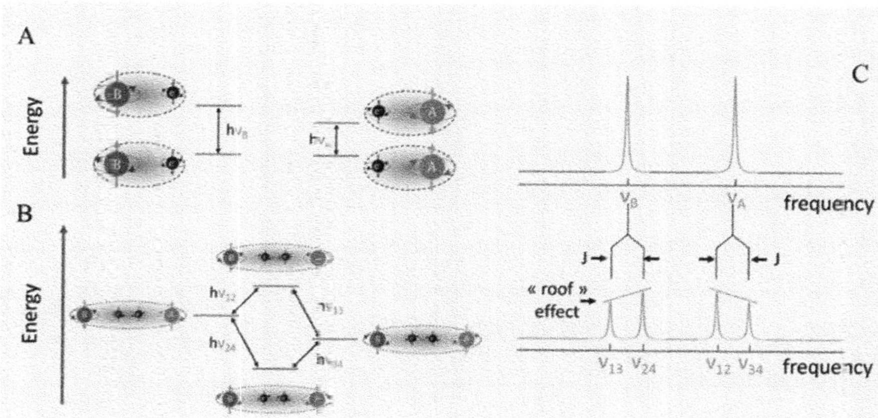

C

Transition $i \leftrightarrow j$	Frequency ν_{ij}	Relative intensity
$1 \leftrightarrow 2$	$(\nu_A + \nu_B)/2 + J/2 - C/2$ $\approx \nu_A + J/2$	$1 + J/C$
$1 \leftrightarrow 3$	$(\nu_A + \nu_B)/2 + J/2 + C/2$ $\approx \nu_B + J/2$	$1 - J/C$
$2 \leftrightarrow 4$	$(\nu_A + \nu_B)/2 - J/2 + C/2$ $\approx \nu_B - J/2$	$1 + J/C$
$3 \leftrightarrow 4$	$(\nu_A + \nu_B)/2 - J/2 - C/2$ $\approx \nu_A - J/2$	$1 - J/C$

Figure 9.3. *Energy diagrams and NMR spectra for (A) two isolated nuclei and (B) a system of two spins A and B linked by a covalent bond. (C) Resonant frequencies ν_{ij} and relative intensities for the AB spins system:* $C = \sqrt{(\nu_A - \nu_B)^2 + J^2} \approx |\nu_A - \nu_B|$ *for* $J \ll |\nu_A - \nu_B|$

Generally, it can be assumed that the *J*-coupling manifests as a splitting of the NMR resonances following rather simple rules:

– equivalent nuclei, that is, those experiencing strictly identical magnetic environments, do not produce distinct resonance lines;

– for an AB_n system with n the number of equivalent nuclei B with a spin *I*, the spectrum of the first order for nucleus A presents $(2nI + 1)$ resonance lines. For $I = 1/2$, the intensities are given by the coefficients of the binomial series $(1 + X)^n$;

– if more than two groups of equivalent nuclei are coupled, successive splittings have to be composed for the considered nuclei group.

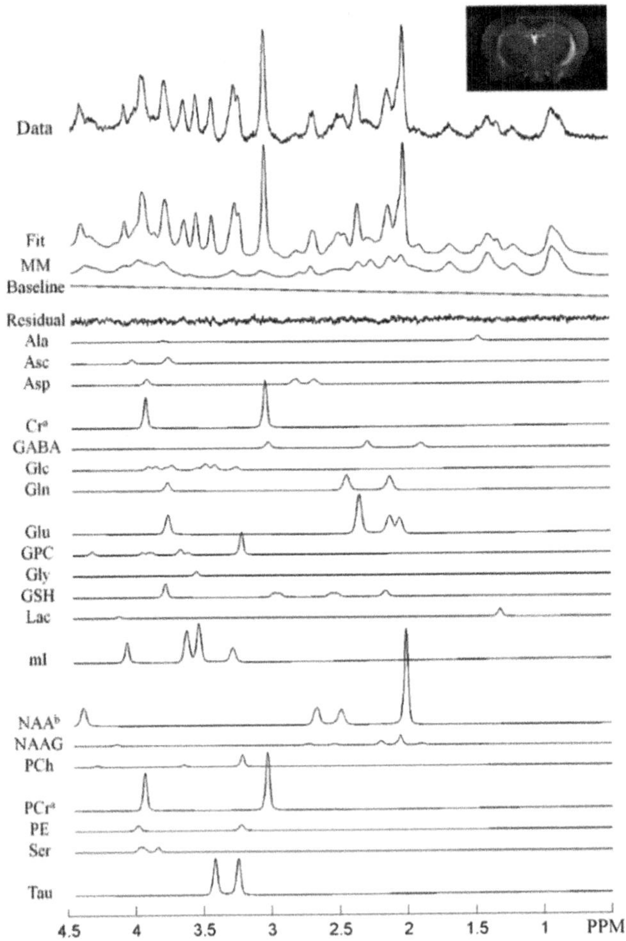

Figure 9.4. *[1]H spectrum acquired in a rat at 17 T and its spectral decomposition*

COMMENT ON FIGURE 9.4. *Abbreviations: macromolecules (MM), alanine (Ala), ascorbate (Asc), aspartate (Asp), creatine (Cr), gamma-aminobutyric acid (GABA), glucose (Glc), glutamine (Gln), glutamate (Glu), glycero-phosphoryl-choline (GPC), glycine (Gly), glutathione (GSH), lactate (Lac), myo-inositol (mI), N-acetyl-aspartate (NAA), N-acetyl-aspartyl-glutamate (NAAG), phosphoryl-choline (PCh), phosphocreatine (PCr), phosphoryl-ethanolamine (PE), serine (Ser) and taurine (Tau) (Lopez-Kolkovsky 2015).*

9.2.3. *Metabolites investigated in MRS*

Metabolites are small (M < 200 Da) and mobile ($10^{-9} < \tau_C < 10^{-8}$ s) molecules participating in the metabolism of our cells and whose concentration is sufficient to be detected ([Met] > 10^{-3} mol/L) in a reasonable time. These metabolites and their concentrations depend on the investigated species and organ. In a human or mouse brain, around 20 metabolites are considered detectable using ^{1}H MRS (Figure 9.4). Among the most prominent are N-acetyl-aspartate, a marker of neural density or vitality; creatine and its phosphorylated form, phosphocreatine, an energy buffer; the choline compounds, intermediaries of membranal metabolism; glutamate and GABA, the main excitatory and inhibitory neurotransmitters, respectively; energetic substrates such as glucose and lactate; osmolytes like myo-inositol and taurine; or antioxidants such as glutathione and ascorbate (vitamin C). MRS identifies these metabolites as markers of abnormal metabolism when unusually absent or concentrated in tissues. This can be particularly useful in oncology (Julià-Sapé 2019), neurology (Rothman 2019), diabetology or myology (Kšŝák 2021).

9.2.4. *Principle of signal localization*

In vivo MRS provides a biochemical analysis of a volume of interest (VOI) or voxel thanks to different methods of 3D localization or spatial encoding of the NMR signal. These methods are based on the same principles of slice selection or phase encoding employed in MRI (see section 1.5.1). Two approaches can be distinguished: *single voxel spectroscopy* (SVS) and *chemical shift imaging* (CSI).

9.2.4.1. *Single voxel spectroscopy*

SVS aims to acquire a global NMR spectrum from the organ or structure under investigation. The most common SVS sequences are OVS (outer volume suppression), ISIS (image selected in vivo spectroscopy) (Ordidge 1986), STEAM (STimulated Echo Acquisition Mode) (Frahm 1987) and PRESS (Point RESolved Spectroscopy) (Bottomley 1987). Figures 9.5 and 9.6 illustrate the chronograms and present the principles of these spatial localization sequences.

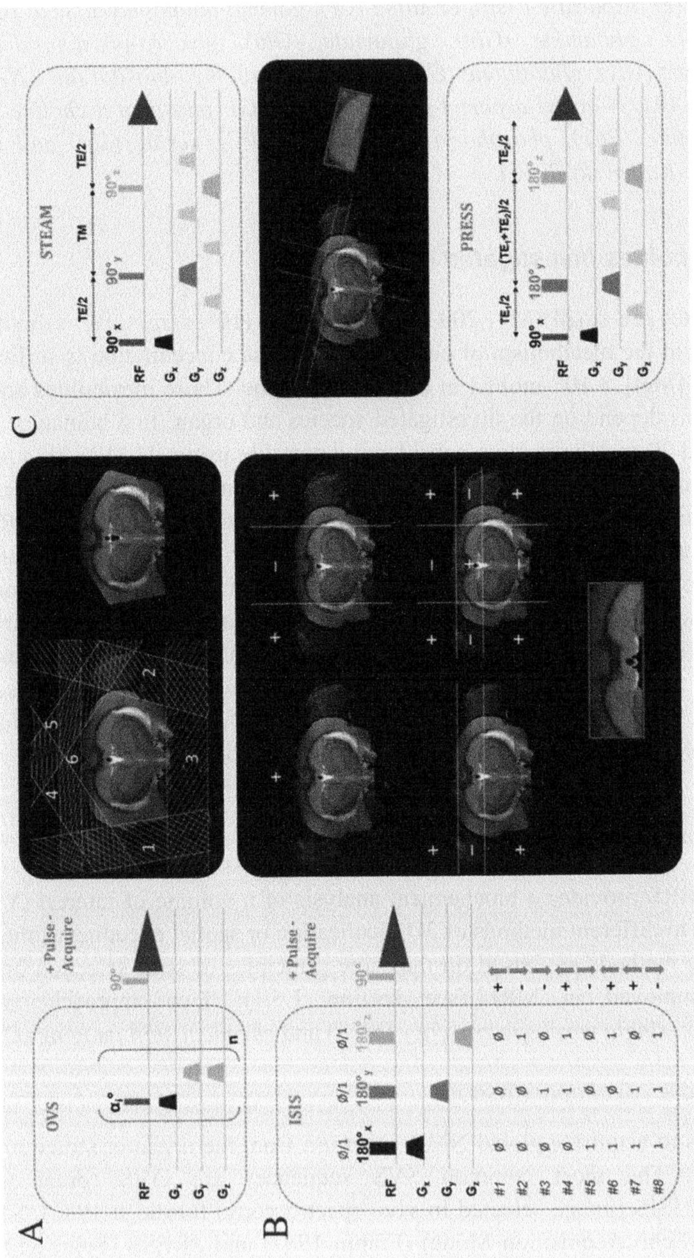

Figure 9.5. *Main MRS signal localization sequences*

COMMENT ON FIGURE 9.5.– *(A) Signal pre-saturation bands are positioned to excite and then dephase the signals outside the voxel. (B) The signal is localized by means of three spatially selective inversion pulses, executed with a pattern of eight scans such that the intra-voxel signal is summed up (while canceling out the signals outside the voxel). (C) The STEAM and PRESS sequences corresponding to the application of three spatially selective pulses define a parallelepiped where an echo (at TE + TM for STEAM) or a double spin echo (at TE = TE_1 + TE_2 for PRESS) is stimulated and can be recorded.*

Other localization sequences have been proposed, such as LASER (Localization by Adiabatic SElective Refocusing) (Garwood and DelaBarre 2001), semi-LASER (Öz and Tkáč 2011) or SPECIAL (SPin-ECho full-Intensity Acquired Localized) (Mlynárik 2006). These sequences employ pairs of adiabatic refocusing pulses to generate spin-echoes despite strong non-uniformities of the $\boldsymbol{B_1}$ field, in particular when employing a surface coil, or at very high magnetic fields (see Chapters 2 and 12). In addition, using adiabatic pulses has the benefit of large bandwidths, which reduce chemical shift artifacts (see section 9.5).

In practice, multiple localization sequences can be combined together. In particular, OVS bands can be placed at the level of moving organs or the scalp (the corresponding RF pulses operating at the resonance frequency of lipids) before STEAM or PRESS sequences to reduce the contamination of the spectra by undesired signals originating from outside of the voxel.

9.2.4.2. *Chemical shift imaging*

NMR spectroscopic imaging or CSI provides a matrix of spectra from a volume of interest by combining a spatial localization sequence with a phase encoding pattern (see section 1.5.1) that preserves spectroscopic information.

As in conventional MRI, a phase encoding scheme is charted across the Fourier or k-space typically along a Cartesian grid with phase-modulated NMR signals $S(k_x, k_y, t)$:

$$S(k_x, k_y, t) = \iiint \rho(x, y, \delta)\, e^{-i(k_x.x + k_y.y + \delta.B_0 t)} dx dy d\delta \qquad [9.4]$$

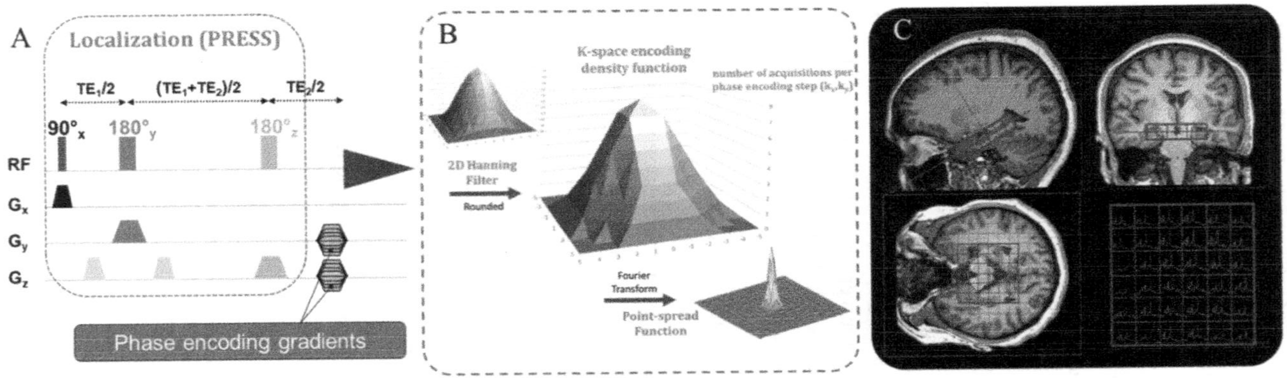

Figure 9.6. *Generic 2D chemical shift imaging (CSI) sequence. By combining a spatial localization sequence (A) with a phase encoding scheme (B), one can acquire and reconstruct a matrix of spectra (C) from which metabolic images can be computed*

Applying a Fourier transform first in space and then in the time domain enables the reconstruction of a matrix of NMR spectra corresponding to each pixel of the spectroscopic image. It should be noted that the actual spatial resolution of the spectroscopic image is estimated via the point spread function (PSF). Due to the modest size of the phase encoding matrix, the PSF can be improved by applying a Hanning-type apodization filter a posteriori, or, preferably, by employing a density-optimized k-space encoding pattern (see Figure 9.6(B)).

9.2.5. *Signal editing, suppression and inversion*

9.2.5.1. *Water signal suppression – metabolic cycling*

In ^{1}H MRS, the water signal is several orders of magnitude larger than the signals from the different metabolites of interest. Therefore, to allow their detection, several techniques exist to suppress the water signal. This is usually achieved by including a presaturation module composed of a train of frequency-selective RF pulses with the role of exciting the water signal and then dephasing it immediately before a SVS or CSI sequence. Typical methods are CHESS, WET or VAPOR (Ogg 1994; Tkáč 1999). Another approach, the so-called metabolite cycling, consists of a selective inversion of the water signal (Giapitzakis 2018). Adding two spectra acquired with and without inversion provides a metabolic profile without the residual water signal – if a perfect inversion is indeed achieved.

9.2.5.2. *Spectral editing*

As illustrated in Figure 9.4, several resonances can overlap (especially at low magnetic fields) and some metabolites such as lactate, GABA, or glutathione are hard to detect and quantify in a rigorous way. For these metabolites, it is recommended to use spectral-editing sequences or J-difference editing (Mescher 1998; Harris 2017). Let us consider an AB spin system with a J-coupling term J_{AB}. Due to this coupling, after a spin-echo, the resonances exhibit a phase $\varphi = \pi J_{AB} TE$. If $TE = 1/J_{AB}$, then $\varphi = \pi$. Spectral editing consists of canceling out this phase for spin B via a selective inversion of the transverse magnetization of spin A at TE/4 and 3TE/4 (Figure 9.7). Since these inversions are neutral for non-coupled spins (except for spins resonating at the frequency of spin A), subtracting two spectra with and without inversion provides a visualization of the resonances of spin B without the interference of the resonances of non-coupled spins.

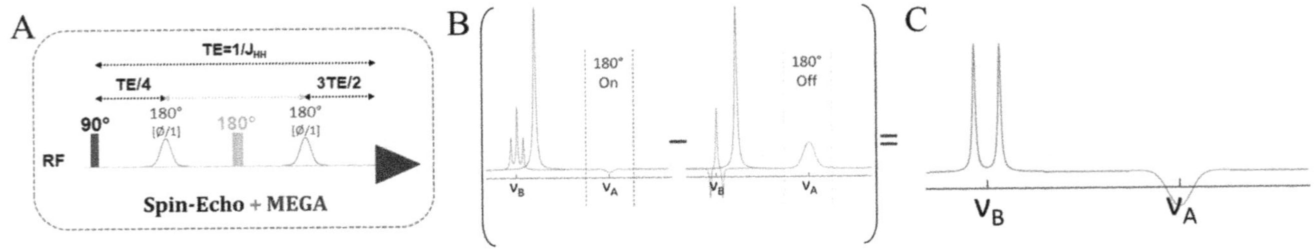

Figure 9.7. *Schematics of the spectral editing method MEGA-SE (A). The two selective inversions of spins A (in orange, at the frequency ν_A) refocuse the phase of spins B (in blue, at the frequency ν_B) due to the J_{AB} coupling. By repeating the measurement without the frequency-selective inversions and subtracting the two spectra (B), the resonance spectra of spins B are better resolved (C) than previously, when they were masked by the signal of non-coupled spins (singlet in gray)*

9.2.6. *Experimental considerations in MRS*

9.2.6.1. B_0 shimming

A critical condition for acquiring high-quality spectra is the generation of a uniform $\boldsymbol{B_0}$ field in the spectroscopic voxel. The homogenization (or shimming) of the $\boldsymbol{B_0}$ field is performed by adjusting the currents in the so-called shim coils that generate magnetic fields following spherical harmonic functions of the first and second order (Gruetter and Tkáč 2000). The shimming efficacy can be verified by measuring the full width at half maximum of the water peak $\Delta\nu_{1/2} = {}^{1}/_{\pi T_2} + \gamma\Delta B_0$. Ideally, $\Delta\nu_{1/2}$ should be of the order of 0.04 ppm, which yields thin and high-intensity spectral lines.

9.2.6.2. *Chemical shift artifact*

The chemical shift displacement error originates from the fact that for two resonances separated by δ, their signals originate from two different planes. This distance between those two planes is proportional to δ/BW_{RF}, with BW_{RF} the bandwidth of the spatially selective pulse. In the case of an MRS sequence with several spatially selective pulses, these co-localization errors accumulate and can hinder the interpretation of the spectrum. It is therefore advisable to apply RF pulses with a large bandwidth and to use an operating frequency at the center of the frequency range or at the frequency of the investigated metabolite (rather than the water frequency).

9.3. Processing and quantification of MRS signals

The main objective of analyses of spectra acquired in vivo (Figure 9.8) is to detect the metabolites in the sample and "quantify" their concentrations.

9.3.1. *Good practices for preprocessing MRS/CSI data*

Before proceeding with the quantification step, it is often useful to "prepare" the signals. Acquired spectroscopy data cannot elude practical imperfections such as eddy currents, frequency drifts or subject motion. Before the quantification step, the preliminary step that will improve the quantification and the quality of the spectra (width at half maximum, signal-to-noise ratio [SNR]) is called the signal preprocessing step. The main preprocessing aspects are described below.

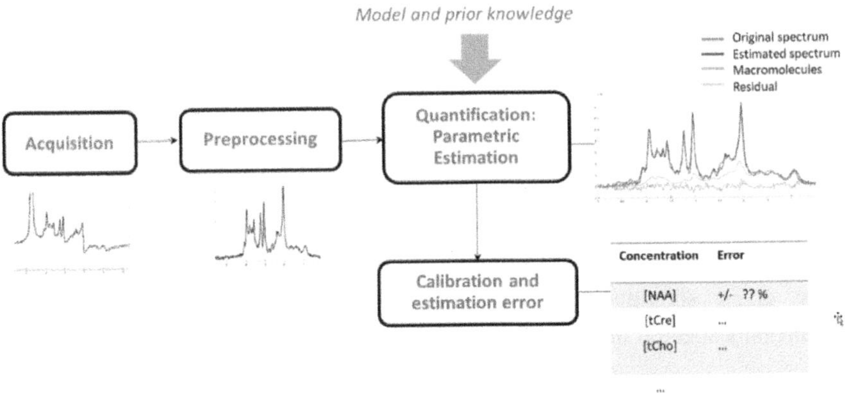

Figure 9.8. *Overview of the steps and concepts for the analysis of in vivo NMR spectroscopy signals leading to the determination of metabolite concentrations*

9.3.1.1. *Correction of zero- and first-order phase*

The complex spectra obtained from the acquisition chain need to be "re-phased" to observe and analyze their real part (see section 9.2.1) that corresponds to the absorption spectrum. Conventionally, a spectrum is said to be phased when the lines (especially for singlets) of its real part are all positive (Figure 9.9(Ai)). For multiplets, some resonances can be negative because of the scalar coupling (Figure 9.7(B)). The phases to be corrected ($-\varphi_c$) have multiple causes: phase difference between transmission and reception, unbalanced delays in the sequence, imperfections in the digitization of the RF pulses, digital-to-analog conversion, differences between RF coil elements and different cable lengths. These result in two phase terms: zero-order and first-order phases that can be corrected either manually or automatically.

9.3.1.2. *Eddy-current correction*

When the signals are acquired, residual eddy currents (see section 1.5.2.1) and non-uniformities of the magnetic field distort the envelope of the NMR signal's decay over time. In the frequency domain, this manifests as an alteration of the lines, which ideally should be Lorentzian (see section 9.2.1 and Figure 9.9(Aii)). The distortions due to eddy currents can be reduced or corrected in a preprocessing step.

Supposing that these distortions are identical for all the resonance lines, it is possible to estimate the deformation of a reference signal, such as the water signal (spectrum without water suppression), and to correct the metabolites signal by applying an opposite phase modulation (De Graaf 1990).

9.3.1.3. *Correction of the frequency drift*

Frequency drifts are often observed during an acquisition: this phenomenon corresponds to a gradual change of the $\boldsymbol{B_0}$ field due to the warm-up of the ferromagnetic components providing passive shimming, or to the temperature variation in the sample. To correct this drift, frequency variations can be determined for all the spectra before averaging, by following a reference peak (water, or a major resonance component such as creatine), or by estimating the frequency shift of the complex signal in the time domain, which is then applied for each signal.

9.3.1.4. *A posteriori suppression of water residual*

When the magnetic field has a good uniformity, water suppression during the acquisition is effective. This is often the case for SVS acquisitions, but it cannot be guaranteed for CSI scans. The most effective and used methods for suppressing the residual water peak in post-acquisition are those based on singular value decomposition (SVD). These methods are based on linear algebra properties, with the most known being those based on the linear prediction method and those employing a state space model with SVD of a Hankel matrix (HSVD, HLSVD) as used in automatic control and identification. The Hankel matrix is obtained by positioning each signal sample in such a way that all the values are constant along ascending diagonals. The sequence of signal samples is described by a simple model in terms of complex amplitudes ($c'_k = c_k exp\, j\phi_k$) and poles ($z_k = exp(-\alpha_k + j2\pi f_k)t_e$) of the signal according to the expression $\hat{y}_n = \sum_{k=1}^{K} c'_k z_k^n, n = 0, \ldots, N-1$. The SVD of the Hankel matrix enables the determination of complex poles and amplitudes of the expression $\hat{\boldsymbol{y}}_n$. This is a purely mathematical description and the signal energy distribution by components does not necessarily represent the distribution by metabolites (Figure 9.4). To suppress the residual water signal, thanks to the mathematical model of the signal in an interval [ν_1; ν_2] centered at the water signal, the corresponding components are subtracted from the spectrum (Figure 9.9(Bi, Bii)).

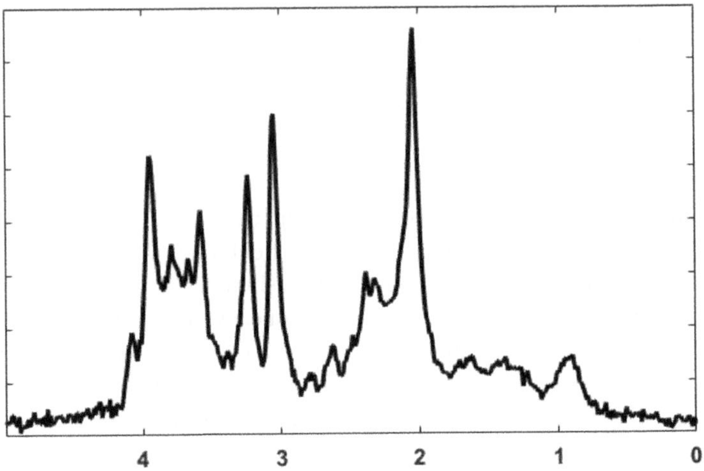

i

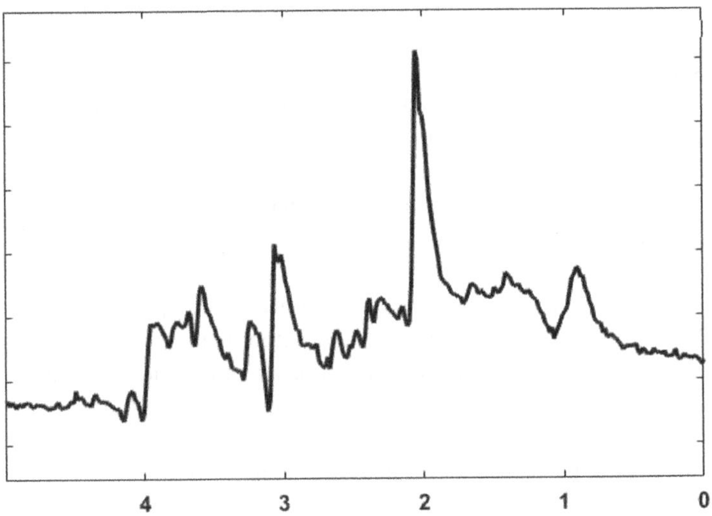

ii

A

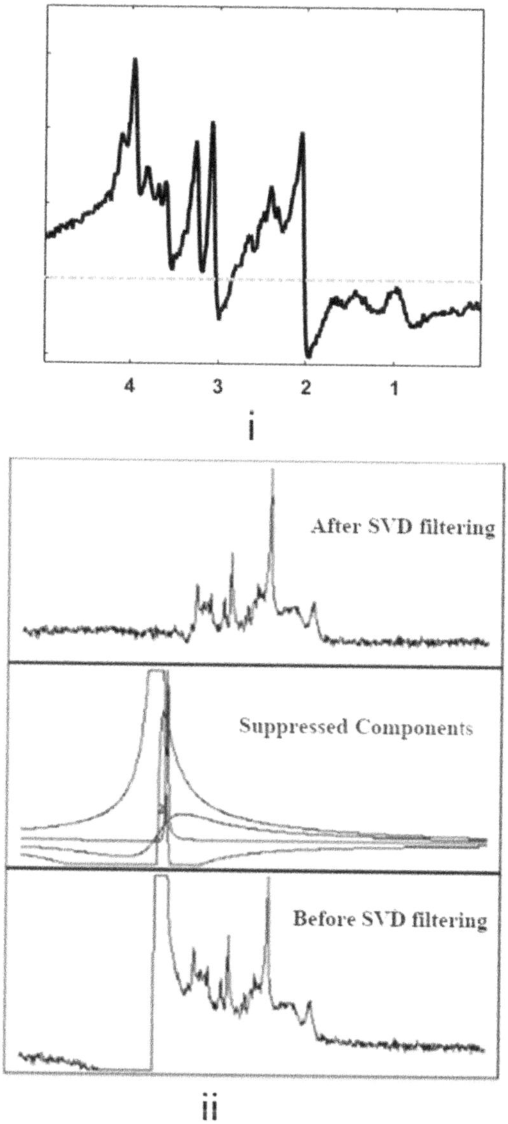

B

Figure 9.9. *(A) Examples of (i) a phased spectrum and (ii) a spectrum affected by eddy currents. (B) (i) Spectrum affected by a zero-order phase; (ii) example of water suppression, after decomposition of the signal via HLSVD: below, a spectrum with water residual; in the middle, the components modeling the water residual via HLSVD; above, spectrum after removing the water components*

9.3.2. *Quantification method*

At zero (or very short) echo time, the area under the curve of the real part of a phased spectrum is proportional to the number of spins contributing to this signal, and therefore, for a given volume element, to the concentration of the corresponding molecule or chemical group. The main quantification operation consists of determining the relative proportions of the spectral components originating from different chemical groups or molecules, which are characterized by their chemical shifts. When the spectra are sufficiently resolved as in high-resolution NMR, the measurement of the area under the curve of the resonance peaks can be done via a simple integral. This approach is increasingly difficult to implement in vivo due to the variable uniformity conditions of the magnetic field that broaden the lines and the spectral overlap that impedes distinguishing neighboring resonances. The acquired signal is usually described by a parametric function and the quantification methods consist of determining these parameters. These methods perform this correction in the time or frequency domains and may or may not require a model function and a priori knowledge from the user. Once a mathematical model (i.e. a model function) is adopted for describing a spectroscopic signal, the implemented quantification algorithms consist of determining the unknown parameters of the model function.

9.3.2.1. *Model function*

Most methods proposed in the literature are based on the minimization of the distance between acquired (or preprocessed) data and a mathematical model to determine the optimal parameters.

Depending on the complexity of the spectrum to be analyzed, different models can be employed:

– a sum of Lorentz-shaped lines: $y_n = \sum_{k=1}^{M_p} a_k e^{j\phi_k} e^{(-d_k + j2\pi f_k)t_n}$;

– a sum of Gaussian-shaped lines: $y_n = \sum_{k=1}^{M_p} a_k e^{j\phi_k} e^{(-g_k t_n + j2\pi f_k)t_n}$;

– a sum of Voigt-shaped lines (Bruce 2000) that approximate the Gaussian broadening of resonant frequencies whose lines are ideally Lorentzian shaped.

The models above are expressed in the time domain, but when an analytical expression is available they can also be written in the frequency domain (e.g. $Y_n = \sum_{k=1}^{M_p} \frac{a_k e^{j\phi_k} d_k}{d_k^2 + 4\pi^2 (f_n - f_k)^2}$, for Lorentzian lines). In each case, the signal is described as a sum of M_p resonances with an amplitude a_k (proportional to the area under the curve in the frequency domain), and characterized by their frequencies ν_k (chemical shift), relative phases ϕ_k and damping factors d_k (Lorentzian case) or g_k (Gaussian case). The latter two are related to the effective transverse relaxation time T_2* and to the non-uniformities of the static field (see section 9.2.6.2). These descriptions are useful whenever the acquired spectrum presents lines that are simple or easy to model, such as in ^{1}H spectroscopy with long echo times (TE = 144 ms), ^{31}P (Figure 9.14), or ^{13}C spectra (Figure 9.15).

In the case of signals acquired at short echo times, the recommended model is a weighted sum of simulated or acquired in vitro metabolite spectra. An example of the model function used in the LCModel method (Provencher 1993), which is the most widely used quantification method in the community, performing the minimization in the frequency domain, is the following:

$$Y_n = e^{i\phi_0+\nu_n\phi_1}\left[\sum_{j=1}^{N_B}\beta_j B_j(\nu_n) + \sum_{l=1}^{N_M} C_l \sum_{k=-N_S}^{N_S} S_k M_l(\nu_{n-k};\ \gamma_l, \epsilon_l)\right] \quad [9.5]$$

B_j corresponds to a B-spline modeling of the baseline, ϕ_0 and ϕ_1 are the adjustable phases of the zero and first order, C_l is the parameter of the metabolites proportion (directly related to the concentration), S_k is the convolution with an arbitrary line shape that has to be determined, γ_l are the frequency shifts, ϵ_l is the line broadening due to shorter T_2 or T_2^*.

In this case, the N_M signals of M_l metabolites are known and considered as a priori knowledge. They can be obtained from in vitro measurements or simulations based on required quantum mechanics (see section 9.3.2.2).

The model functions can be more or less complex. The more parameters have to be estimated, the more probability there is that these parameters are correlated among each other: the optimization algorithm will then have to restrict the parameter search to allowed intervals of values and/or penalize the minimization. Several solutions have been proposed and have been reviewed by the community (https://mrshub.org/).

The minimization of the distance between the function model and the acquired data is most commonly solved using iterative algorithms such as Gauss–Newton or Levenberg–Marquardt, but these methods tend to fall into local minima and a way to avoid this pitfall is to reiterate the optimization process with varying initial parameters. In a more marginal way, Bayesian approaches have been proposed and provide a global optimization of the problem. They are based on Markov chain Monte Carlo (MCMC) methods and the Metropolis–Hasting algorithm.

9.3.2.2. *Generation of the decomposition basis*

The metabolite spectra used as a priori knowledge and the decomposition basis of the NMR spectrum are obtained either experimentally or via numerical simulations. While it can be complicated to acquire experimental spectra (which involves the preparation of dedicated test objects, control of physicochemical parameters, etc.), it is often preferable to calculate the spectra of each metabolite by simulating the corresponding spins system and its evolution during the considered NMR sequence. For this purpose, the formalism of the "density operator" is used by many free simulation programs (e.g. Spinach, (py)GAMMA, SIMPSON).

Without going into the details of the required quantum mechanical considerations, the density operator, or density matrix, is a mathematical object defined by John von Neumann in 1927 that combines all the statistically possible quantum states in a single matrix. This formalism links the statistical approach with the quantum one. It gives access to all the average macroscopic values of a given observable. The time evolution of the density operator is described by Liouville–von Neuman's equation. This equation is equivalent to Schrödinger's equation of wave functions:

$$\hat{\sigma}(t) = \exp(-i\widehat{H}t)\hat{\sigma}(0)\exp(i\widehat{H}t) \quad [9.6]$$

For each event of a sequence, the corresponding Hamiltonians ($\widehat{H}$) have to be determined. Thus, a pulse execution corresponds to a Hamiltonian that describes the interaction between the spin and the radiofrequency field: $\widehat{H}_1 = \omega_1 \hat{I}_q$ where q denotes the phase of the radiofrequency pulse. During the inter-pulse delays, the Hamiltonian of the spin system is active and brings into play the interactions to which the considered spins are subjected. These interactions are as follows: (i) the Zeeman interaction (between the spins system and the static magnetic field), described as the product between the chemical shift and the z-component (if the B_0 field is oriented along z) of the operator of the intrinsic kinetic moment ($\widehat{I_z}$); (ii) the scalar couplings (see section 9.2.2.1); the other interactions (dipolar, quadripolar) important in NMR of solids are neglected here. The dipolar coupling in a solution is considered to be completely canceled out by the averaging due to the isotropic molecular motions and fluctuations. Finally, the signal is "measured" by determining the transverse components of the spins system. All these steps are programmed to predict the evolution of the spins system under the effect of the magnetic fields B_0 and $B_1(t)$. Due to the many matrix operations to be executed for simulating a complex sequence with several radiofrequency pulses and large density matrices corresponding to systems with several spins, intensive numerical computation becomes quickly necessary.

9.3.2.3. *Modelization of the signal from macromolecules*

The NMR spectra of the ^{1}H of the brain measured at short echo times contain signals coming from mobile macromolecules (MM) (Behar 1993). These signals originate from (semi-)mobile protons in proteins, as well as in lipids in cytosolic suspensions, particularly visible in some pathological cases (such as tumors or multiple sclerosis). Since these protons have shorter T_1 and T_2 relaxation times (and a lower apparent diffusion coefficient) than the protons in metabolites with a lower molecular weight, their resonances are wider and their sum leads to a modulation of the baseline, which disappears for long echo times. Thus, during spectral decomposition, it is important to take into account their contributions in order to not bias the quantification of the metabolites (Cudalbu 2021). For this reason, it is recommended to acquire an experimental spectrum of these macromolecules by taking advantage of their difference in T_1 relaxation times, in particular, thanks to (double) inversion-recovery signal preparation blocks (De Graaf 2006) which remove the contribution of the metabolites. Another option is to model the experimental spectrum of the MM. Since the composition, amplitudes and relaxation time of the different macromolecules vary with experimental conditions (species, B_0, *TE*, etc.), it is advisable to measure the spectra of MM (and, eventually, optimize their modeling) specifically for each study.

9.3.2.4. *The case of chemical shift imaging data*

The goal of processing CSI data (see section 9.2.4.3) is to obtain maps of the concentrations of metabolites, also called metabolic images. Most software programs and processing and quantification methods applicable to SVS data can be applied to CSI data, simply by analyzing each spectrum of the matrix independently. However, taking into account anatomic information in the metabolic maps reconstruction process improves the interpretation of the metabolic maps by smoothening these maps within the different structures. These methods, not yet available in clinical routine, are based on optimization strategies that constrain – either via subsequent iterations or via a cost term – the phases, line widths and frequency shifts to be close whenever the voxels belong to a homogeneous region on an anatomical image (Maudsley 2006; Kelm 2012).

9.3.2.5. *Calibration, external versus internal references*

Once the relative amplitudes of each biochemical component contributing to the signal are obtained, the “absolute concentrations”, most often expressed in mmol/L, have to be retrieved. Generally, the concentration [m] of a metabolite **m** can be obtained from the estimated relative amplitude $\boldsymbol{a_m}$ and the amplitude of a reference signal $\boldsymbol{a_{ref}}$ according to the following expression:

$$[m] = \frac{a_m}{a_{ref}}[ref] \times correction(T_1, T_2, NA, \text{nb of equivalent nuclei}) \qquad [9.7]$$

The reference signal corresponds either to (i) an external reference, a sample of a component with a known concentration $[ref]$ located outside the investigated object but still within the volume sensed by the coil, or to (ii) an internal reference, a metabolite whose concentration $[ref]$ is considered to be stable and known in the tissues (e.g. water or creatine + phosphocreatine). The amplitude $\boldsymbol{a_{ref}}$ of this reference component will be obtained with the same acquisition sequence as for $\boldsymbol{a_m}$. The main correction factors are the ones related to the differences in relaxation times between the reference and the metabolite of interest, the number of accumulations NA, and the difference in the number of equivalent nuclei between the reference metabolite and the investigated metabolite. To be precise, other effects should be taken into account such as the nOE (nuclear Overhauser Effect), diffusion weighting, or the effect of the RF pulse. These numerous correction terms show how difficult it is to estimate a truly "absolute" concentration. It is also possible to synthesize an electronic reference signal (ERETIC method) (Heinzer-Schweizer 2010), which is added to the acquired signal whose amplitude and phase are precisely set. Most of all, when exploiting the quantification results, it is useful to ask oneself which main factors or parameters could be affected by the investigated phenomenon or pathology and to try to take them into account for the quantitative analysis as much as possible.

9.3.2.6. *Estimation errors: Cramér–Rao bounds and residuals*

The relative amplitudes obtained at the end of the quantification process are estimations, with which a measurement uncertainty estimation can be associated to determine the reliability of the results. Cramér–Rao's theory determines the lower bound of the variances associated with the estimated parameters – supposing that the estimators are not biased. This bound is independent from the employed quantification method and represents an accuracy standard to which the quantification results can be compared. The calculation of the Cramér–Rao lower bounds (CRLB) requires the computation of Fisher's information matrix, which is defined as the variance associated with the maximum likelihood. If the only stochastic variable in our description is the measurement noise, the partial derivatives of the log-likelihood function are the partial derivatives of the chosen model function $\widehat{\boldsymbol{F}}$ with respect to the parameters p: $I_{i,j} = \sum_{k=0}^{N} \left(\frac{\partial \hat{F}(t_k,p)}{\partial p_i}\right)^* \left(\frac{\partial \hat{F}(t_k,p)}{\partial p_j}\right)$, where $\widehat{\boldsymbol{F}}$ is the model function describing the signal (a discrete function of time, with $t_k = k\Delta te$, Δte being the sampling step) and $\boldsymbol{p}$ is a vector of parameters (typically amplitude, frequency variation, phase variation, damping factor, etc.). This matrix is a measure of the information on the parameters carried by the measured signal. Calculating the Cramér–Rao bounds consists of considering, for each parameter, every diagonal element of the inverse Fisher's matrix. For any unbiased estimator of parameters $\boldsymbol{p}$, its variance is greater than the Cramér–Rao lower bound (Fréchet–Darnois–Cramér–Rao inequality). Studying these bounds is useful for designing an experiment and sampling strategies (Bolliger 2013). The covariance matrix (considering not only the diagonal of the inverse Fisher's matrix but also the cross-terms) helps understand the correlations between parameters (Ratiney 2004). The quantification results are often provided with the related Cramér–Rao bounds (as a percentage of estimated amplitudes). It should be noted that there is no guarantee that the estimator variances reach the lower bound or that the estimators are unbiased (starting hypothesis). Some studies use relative bounds as an exclusion criterion for filtering the results. This approach is dangerous and could bias the estimations of the average metabolite concentrations in a given population when the concentrations are low (Kreis 2016).

To evaluate the quantification quality, inspecting the residual signals (resulting from the difference between the acquired signal/spectrum and the modeled one) enables the detection of systematic errors (under- or over-estimation of metabolites). In fact, in the case of perfect adjustments, the residual signal must contain only noise samples.

9.4. Chemical exchange saturation transfer imaging

In most biological systems, the exchanges between different chemical species play a major role in several reactions and any physicochemical change in the medium can have a significant effect on these exchanges. The effect of chemical exchanges on the NMR spectra has been reported since 1951 (Liddel 1951) and a mathematical framework has been proposed by modifying the Bloch equations to include the evolution of the magnetization whenever two molecules exchange protons (McConnell 1958). Since then, the technique has rapidly developed for investigations of chemical compounds followed by in vivo applications proposed at the end of the 1980s. In the 2000s, the technique was proposed as a new imaging contrast under the term CEST (chemical exchange dependent saturation transfer) (Ward 2000). The CEST approach has then evolved and diversified, with rather varied applications such as the detection of macromolecules (Wolff 1986) or endogenous metabolites (Cai 2012) with high sensitivity, or exogenous contrast agents (e.g. Lipo/ParaCEST agents) (Aime 2005; van Zijl 2011).

9.4.1. *General principle*

The general principle of CEST is based on the observation of the saturation transfer between two or more groups of exchanging protons. Let us consider two groups of such protons, A and B, representing, respectively, protons of free water (solvent, corresponding to the protons observed in conventional MRI), and bound protons of a solute (not directly observable via MRI due to their low concentration or too-short T_2*) (Figure 9.10). An RF pulse is applied at the resonant frequency of B protons, destroying their magnetization. Due to the chemical exchange, a part of the saturation is transferred from the solute to the solvent, leading to a decreased signal of A protons. Indirect observation of B protons is thus made possible via the decrease in the free water signal resulting from the saturation transfer from one proton group to another.

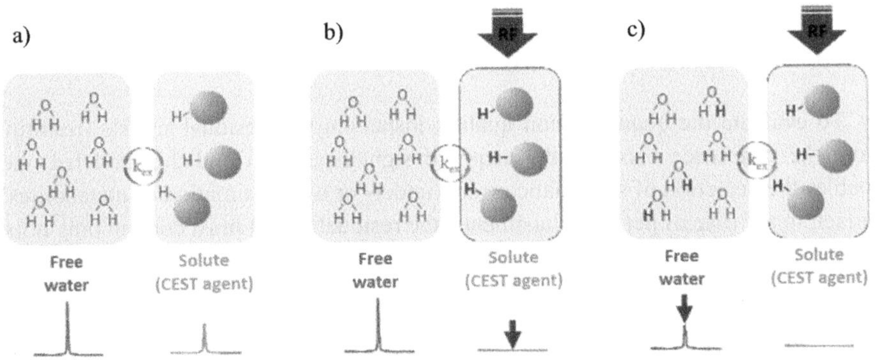

Figure 9.10. *(a) System at the initial state: no saturation has been applied. (b) Saturation applied at the frequency of resonance of the CEST agent's protons. The NMR signal of the solute protons decreases until it reaches zero (red arrow). (c) Transfer of saturated protons (represented in red) to free water results in a decrease in the water's NMR signal (red arrow)*

9.4.2. *Conditions for CEST effect*

To describe the evolution of magnetization in the presence of proton exchange, let us consider again the system with two proton species, A and B. These two pools of protons are characterized by their magnetization (M_{0A} and M_{0B}), longitudinal ($R_{1A} = 1 / T_{1A}$ and $R_{1B} = 1 / T_{1B}$) and transverse ($R_{2A} = 1 / T_{2A}$ and $R_{2B} = 1 / T_{2B}$) relaxation rate as well as by intrinsic resonance frequency (ω_A and ω_B). These populations are in exchange with rates denoted as k_{AB} (from A to B) and k_{BA}

(from B to A). After applying an RF pulse along the Ox-axis, the Bloch–McConnell equations are written as:

$$\frac{dM_{xA}}{dt} = -\Delta\omega_A M_{yA} - (R_{2A} + k_{AB})M_{xA} + k_{BA}M_{xB}$$

$$\frac{dM_{yA}}{dt} = \Delta\omega_A M_{xA} - (R_{2A} + k_{AB})M_{yA} + \omega_1 M_{zA} + k_{BA}M_{yB}$$

$$\frac{dM_{zA}}{dt} = -\omega_1 M_{yA} - R_{1A}(M_{zA} - M_{0A}) - k_{AB}M_{zA} + k_{BA}M_{zB}$$

$$\frac{dM_{xB}}{dt} = k_{AB}M_{xA} - (R_{2B} + k_{BA})M_{xB} - \Delta\omega_B M_{yB}$$

$$\frac{dM_{yB}}{dt} = k_{AB}M_{yA} + \omega_B M_{xB} - (R_{2A} + k_{BA})M_{yB} + \omega_1 M_{zB}$$

$$\frac{dM_{zB}}{dt} = -k_{AB}M_{zA} - \omega_1 M_{yB} - R_{1B}(M_{zB} - M_{0B}) + k_{BA}M_{zB} \quad [9.8]$$

with M_{xA}, M_{yA}, M_{zA} and M_{xB}, M_{yB}, M_{zB}, the magnetizations in the rotating frame; M_{0A} and M_{0B}, the equilibrium magnetizations; $\Delta\omega_A$ and $\Delta\omega_B$, the differences between the resonance frequencies of each group of protons A and B and the frequency of the applied saturation RF pulse $\omega_1 = \gamma B_1$, where B_1 is its amplitude in teslas.

After applying a non-frequency-selective excitation pulse (e.g. a 90° pulse), A and B spins are tipped to the transverse plane. At $t = 0$, the magnetization of each pool is described by: $M_A = \begin{pmatrix} 0 \\ M_{0A} \\ 0 \end{pmatrix}$ and $M_B = \begin{pmatrix} 0 \\ M_{0B} \\ 0 \end{pmatrix}$. After the perturbation, the evolution of the magnetizations in the transverse plane will be defined by the following equations:

$$\frac{dM_{xA}}{dt} = -\Delta\omega_A M_{yA} - (R_{2A} + k_{AB})M_{xA} + k_{BA}M_{xB}$$

$$\frac{dM_{yA}}{dt} = \Delta\omega_A M_{xA} - (R_{2A} + k_{AB})M_{yA} + \omega_1 M_{zA} + k_{BA}M_{yB}$$

$$\frac{dM_{xB}}{dt} = k_{AB}M_{xA} - (R_{2B} + k_{BA})M_{xB} - \Delta\omega_B M_{yB}$$

$$\frac{dM_{yB}}{dt} = k_{AB}M_{yA} + \omega_B M_{xB} - (R_{2A} + k_{BA})M_{yB} \quad [9.9]$$

This system can be re-written in a matrix form by considering the complex transverse magnetization $M_T = M_y - iM_x$:

$$\frac{d}{dt}\begin{pmatrix} M_{TA} \\ M_{TB} \end{pmatrix} = \begin{pmatrix} i\Delta\omega_A - (R_{2A} + k_{AB}) & k_{BA} \\ k_{AB} & i\Delta\omega_B - (R_{2B} + k_{BA}) \end{pmatrix} \begin{pmatrix} M_{TA} \\ M_{TB} \end{pmatrix} \quad [9.10]$$

The analytical solutions of this system that characterize the evolution over time of the transverse magnetizations in the presence of chemical exchanges are: $M_{TA}(t) = c_{1A}.e^{\lambda_1 t} + c_{2A}.e^{\lambda_2 t}$ and $M_{TB}(t) = c_{1B}.e^{\lambda_1 t} + c_{2B}.e^{\lambda_2 t}$ with λ_1 and λ_2 the eigenvalues of the matrix.

Let us consider the case where the concentrations of A and B are equal ($M_{0A} = M_{0B}$). At equilibrium, the flows of protons are equal, hence $k_{AB} = k_{BA}$ and, as a consequence, $k_{AB}.M_{0A} = k_{BA}.M_{0B}$. Thus, it is possible to determine the analytical solutions by neglecting the transverse relaxations:

$$\lambda_1 = i\left(\frac{\Delta\omega_A + \Delta\omega_B}{2}\right) - k_{AB} + W, \lambda_2 = i\left(\frac{\Delta\omega_A + \Delta\omega_B}{2}\right) - k_{AB} - W$$

$$c_{1A} = \frac{M_{0A}}{2W}\left(i\left(\frac{\Delta\omega_A - \Delta\omega_B}{2}\right) + k_{AB} + W\right), \quad c_{2A} = \frac{M_{0A}}{2W}\left(-i\left(\frac{\Delta\omega_A - \Delta\omega_B}{2}\right) + k_{AB} + W\right)$$

$$c_{1B} = \frac{M_{0B}}{2W}\left(i\left(\frac{\Delta\omega_A - \Delta\omega_B}{2}\right) + k_{AB} + W\right), \quad c_{2B} = \frac{M_{0B}}{2W}\left(-i\left(\frac{\Delta\omega_A - \Delta\omega_B}{2}\right) + k_{AB} + W\right) \quad [9.11]$$

with $W = \sqrt{(k_{AB})^2 - \left(\frac{\Delta\omega_A - \Delta\omega_B}{2}\right)^2}$.

Therefore, the measured signal will be equivalent to the sum of transverse magnetizations of each protons population: $M_{TA}(t) + M_{TB}(t)$.

In order to better understand the effects of the chemical exchange on the observation of different pools of protons, let us consider two exchange regimes.

In the case of slow exchanges between the two groups of protons ($k_{AB} \ll |\Delta\omega_A - \Delta\omega_B|$), the different terms of the analytical solutions can be simplified:

$$W \approx \frac{\Delta\omega_A - \Delta\omega_B}{2}, \lambda_1 \approx i\Delta\omega_A - k_{AB}, \lambda_2 \approx i\Delta\omega_B - k_{AB}, c_{1A} \approx M_{0A}$$

$$c_{1B} \approx M_{0B}, c_{2A} \approx c_{2B} \approx 0 \quad [9.12]$$

With these estimations, the signal is expressed as $S(t) = M_{TA}(t) + M_{TB}(t) = M_{0A}e^{(i\Delta\omega_A - k_{AB})t} + M_{0B}e^{(i\Delta\omega_B - k_{AB})t}$. The Fourier transform of this signal corresponds to a spectrum with two peaks with intensities M_{0A} and M_{0B} centered at $\Delta\omega_A$ and $\Delta\omega_B$ and with a width at half maximum of $2k_{AB}$ (Figure 9.11).

In the case of fast exchanges ($k_{AB} \gg |\Delta\omega_A - \Delta\omega_B|$), the solutions become:

$$W \approx k_{AB}\left(1 - \frac{(\Delta\omega_A - \Delta\omega_B)^2}{8(k_{AB})^2}\right),\ \lambda_1 \approx i\frac{(\Delta\omega_A - k_{AB})}{2} - k_{AB} + W$$

$$\lambda_2 \approx i\frac{(\Delta\omega_A - k_{AB})}{2} - k_{AB} - W,\ c_{1A} \approx M_{0A},\ c_{1B} \approx M_{0B},\ c_{2A} \approx c_{2B} \approx 0 \quad [9.13]$$

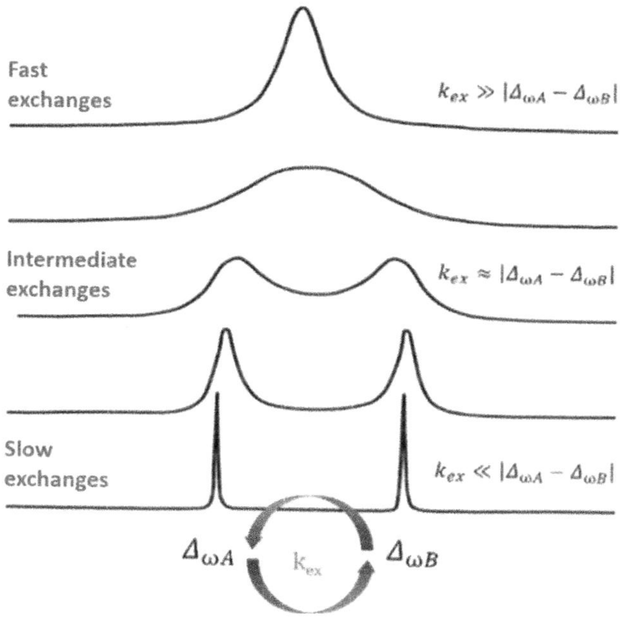

Figure 9.11. *Conditions for observing the CEST effect*

The measured signal is thus defined by:

$$S(t) = M_{TA}(t) + M_{TB}(t) = M_{0A}e^{\left(\frac{i(\Delta\omega_A - k_{AB})}{2} - \frac{(\Delta\omega_A - \Delta\omega_B)^2}{8k_{AB}}\right)t} + M_{0B}e^{\left(\frac{i(\Delta\omega_A - k_{AB})}{2} + \frac{(\Delta\omega_A - \Delta\omega_B)^2}{8k_{AB}}\right)t}$$

The observed spectrum will be composed of a single peak with an intensity $M_{0A} + M_{0B}$ centered at $\frac{\Delta\omega_A - \Delta\omega_B}{2}$ and with a width at half maximum of $\frac{(\Delta\omega_A - \Delta\omega_B)^2}{4(k_{AB})^2}$.

Since the magnetization transfer is only possible between two populations of protons with different frequencies, it is clear that there is a condition for observing the CEST effect which depends on the difference between the chemical shifts between the two groups and on their exchange rates, that is, $k_{AB} \ll |\Delta\omega_A - \Delta\omega_B|$.

9.4.3. *Saturation transfer*

Let us suppose that applying an RF pulse selectively saturates the B protons without affecting the A protons. Three hypotheses can be considered: complete, partial, or weak saturation of B protons.

In the case of complete saturation of B protons, the magnetization of the system will evolve according to the Bloch–McConnell equations until the transfer flow becomes zero, that is, until an equilibrium state is reached where the number of protons exchanged by each pool is identical. When the equilibrium is achieved, the magnetization of pool B becomes zero, $M_{xB} = M_{yB} = M_{zB} = 0$, leading to a simplification of the equations above where all the time dependencies are suppressed. From these hypotheses, solving the Bloch–McConnell equations yields:

$$\frac{M_{zA}(t)}{M_{0A}} = \frac{R_{1A}}{R_{1A} + k_{AB}} + \left(1 - \frac{R_{1A}}{R_{1A} + k_{AB}}\right) e^{-(R_{1A} + k_{AB})t} \qquad [9.14]$$

From this expression, we can retrieve a simple value of the proton transfer ratio (PTR), also called the saturation rate, for a complete saturation: $PTR = 1 - \frac{M_{zA}}{M_{0A}} = \frac{M_{0A} - M_{zA}}{M_{0A}} = \frac{k_{AB}}{R_{1A} + k_{AB}}$. As we can see, the efficacy of the magnetization transfer, represented by PTR, depends on the longitudinal relaxation times of the A protons as well as on the exchange rate between the A and B protons. Thus, there is a sort of equilibrium between the magnetization recovered via the longitudinal relaxation and its destruction by the magnetization transfer via the exchange of protons with the pool of B protons.

In practice, a trade-off has to be achieved to control the energy deposited in tissues as heat by limiting the duration ($<5\ T_{1B}$) and intensity of the saturation block.

As a result, the saturation of the B protons is often partial. By neglecting the frequency evolution terms, the Bloch–McConnell equation system becomes:

$$\frac{dM_{yA}}{dt} = R_{2A}M_{yA} - k_{AB}M_{yA} + k_{BA}M_{yB}$$

$$\frac{dM_{zA}}{dt} = -R_{1A}(M_{zA} - M_{0A}) - k_{AB}M_{zA} + k_{BA}M_{zB}$$

$$\frac{dM_{yB}}{dt} = -R_{2A}M_{yB} - k_{BA}M_{yB} + k_{AB}M_{yA} - \omega_1 M_{zB}$$

$$\frac{dM_{zB}}{dt} = -R_{1B}(M_{zB} - M_{0B}) + k_{AB}M_{zA} - k_{BA}M_{zB} + \omega_1 M_{yB} \qquad [9.15]$$

At equilibrium, the time derivatives cancel out and we can thus solve the system:

$M_{zB} - M_{0B} = \frac{\omega_1^2 M_{0B}}{\omega_1^2+pq}$, $M_{yB} = \frac{\omega_1 q M_{0B}}{\omega_1^2+pq}$, $M_{zB} - M_{0B} = \frac{\omega_1^2 M_{0B}}{\omega_1^2+pq}$,

$M_{yB} = \frac{\omega_1 q M_{0B}}{\omega_1^2+pq}$, with $p = R_{2B} + k_{BA} - \frac{k_{AB}k_{BA}}{R_{2A}+k_{AB}}$ and $q = R_{1B} + k_{BA} - \frac{k_{AB}k_{BA}}{R_{1A}+k_{AB}}$

If the saturation is applied for a sufficiently long time such that complete saturation of the solute protons is achieved, PTR is equal to:

$$PTR(\Delta\omega_B) = \frac{k_{AB}}{R_{1A}+k_{AB}} \frac{\omega_1^2}{\omega_1^2+pq+\frac{p}{q}\Delta\omega_B^2} \qquad [9.16]$$

The saturation ratio α of the pool B can be obtained as: $\alpha(\Delta\omega_B) = \frac{\omega_1^2}{\omega_1^2+pq+\frac{p}{q}\Delta\omega_B^2}$.

In the case of weak saturation, the magnetization of the solute protons will relax to equilibrium almost immediately after saturation, with very little effect on the signal of free water. We can thus approximate the magnetization of free water ($M_{zA}(0) = M_{0A}$) and derive the proton transfer as a function of the saturation time t_{sat}: $PTR(t_{sat}) = \frac{\alpha.k_{AB}}{R_{1A}+k_{AB}}\left(1 - e^{-t_{sat}(R_{1A}+k_{AB})}\right)$. Knowing that to abide by the magnetization flow between the two pools of protons, the exchange rates must satisfy the condition $k_{AB}M_{zB} = k_{BA}M_{zA}$; we can express PTR as a function of the saturation time and of the magnetizations M_{zA} and M_{zB} of the two proton pools: $PTR(t_{sat}) = \frac{\alpha.k_{BA}}{R_{1A}+k_{AB}} \frac{M_{zB}}{M_{zA}}\left(1 - e^{-t_{sat}(R_{1A}+k_{AB})}\right)$. The PTR, and thus the CEST effect, depends on the duration of the applied RF pulse (t_{sat}), the longitudinal relaxation times T_{1A}, the ratio $\frac{M_{zB}}{M_{zA}}$ proportional to the ratio of the proton concentrations $\left(\frac{[\text{solute}]}{[\text{free water}]}\right)$, the exchange rate k_{BA}, and finally the amplitude of the pulse (ω_1) which is a fundamental parameter regarding the saturation efficacy (α).

It can be noticed that in the case of weak saturation, the *PTR* increases with saturation intensity B_1. This is valid until B_1 becomes too large because the saturation regime changes and the saturation will affect not only the solute protons but also a part of free water protons. Therefore, this so-called direct saturation (also called spillover effect) should be limited as much as possible while trying to achieve the maximum CEST effect. It is possible to determine the optimal saturation power, for which the contribution of the saturation of pool B is maximum, satisfying the relationship (Woessner 2005): $k_{BA} = \omega_{1opt} = 2\pi\gamma B_{1opt}$.

9.4.4. Characterization of the magnetization transfer

In order to characterize the CEST effect of a contrast agent or a molecule under investigation (B protons), it is worth measuring the longitudinal magnetization M_{ZA} of the observable group of protons (A protons) as a function of the applied saturation frequency. In practice, the longitudinal magnetization measured at a given saturation frequency is normalized by the magnetization without saturation M_{0A}. The evolution of this normalized signal M_{ZA}/M_{0A} is monitored as a function of saturation frequency to obtain a Z-spectrum (Grad 1991), as illustrated in Figure 9.12.

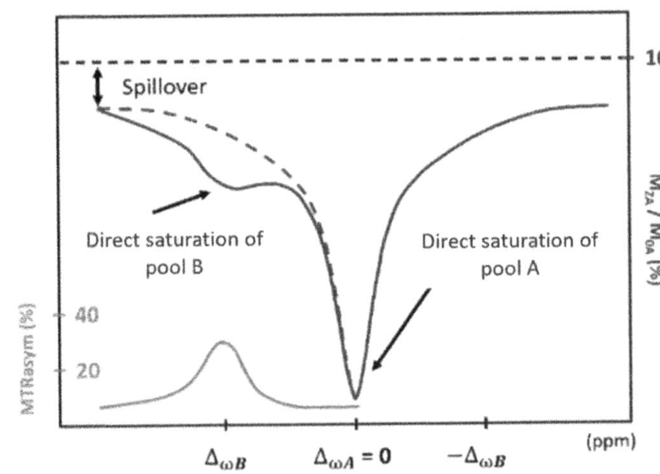

Figure 9.12. *Example of a typical Z-spectrum and MTRasym for a two-compartment model*

The Z-spectrum exhibits two minima: an absolute minimum corresponding to the direct saturation of pool A protons (free water) and a local minimum observed at the saturation frequency of B protons (solute). Another observation is that when the saturation is applied off-resonance, the maximum magnetization fraction M_{zA}/M_{0A} is not equal to 100%. This is due to the direct saturation of the observed protons. To a first approximation, this effect is symmetric with respect to the free water frequency. Consequently, this contribution, non-specific to the desired CEST effect, can be removed by calculating the MTRasym (asymmetrical magnetization transfer ratio; Figure 9.11) defined by the following equation:

$$MTRasym(\delta_{sat}) = \frac{M_{zA}(-\Delta\omega_B) - M_{zA}(\Delta\omega_B)}{M_{0A}} \qquad [9.17]$$

To optimize the detection of a molecule in a CEST scan, several parameters of the saturation pulse should be considered: the saturation frequency $\Delta\omega_B$, which has to be applied over a frequency range centered at the water frequency and radiating at the frequency of the investigated molecule; the duration of the saturation t_{sat} – the slower the exchanges, the longer it will take for the saturation to be transferred to free water; thus, to maintain the protons saturated for the exchange duration, t_{sat} will have to be adapted depending on the exchange rate; saturation intensity B_1: the faster are the exchanges, the more intense it must be, although without generating direct saturation effects. Many applications of CEST imaging exist. Only a few of them are illustrated in Figure 9.13. CEST imaging is an extremely active research domain and the increase of scan protocols across the world, including in the clinical domain, suggests that CEST imaging will soon be accessible in clinical routine in the entire community.

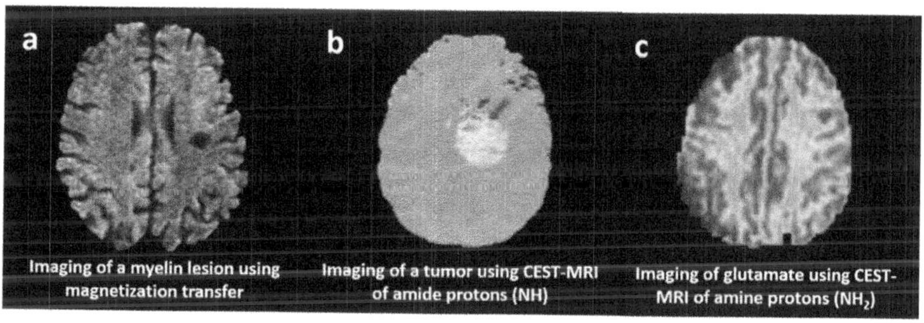

Figure 9.13. *Examples of CEST-MRI applications for myelin imaging (a) (Grossman 1994), tumor imaging (b) (Zhao 2008) and glutamate imaging (c) (Cai 2012)*

9.5. Non-proton nuclei MR spectroscopy or imaging

9.5.1. *Nuclei of interest in metabolic MRS/MRI*

Beyond the proton (^1H), NMR enables the detection and mapping of several other stable isotopes of nuclei relevant to biomedical research. Due to their gyromagnetic ratios γ and natural abundance lower than those of ^1H, these non-proton or exotic (denoted as X) nuclei distinguish themselves by their lower Larmor frequency and a much lower macroscopic magnetization. Nevertheless, MR spectroscopy and imaging of these exotic nuclei are promising tools to investigate normal and pathological metabolism. Notably, their sensitivity and specificity keep on improving, in particular thanks to the ongoing advances in MRI scanners at high and ultra-high magnetic fields (Ladd 2018; Choi 2020; Hu 2020). Among these X-nuclei, some are naturally abundant isotopes in tissues such as ^{23}Na, ^{31}P, ^{35}Cl or ^{39}K; on the other hand, others are minor isotopes of atoms that are ubiquitous in biochemistry such as ^{13}C, ^{15}N or ^{17}O; and finally, there are also exogenous nuclei such as ^{19}F, ^7Li, ^{129}Xe or ^3He. While the latter ones are most often used as contrast agents in molecular MRI (except for lithium, which is prescribed to some patients with bipolar or depressive disorders), the endogenous nuclei allow for the probing of the brain metabolism in a non-invasive and non-ionizing way.

9.5.1.1. *Sensitivity differences*

In order to grasp the relative sensitivities associated with X-nuclei MRS/MRI, it is useful to contemplate the equation of the SNR (Zhu 2005):

$$SNR \propto \gamma^2 [X] V_{oxel} \sqrt{AT} . B_0{}^{\beta} \sqrt{Q.T_2^* / T_1}, \sim 7/4 \qquad [9.18]$$

where V_{oxel} is the volume of the voxel, Q is the loaded quality factor of the receive coil and AT is the acquisition time of the NMR signal. Besides the nonlinear dependence on B_0 intensity, we can note that the *SNR* has a quadratic dependence on the gyromagnetic ratio. Consequently, the nuclei with lower gyromagnetic ratios are also intrinsically less sensitive (see Table 9.1). A second factor is the volumetric density *[X]*, which is directly related to the natural abundance of the considered X nucleus. Because of it, to detect rare isotopes (such as ^{15}N, ^{17}O or ^{13}C), their fractional isotopic enrichment must be artificially increased. A third term is $\sqrt{T_2^* / T_1}$; this ratio represents the available amount of signal per unit of time. The nuclei with a spin >1/2 have bi-exponential transverse and longitudinal relaxations with fast and slow components related to the interaction between their non-zero quadripolar nuclear electrical moment with the complex biological environment. Therefore, for these nuclei (e.g. ^{23}Na, ^{17}O, etc.) it is crucial to minimize the echo times for the successful detection of the short components and to employ short repetition times to exploit their short T_1.

9.5.2. *Applications overview*

9.5.2.1. ^{23}*Na MRI*

Sodium-23 is the second most concentrated nucleus in the brain. The Na^+ cation plays a fundamental role in osmotic balance and in neuron's transmembranar depolarization/hyperpolarization phenomena occurring during neurotransmission (action potential generation and propagation via saltatory conduction in nerves). Maintaining or re-establishing the transmembranar concentration gradient implies, in particular, an energy-wise expensive action of the Na^{+}/K^{+}-ATPase pump. Moreover, a normal intracellular concentration of sodium (ISC = 14 mmol/L) is considered a positive indication of cellular viability and integrity (Fleysher 2013). However, distinguishing the intra- and extra-cellular sodium is not always possible. For this reason, an increase in tissue sodium concentration (TSC; Figure 9.14) has been suggested as an early biomarker of pathology progression in the context of several cerebral diseases (stroke, Alzheimer's, Huntington's, multiple sclerosis, glioblastoma) (Shah 2016). In addition, propositions to exploit the multiple coherences of the ^{23}Na signal have been made to distinguish between more or less alive cells (Hoesl 2019). Thanks to the development of MRI sequences with ultrashort echo times (TE < 1 ms) and their combination with non-Cartesian k-space sampling schemes such as twisted projection imaging (Boada 1997), sodium images of the human brain can be acquired at 3-mm isotropic resolution in a few minutes.

9.5.2.2. ^{31}*P MRS*

Phosphorus-31 (^{31}P) is present in all living organisms in the form of phosphate ions ($H_2PO_4/HPO_4^-/PO_4^{2-}$) as well as in some phosphorylated metabolites: on the one hand, biomolecules acting as energy storage for our cells, such as adenosine triphosphate (ATP) and phosphocreatine (PCr) and, on the other hand, intermediates of membrane metabolism, such as phosphomonoesters (PME = PCh + PE) and phosphodiesters (PDE = GPC + GPE). Therefore, in vivo ^{31}P MRS enables direct studies of energy synthesis and membrane metabolism (via the PDE/PME ratio) or the intracellular redox potential (via the NAD^+/NADH ratio) (Zhu 2009; Kim 2017). Since the ^{31}P NMR sensitivity is about 7% of the one for ^{1}H, spatial resolutions for ^{31}P MRS are quite modest. So far, these phosphorylated metabolites have been mapped at spatial resolutions as low as 10–20 mm in humans at 7 T (Lu 2013; Rink 2017). In combination with saturation transfer methods (similar to CEST), ^{31}P MRS allows for probing the creatine kinase ($PCr + ADP^- + H^+ \leftrightarrow Cr + ATP$) or the ATP synthesis/hydrolysis ($ATP \leftrightarrow ADP + Pi$) fluxes (Chen 2018).

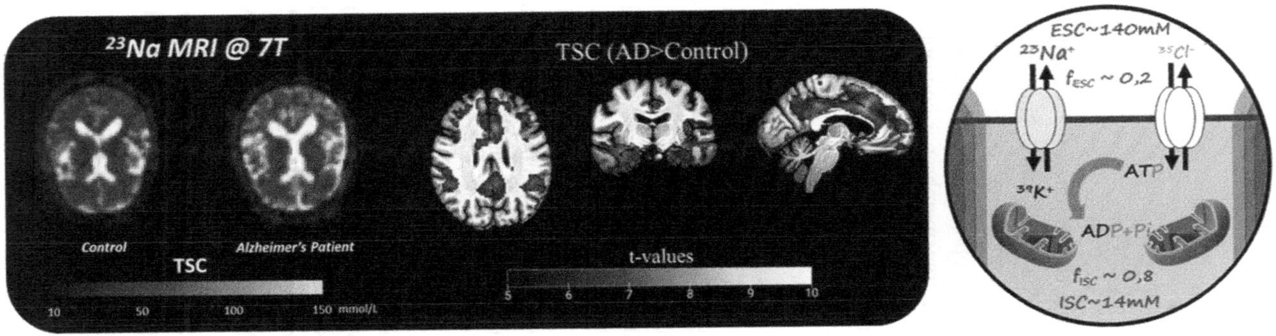

Figure 9.14. ^{23}*Na MRI can detect increases in tissue sodium concentration (TSC =* f_{ISC}**ISC +* f_{ESC}**ESC,* f_{ISC} *~ 0.8;* f_{ESC} *~ 0.2; ESC = 140 mmol/L) in different cortical regions in Alzheimer's disease (AD) patients compared to elderly control subjects (Haeger 2021)*

9.5.2.3. ^{13}C MRS

^{13}C MRS also probes the energetic metabolism with the peculiarity of being able to distinguish between neuronal and glial contributions to the Krebs cycle (Rothman 2011; Valette 2017). In particular, it enables the in vivo evaluation of the recycling flow of glutamate and GABA, a measure of their respective neurotransmissions (Patel 2015). For this purpose, one or several energetic substrates (typically glucose, acetate, or lactate) labeled with ^{13}C must be perfused to acquire fractional enrichment curves of glutamate, glutamine, or GABA that are then adjusted numerically to metabolic models (Tiret 2015).

For rapid metabolic processes such as the activity of lactate dehydrogenase (Pyruvate + NADH ↔ Lactate +NAD^+), hyperpolarized molecules labeled with ^{13}C can be used (Wang 2019). Thanks to hyperpolarization, the polarization reaches about 40% for a few seconds (~T_1s), and images of abnormal metabolic activity in tumors can be acquired rapidly.

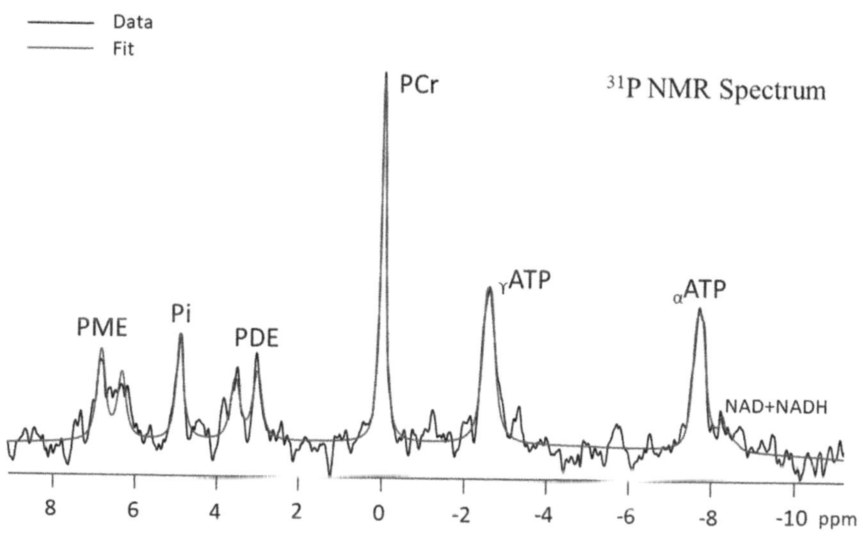

Figure 9.15. *Typical ^{31}P NMR spectrum acquired in vivo from a healthy human volunteer at 7 T*

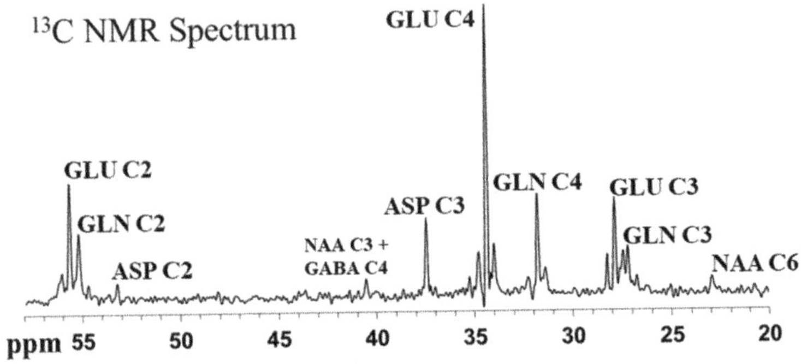

Figure 9.16. *^{13}C NMR spectrum acquired in vivo from a healthy human volunteer at 4T after a 2-h infusion of ^{13}C-labeled glucose*

9.6. Conclusion

It would be impossible to describe and explain in this chapter the many techniques and applications that constitute the field of in vivo NMR spectroscopy and metabolic imaging. In this chapter, we focused on brain applications, yet there are many other exciting applications in oncology, diabetology and myology. It is equally important to stress the ongoing development of these methods and the forthcoming realization of their actual potential in biomedical research thanks to the advent of ultrahigh-magnetic field MRI scanners, on the one hand, and, on the other hand, hyperpolarization approaches at low magnetic fields. Finally, interested readers are encouraged to read the references cited in these pages and to continue their research.

9.7. References

Ackerman, J.J., Grove, T.H., Wong, G.G., Gadian, D.G., Radda, G.K. (1980). Mapping of metabolites in whole animals by 31 P NMR using surface coils. *Nature*, 283(5743), 167–170.

Aime, S., Delli Castelli, D., Terreno, E. (2005). Highly sensitive MRI chemical exchange saturation transfer agents using liposomes. *Angewandte Chemie International Edition*, 44(34), 5513–5515.

Behar, K.L. and Ogino, T. (1993). Characterization of macromolecule resonances in the 1H NMR spectrum of rat brain. *Magnetic Resonance in Medicine*, 30(1), 38–44.

Bloch, F. (1946). Nuclear induction. *Physical Review*, 70(7/8), 460.

Boada, F.E., Gillen, J.S., Shen, G.X., Chang, S.Y., Thulborn, K.R. (1997). Fast three dimensional sodium imaging. *Magnetic Resonance in Medicine*, 37(5), 706–715.

Bolliger, C.S., Boesch, C., Kreis, R. (2013). On the use of Cramer–Rao minimum variance bounds for the design of magnetic resonance spectroscopy experiments. *Neuroimage*, 83, 1031–1040.

Bottomley, P.A. (1987). Spatial localization in NMR spectroscopy in vivo. *Annals of the New York Academy of Sciences*, 508(1), 333–348.

Bruce, S.D., Higinbotham, J., Marshall, I., Beswick, P.H. (2000). An analytical derivation of a popular approximation of the Voigt function for quantification of NMR spectra. *Journal of Magnetic Resonance*, 142(1), 57–63.

Cai, K., Haris, M., Singh, A., Kogan, F., Greenberg, J.H., Hariharan, H., Detre, J.A., Reddy, R. (2012). Magnetic resonance imaging of glutamate. *Nature Medicine*, 18(2), 302–306.

Chen, C., Stephenson, M.C., Peters, A., Morris, P.G., Francis, S.T., Gowland, P.A. (2018). 31P magnetization transfer magnetic resonance spectroscopy: Assessing the activation induced change in cerebral ATP metabolic rates at 3 T. *Magnetic Resonance in Medicine*, 79(1), 22–30.

Choi, C.H., Hong, S.M., Felder, J., Shah, N.J. (2020). The state-of-the-art and emerging design approaches of double-tuned RF coils for X-nuclei, brain MR imaging and spectroscopy: A review. *Magnetic Resonance Imaging*, 72, 103–116.

Cudalbu, C., Behar, K.L., Bhattacharyya, P.K., Bogner, W., Borbath, T., de Graaf, R.A., Gruetter, R., Henning, A., Juchem, C., Kreis, R. et al. (2021). Contribution of macromolecules to brain 1H MR spectra: Experts' consensus recommendations. *NMR in Biomedicine*, 34(5), e4393.

Ernst, R.R. and Anderson, W.A. (1966). Application of Fourier transform spectroscopy to magnetic resonance. *Review of Scientific Instruments*, 37(1), 93–102.

Fleysher, L., Oesingmann, N., Brown, R., Sodickson, D.K., Wiggins, G.C., Inglese, M. (2013). Noninvasive quantification of intracellular sodium in human brain using ultrahigh-field MRI. *NMR in Biomedicine*, 26(1), 9–19.

Frahm, J., Merboldt, K.D., Hänicke, W. (1987). Localized proton spectroscopy using stimulated echoes. *Journal of Magnetic Resonance*, 72(3), 502–508.

Garwood, M. and DelaBarre, L. (2001). The return of the frequency sweep: Designing adiabatic pulses for contemporary NMR. *Journal of Magnetic Resonance*, 153(2), 155–177.

Giapitzakis, I.A., Avdievich, N., Henning, A. (2018). Characterization of macromolecular baseline of human brain using metabolite cycled semi-LASER at 9.4 T. *Magnetic Resonance in Medicine*, 80(2), 462–473.

de Graaf, A.A., Van Dijk, J., Boé, W. (1990). Quality: Quantification improvement by converting lineshapes to the Lorentzian type. *Magnetic Resonance in Medicine*, 13(3), 343–357.

de Graaf, R.A., Brown, P.B., McIntyre, S., Nixon, T.W., Behar, K.L., Rothman, D.L. (2006). High magnetic field water and metabolite proton T_1 and T_2 relaxation in rat brain in vivo. *Magnetic Resonance in Medicine*, 56(2), 386–394.

Grad, J., Mendelson, D., Hyder, F., Bryant, R.G. (1991). Applications of nuclear magnetic cross-relaxation spectroscopy to tissues. *Magnetic Resonance in Medicine*, 17(2), 452–459.

Grossman, R.I., Gomori, J.M., Ramer, K.N., Lexa, F.J., Schnall, M.D. (1994). Magnetization transfer: Theory and clinical applications in neuroradiology. *Radiographics*, 14(2), 279–290.

Gruetter, R. and Tkáč, I. (2000). Field mapping without reference scan using asymmetric echo-planar techniques. *Magnetic Resonance in Medicine*, 43(2), 319–323.

Haeger, A., Coste, A., Lerman-Rabrait, C., Lagarde, J., Schulz, J.B., Vignaud, A., Sarazin, M., Bottlaender, M., Reetz, K., Romanzetti, S. et al. (2020). Quantitative sodium imaging using ultra-high field magnetic resonance imaging in patients with Alzheimer's disease: Neuroimaging/optimal neuroimaging measures for tracking disease progression. *Alzheimer's & Dementia*, 16, e042107.

Harris, A.D., Saleh, M.G., Edden, R.A. (2017). Edited 1H magnetic resonance spectroscopy in vivo: Methods and metabolites. *Magnetic Resonance in Medicine*, 77(4), 1377–1389.

Heinzer-Schweizer, S., De Zanche, N., Pavan, M., Mens, G., Sturzenegger, U., Henning, A., Boesiger, P. (2010). In-vivo assessment of tissue metabolite levels using 1H MRS and the Electric REference To access In vivo Concentrations (ERETIC) method. *NMR in Biomedicine*, 23(4), 406–413.

Hoesl, M.A.U., Kleimaier, D., Hu, R., Malzacher, M., Nies, C., Gottwald, E., Schad, L.R. (2019). (23) Na Triple-quantum signal of in vitro human liver cells, liposomes, and nanoparticles: Cell viability assessment vs. separation of intra- and extracellular signal. *Journal of Magnetic Resonance Imaging: JMRI*, 50(2), 435–444.

Hoult, D.I., Busby, S.J., Gadian, D.G., Radda, G.K., Richards, R.E., Seeley, P.J. (1974). Observation of tissue metabolites using 31P nuclear magnetic resonance. *Nature*, 252(5481), 285–287.

Hu, R., Kleimaier, D., Malzacher, M., Hoesl, M.A.U., Paschke, N.K., Schad, L.R. (2020). X-nuclei imaging: Current state, technical challenges, and future directions. *Journal of Magnetic Resonance Imaging: JMRI*, 51(2), 355–376.

Julià-Sapé, M., Candiota, A.P., Arús, C. (2019). Cancer metabolism in a snapshot: MRS(I). *NMR in Biomedicine*, 32(10), e4054.

Kelm, B.M., Kaster, F.O., Henning, A., Weber, M.A., Bachert, P., Boesiger, P., Hamprecht, F.A., Menze, B.H. (2012). Using spatial prior knowledge in the spectral fitting of MRS images. *NMR in Biomedicine*, 25(1), 1–13.

Kim, S.Y., Cohen, B.M., Chen, X., Lukas, S.E., Shinn, A.K., Yuksel, A.C., Li, T., Du, F., Öngür, D. (2017). Redox dysregulation in schizophrenia revealed by in vivo NAD+/NADH measurement. *Schizophrenia Bulletin*, 43(1), 197–204.

Kreis, R. (2016). The trouble with quality filtering based on relative Cramér-Rao lower bounds. *Magnetic Resonance in Medicine*, 75(1), 15–18.

Krššák, M., Lindeboom, L., Schrauwen-Hinderling, V., Szczepaniak, L.S., Derave, W., Lundbom, J., Befroy, D., Schick, F., Machann, J., Kreis, R. et al. (2021). Proton magnetic resonance spectroscopy in skeletal muscle: Experts' consensus recommendations. *NMR in Biomedicine*, 34(5), e4266.

Ladd, M.E., Bachert, P., Meyerspeer, M., Moser, E., Nagel, A.M., Norris, D.G., Schmitter, S., Speck, O., Straub, S., Zaiss, M. (2018). Pros and cons of ultra-high-field MRI/MRS for human application. *Progress in Nuclear Magnetic Resonance Spectroscopy*, 109, 1–50.

Liddel, U. and Ramsey, N.F. (1951). Temperature dependent magnetic shielding in ethyl alcohol. *The Journal of Chemical Physics*, 19(12), 1608.

Lopez-Kolkovsky, A.L., Mériaux, S., Boumezbeur, F. (2016). Metabolite and macromolecule T_1 and T_2 relaxation times in the rat brain in vivo at 17.2 T. *Magnetic Resonance in Medicine*, 75(2), 503–514.

Lu, A., Atkinson, I.C., Zhou, X.J., Thulborn, K.R. (2013). PCr/ATP ratio mapping of the human head by simultaneously imaging of multiple spectral peaks with interleaved excitations and flexible twisted projection imaging readout trajectories at 9.4 T. *Magnetic Resonance in Medicine*, 69(2), 538–544.

Maudsley, A.A., Darkazanli, A., Alger, J.R., Hall, L.O., Schuff, N., Studholme, C., Yu, Y., Ebel, A., Frew, A., Goldgof, D. et al. (2006). Comprehensive processing, display and analysis for in vivo MR spectroscopic imaging. *NMR in Biomedicine*, 19(4), 492–503.

McConnell, H.M. (1958). Reaction rates by nuclear magnetic resonance. *The Journal of Chemical Physics*, 28(3), 430–431.

Mescher, M., Merkle, H., Kirsch, J., Garwood, M., Gruetter, R. (1998). Simultaneous in vivo spectral editing and water suppression. *NMR in Biomedicine: An International Journal Devoted to the Development and Application of Magnetic Resonance In Vivo*, 11(6), 266–272.

Mlynárik, V., Gambarota, G., Frenkel, H., Gruetter, R. (2006). Localized short-echo-time proton MR spectroscopy with full signal-intensity acquisition. *Magnetic Resonance in Medicine*, 56(5), 965–970.

Moon, R.B. and Richards, J.H. (1973). Determination of intracellular pH by 31P magnetic resonance. *The Journal of Biological Chemistry*, 248(20), 7276–7278.

Odeblad, E. and Lindstrom, G. (1955). Some preliminary observations on the proton magnetic resonance in biologic samples. *Acta Radiologica*, 43(6), 469–476.

Odeblad, E., Bhar, B.N., Lindstrom, G. (1956). Proton magnetic resonance of human red blood cells in heavy-water exchange experiments. *Archives of Biochemistry and Biophysics*, 63(1), 221–225.

Ogg, R.J., Kingsley, P.B., Taylor, J.S. (1994). WET, a T_1- and B_1-insensitive water-suppression method for in vivo localized 1H NMR spectroscopy. *Journal of Magnetic Resonance. Series B*, 104(1), 1–10.

Ordidge, R.J., Connelly, A., Lohman, J.A. (1986). Image-selected in vivo spectroscopy (ISIS). A new technique for spatially selective NMR spectroscopy. *Journal of Magnetic Resonance*, 66(2), 283–294.

Oz, G. and Tkáč, I. (2011). Short-echo, single-shot, full-intensity proton magnetic resonance spectroscopy for neurochemical profiling at 4 T: Validation in the cerebellum and brainstem. *Magnetic Resonance in Medicine*, 65(4), 901–910.

Patel, A.B., de Graaf, R.A., Rothman, D.L., Behar, K.L. (2015). Effects of γ-aminobutyric acid transporter 1 inhibition by tiagabine on brain glutamate and γ-aminobutyric acid metabolism in the anesthetized rat in vivo. *Journal of Neuroscience Research*, 93(7), 1101–1108.

Proctor, W. and Yu, F. (1950). The dependence of a nuclear magnetic resonance frequency upon chemical compound. *Physical Review*, 77(5), 717.

Provencher, S.W. (1993). Estimation of metabolite concentrations from localized in vivo proton NMR spectra. *Magnetic Resonance in Medicine*, 30(6), 672–679.

Purcell, E.M., Torrey, H.C., Pound, R.V. (1946). Resonance absorption by nuclear magnetic moments in a solid. *Physical Review*, 69(1/2), 37.

Rabi, I.I., Zacharias, J.R., Millman, S., Kusch, P. (1938). A new method of measuring nuclear magnetic moment. *Physical Review*, 53(4), 318.

Ratiney, H., Coenradie, Y., Cavassila, S., van Ormondt, D., Graveron-Demilly, D. (2004). Time-domain quantitation of 1H short echo-time signals: Background accommodation. *Magma*, 16(6), 284–296.

Rink, K., Benkhedah, N., Berger, M.C., Gnahm, C., Behl, N.G.R., Lommen, J.M., Stahl, V., Bachert, P., Ladd, M.E., Nagel, A.M. (2017). Iterative reconstruction of radially-sampled (31)P bSSFP data using prior information from (1)H MRI. *Magnetic Resonance Imaging*, 37, 147–158.

Rothman, D.L., De Feyter, H.M., de Graaf, R.A., Mason, G.F., Behar, K.L. (2011). 13C MRS studies of neuroenergetics and neurotransmitter cycling in humans. *NMR in Biomedicine*, 24(8), 943–957.

Rothman, D.L., de Graaf, R.A., Hyder, F., Mason, G.F., Behar, K.L., De Feyter, H.M. (2019). In vivo 13C and 1H-[13C] MRS studies of neuroenergetics and neurotransmitter cycling, applications to neurological and psychiatric disease and brain cancer. *NMR in Biomedicine*, 32(10), e4172.

Shah, N.J., Worthoff, W.A., Langen, K.J. (2016). Imaging of sodium in the brain: A brief review. *NMR in Biomedicine*, 29(2), 162–174.

Shaw, T. and Elsken, R. (1950). Nuclear magnetic resonance absorption in hygroscopic materials. *The Journal of Chemical Physics*, 18(8), 1113–1114.

Tiret, B., Shestov, A.A., Valette, J., Henry, P.G. (2015). Metabolic modeling of dynamic (13)C NMR isotopomer data in the brain in vivo: Fast screening of metabolic models using automated generation of differential equations. *Neurochemical Research*, 40(12), 2482–2492.

Tkác, I., Starcuk, Z., Choi, I.Y., Gruetter, R. (1999). In vivo 1H NMR spectroscopy of rat brain at 1 ms echo time. *Magnetic Resonance in Medicine*, 41(4), 649–656.

Valette, J., Tiret, B., Boumezbeur, F. (2017). Experimental strategies for in vivo 13C NMR spectroscopy. *Analytical Biochemistry*, 529, 216–228.

Van Zijl, P.C. and Yadav, N.N. (2011). Chemical exchange saturation transfer (CEST): What is in a name and what isn't? *Magnetic Resonance in Medicine*, 65(4), 927–948.

Wang, Z.J., Ohliger, M.A., Larson, P.E.Z., Gordon, J.W., Bok, R.A., Slater, J., Villanueva-Meyer, J.E., Hess, C.P., Kurhanewicz, J., Vigneron, D.B. (2019). Hyper-polarized (13)C MRI: State of the art and future directions. *Radiology*, 291(2), 273–284.

Ward, K.M. and Balaban, R.S. (2000). Determination of pH using water protons and chemical exchange dependent saturation transfer (CEST). *Magnetic Resonance in Medicine*, 44(5), 799–802.

Waugh, J., Wang, C., Huber, L., Vold, R. (1968). Multiple-pulse NMR experiments. *The Journal of Chemical Physics*, 48(2), 662–670.

Woessner, D.E., Zhang, S., Merritt, M.E., Sherry, A.D. (2005). Numerical solution of the Bloch equations provides insights into the optimum design of PARACEST agents for MRI. *Magnetic Resonance in Medicine*, 53(4), 790–799.

Wolff, S.D. and Balaban, R.S. (1989). Magnetization transfer contrast (MTC) and tissue water proton relaxation in vivo. *Magnetic Resonance in Medicine*, 10(1), 135–144.

Zhao, J.M., Har-el, Y., McMahon, M.T., Zhou, J., Sherry, A.D., Sgouros, G., Bulte, J.W.M., van Zijl, P.C.M. (2008). Size-induced enhancement of chemical exchange saturation transfer (CEST) contrast in liposomes. *Journal of the American Chemical Society*, 130(15), 5178–5184.

Zhu, X.H., Zhang, N., Zhang, Y., Zhang, X., Ugurbil, K., Chen, W. (2005). In vivo 17O NMR approaches for brain study at high field. *NMR in Biomedicine*, 18(2), 83–103.

Zhu, X.H., Du, F., Zhang, N., Zhang, Y., Lei, H., Zhang, X., Qiao, H., Ugurbil, K., Chen, W. (2009). Advanced in vivo heteronuclear MRS approaches for studying brain bioenergetics driven by mitochondria. *Methods in Molecular Biology*, 489, 317–357.

10

Physical-model-constrained MRI: Fast Multiparametric Quantification

Benjamin LEPORQ[1], **Thomas CHRISTEN**[2] **and Ludovic DE ROCHEFORT**[3,4]

[1] *CREATIS, CNRS, Inserm, INSA Lyon, Université Claude Bernard Lyon 1, France*

[2] *GIN, Inserm, Université Grenoble Alpes, France*

[3] *CRMBM, CNRS, Marseille, France*

[4] *CEMEREM, AP-HM, Hôpital de la Timone, Marseille, France*

10.1. Introduction

Conventional MRI produces images whose voxels represent signal intensities weighted according to different physical phenomena such as relaxation, diffusion and perfusion. The value of the signal intensity is intrinsically dependent on the chosen acquisition sequence parameters and hardware. Quantitative MRI, on the contrary, seeks to produce maps where the value in each voxel is a quantitative measure of a physical parameter (e.g. T_2 relaxation time) or a parameter with biological, biochemical, functional or molecular meaning. The value of quantitative imaging lies in the objective information that it can provide, regardless of the scan protocol or hardware. Therefore, it is aimed at the research and reproducibility of imaging biomarkers, which are objectively measurable features by definition, as indicators of pathological processes or treatment response.

From a technical point of view, quantitative MRI exploits advanced pulse sequences to measure signals that contain parametric information which has to be quantified. These signals have to be modeled, preferably using physical models, and

The Challenges of MRI,
coordinated by Hélène RATINEY and Olivier BEUF. © ISTE Ltd 2024.

an inverse problem has to be formulated to evaluate the quantitative values of a target parameter. Depending on the complexity of the problem, it can be solved using different numerical methods including optimization, regularization, or dictionary-based techniques in combination with machine learning approaches.

Given the complexity of biological processes, several biomarkers are often required to properly characterize tissues. Besides using several separate quantitative MRI sequences, it is also possible to use a single "multiparametric" acquisition. However, this kind of simultaneous sequence containing multiple measurement dimensions carries the inconvenience of increased scan times (to obtain sufficient information) as well as reconstruction times (model complexity). To reduce them, emerging research works measure several parameters simultaneously using a single fast scan. In this chapter, we will present three different approaches enabling fast multiparametric quantitative imaging.

10.2. Multiparametric MRI based on chemical-shift-sensitive acquisitions

10.2.1. *Signal's origin and chemical-shift-encoded acquisitions*

The absence of a refocusing pulse in gradient echo imaging sequences adds undesired components to the signal, resulting in artifacts. Mostly, these effects are related to the chemical shift and macro- and microscopic inhomogeneities of the magnetic field B_0. As described in Chapter 9, the chemical shift phenomenon is a modification of the resonant frequency of the protons within a molecule due to differences in the electronic environment. The protons of water and those of methylene groups, the main components of lipids, differ between them by a chemical shift of 3.4 ppm (220 and 440 Hz at 1.5 and 3.0 T, respectively). Without a refocusing pulse, a medium containing water and lipids would exhibit a modulation of the signal related to the dephasing of isochromats in the spectroscopic domain (the echo time domain).

As discussed in Chapter 1, the absence of refocusing pulses makes the imaging sequence sensitive to local inhomogeneities of the magnetic field B_0. The latter lead to additional dephasing to the spin-spin relaxation of the T_2 time constant, causing the relaxation to occur with the so-called T_2* time constant. These field inhomogeneities are a superposition of several phenomena such as differences in magnetic susceptibility between the tissues, effects of the readout encoding gradients, shim coils and chemical shifts, among others. Among these mechanisms, magnetic susceptibility χ can contain useful information since it is a characteristic property of the tissues. Magnetic susceptibility represents the ability of a substance to magnetize under the effect of a magnetic field. It is expressed as a proportionality factor between the applied static magnetizing field intensity ***H*** and the induced magnetization ***M***:

$$\mathbf{M} = \chi\mathbf{H} = \frac{\chi\mathbf{B_0}}{\mu_0} \quad [10.1]$$

where μ_0 is the vacuum magnetic permeability ($4\pi \times 10^{-7}$ H·m^{-1}).

We have mentioned that the absence of a refocusing pulse in gradient echo pulse sequences can be a source of artifacts. However, if the latter can be undesirable for obtaining anatomical images for diagnostic purposes, some artifacts also carry a lot of information in terms of tissue characterization. Their common aspect is that they affect the MRI signal in the spectroscopic domain. In order to make use of them, it is thus worth recording the time evolution of the signal. For this purpose, gradient echo pulse sequences with multiple echos are favored.

10.2.2. *Physical models and optimization methods for the quantification*

To extract quantitative information from a signal sampled in the spectroscopic domain t_n, the signal has to be modeled. For this purpose, parametric and physical models can be employed. The physical models are more relevant than the parametric ones since their parameters have a true physical and biological meaning, while parametric models are purely mathematical. The parameters of the models are then estimated by solving an inverse problem using optimization techniques.

The complex signal $\check{S}$ as a function of echo time (t_n) for a gradient echo sequence in a medium with water and lipids can be expressed by the following equation:

$$\check{S}(t_n) = \left(\rho_w e^{-R_{2w}^* t_n} + \sum_{k=1}^{k} \rho_k e^{(2\pi i f_k - R_{2k}^* t_n)t_n}\right) e^{2\pi i \psi t_n} \quad [10.2]$$

where ρ_w represents the proton density of water and lipids, and $R_2{}^*{}_w$ is the transverse relaxation rate of water. Contrary to water, lipids consist of a combination of several spectral components, each characterized by proton density ρ_k, a frequency shift with respect to water f_k and a transverse relaxation rate $R_2{}^*{}_k$. ψ represents the frequency shift due to the inhomogeneities of the B_0 field. The k components of lipids observable in MRI correspond to the different chemical groups composing the triglycerides. Eight of them can be distinguished, as illustrated in Figure 10.1.

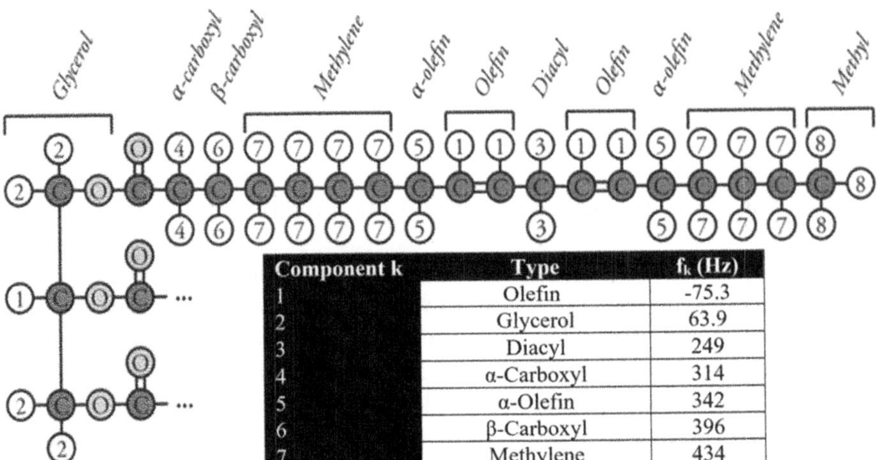

Component k	Type	f_k (Hz)
1	Olefin	-75.3
2	Glycerol	63.9
3	Diacyl	249
4	α-Carboxyl	314
5	α-Olefin	342
6	β-Carboxyl	396
7	Methylene	434
8	Methyl	485

Figure 10.1. *Triglyceride molecule represented with its glycerol group and linoleic acid. The protons of the different chemical groups yield eight specific resonances (k) characterized by a frequency shift fk with respect to the water's resonance*

The model's equation contains 27 parameters. In MR imaging, this type of equation is impossible to solve because the number of unknowns is too large compared to the number of echos. In addition, the problem is ill-conditioned, which requires sampling the frequency domain with a higher temporal resolution than what is achievable. Hence, simplifying strategies have been proposed, consisting of reducing the number of unknowns using a priori knowledge without affecting the estimation of key parameters. In this context, the proton densities of water and lipids are two important parameters because they enable the calculation of the quantitative value of the quantitiy of lipids, the proton density fat fraction (PDFF).

Simplification approaches consist of expressing a single lipid proton density from the proton densities ρ_k of each resonance by introducing weighting coefficients to represent their relative importance (Hines et al. 2009; Leporq et al. 2013). The values of these coefficients have been calibrated using proton spectroscopy measurements of oils and human fatty tissues (Hamilton et al. 2011). These studies have also provided exact measurements of frequency shifts, which can be set in the model. Another approach consists of considering only one transverse relaxation term for water and the different lipid components (Horng et al. 2013). Then, only three unknowns remain in the simplified model, which can be written as:

$$\check{S}(t_n) = \left(\rho_w + \rho_f \sum_{k=1}^{8} C_k e^{2\pi i f_k t_n}\right) e^{2\pi i \check{\psi} t_n} \quad [10.3]$$

where ρ_f is the global fat proton density, C_k is the weighting coefficients of each spectral component, with a sum equal to 1. $\check{\psi}$ becomes a complex term whose imaginary part represents the transverse relaxation rate R_2* and the real part corresponds to the frequency shift related to B_0 field inhomogeneities (ΔB_0) such that:

$$\check{\psi} = \Delta B_0 + iR_2^* \quad [10.4]$$

Such a model enables the estimation of proton densities of water and fat, as well as the common relaxation rate. The fat fraction can be then deduced for each voxel as:

$$\text{PDFF} = \left(\frac{\rho_f}{\rho_w + \rho_f}\right) \times 100 \quad [10.5]$$

The Dixon two-point method with spin echo was the first one to provide a true decomposition of water and fat signals using two echos: a standard echo and a second echo acquired by shifting the refocusing pulse with respect to the echo's center such that the signal is encoded when the water protons and the main lipid component (methylene-CH2) are in phase opposition (Dixon 1984). However, this approach did not allow for accurate PDFF quantification due to confounding factors, such as the integration of all of the lipid spectral components, and it did not take into account the T_2* decay. On the other hand, this approach is limited by "swap artifacts" (inversion of the water and lipid signals) caused by not taking into account the frequency shift related to B_0 inhomogeneities.

More recently, the IDEAL approach (Iterative Decomposition of water and fat with Echo Assymetry and Least-square estimation) has enabled the quantification of PDFF (Reeder et al. 2005, 2007). This method employs several echos and the equation parameters are obtained after linearizing the problem, which optimizes the computation time considerably. At further development stages, different confounding factors have been included, such as the integration of T_2* decay into the model, taking into account all of the lipid spectral components, and the effects of complex Gaussian noise (Liu et al. 2007; Hines et al. 2009). Nevertheless, the problem remains ill-conditioned when the frequency shift related to field inhomogeneities is close to the frequency shift between water and lipids, additionally producing swap artifacts, in particular in the areas with strong field gradients due to magnetic susceptibility. The issue of "chemical ambiguity" can be solved by including a priori knowledge in the optimization procedure (Hernando et al. 2010).

In order to tackle the effects of B_0 field inhomogeneities, research teams have proposed to quantify PDFF and the relaxation time T_2* from the signal's magnitude (O'Regan et al. 2008). This approach provides the advantages of reduced effects of the complex Gaussian noise and robust and accurate quantification of PDFF. However, the loss of information related to the magnitude conversion does not allow for quantification of PDFF greater than 50%. For this reason, such methods cannot be used to investigate adipose tissues and are restricted to steatosis studies (presence of fat in organs).

Although simplifying the signal equation yields a model function that can be exploited for PDFF and T_2* relaxation time quantification in imaging, using a priori knowledge leads to a loss of information. In fact, the pre-calibration of the contribution of the eight lipid spectral components by attributing predetermined parameters supposes that the composition of fatty acids of the triglycerides does not change, which is not the case in practice. On the other hand, determining each component's contribution could help quantify the fatty acid amount in lipids. For this purpose, a research team has proposed an intermediate solution that includes sufficient prior information to solve the system with a suitable sampling of the spectroscopic domain while providing measurements of the lipid composition (Hamilton et al. 2011). The number of protons per triglyceride n_K is quantified for each spectral component as a function of three parameters related to the chemical structure of triglycerides: (i) *ndb*, the average number of double bonds per triglyceride; (ii) *nmidb*, the average number of double bonds per triglyceride interrupted by a methylene group; (iii) *CL*, the average carbon chain length. An illustration is represented in Figure 10.2.

The model function (equation [10.3]) becomes:

$$\check{S}(t_n) = \left(\rho_w . n_w + \rho_f \sum_{k=1}^{8} n_k(ndb, nmidb, CL) e^{2\pi i f_k t_n} \right) e^{2\pi i \psi t_n} \qquad [10.6]$$

It should be noted that this reformulation leads to a change of variables since ρ_w and ρ_f do not represent the proton densities of water and lipids but the number of molecules of water and triglycerides, respectively. n_w is the number of protons per water molecule (i.e. $n_w = 2$).

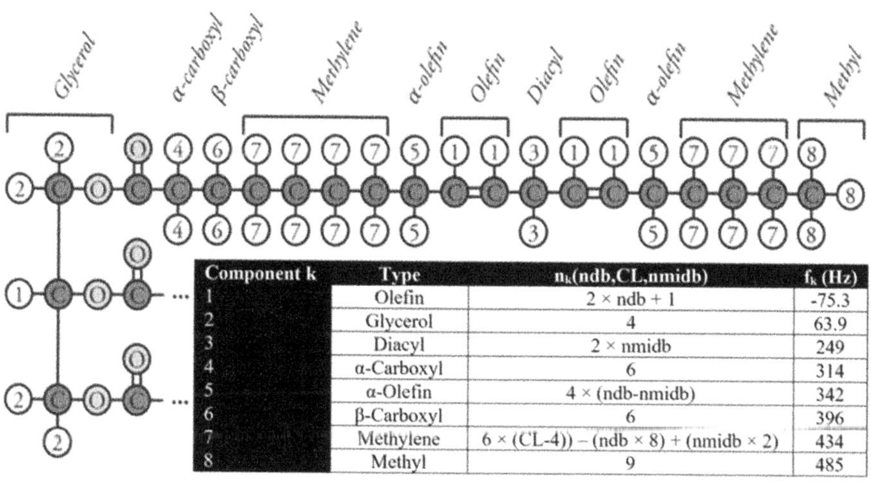

Component k	Type	n_k(ndb,CL,nmidb)	f_k (Hz)
1	Olefin	2 × ndb + 1	-75.3
2	Glycerol	4	63.9
3	Diacyl	2 × nmidb	249
4	α-Carboxyl	6	314
5	α-Olefin	4 × (ndb-nmidb)	342
6	β-Carboxyl	6	396
7	Methylene	6 × (CL-4)) – (ndb × 8) + (nmidb × 2)	434
8	Methyl	9	485

Figure 10.2. *Triglyceride molecule represented with its glycerol group and linoleic acid. The number of protons nk of each spectral component k is expressed as a function of three parameters ndb, nmidb and CL*

Starting from this new model function (equation [10.6]), Peterson and Månsson have modified the IDEAL method to estimate these parameters and deduce from them the fractions of saturated, monounsaturated and polyunsaturated fatty acids simultaneously with the measurement of PDFF and T_2* (Peterson and Månsson 2013). However, the degrees of freedom remain numerous, requiring the acquisition of a large number of echos to solve the system, which can lead to issues in the robustness of parameter estimation.

To reduce the degrees of freedom of the model, Bydder et al. (2011) have shown that there was a heuristic link between the main fatty acids found in vegetal oils and in the *living* (fatty acid chain length comprised between 16 and 20 saturated, monounsaturated, and diunsaturated carbons), enabling *CL* and *nmidb* to be expressed as a function of *ndb*:

$$\mathrm{CL} = 16.8 + 0.25\ \mathrm{ndb}\ \text{and}\ \mathrm{nmidb} = 0.093\ \mathrm{ndb}^2 \qquad [10.7]$$

From this work, an approach was proposed to simultaneously quantify the composition of lipids, adipose tissue, and T_2* without requiring an additional unknown. To do so, Leporq et al. (2014) proposed a segmented approach, focusing first on the temporal evolution of the unwrapped phase of the signal to measure the frequency displacement related to B_0 field inhomogeneities (ΔB_0) (first order dephasing) and the phase at the origin (zero-order dephasing). The phase of the signal is then corrected and the "demodulated" real part images are reconstructed (Leporq et al. 2014). This simplifies the model by neglecting the imaginary part of the signal and the dephasing term related to the field inhomogeneities as:

$$\mathrm{real}(\mathrm{S}(\mathrm{t_n})) = \left(\rho_w . n_w + \rho_f \sum_{k=1}^{8} n_k(\mathrm{ndb}, \mathrm{nmidb}, \mathrm{CL}) e^{2\pi i f_k t_n} \right) e^{-R_2^* t_n} \qquad [10.8]$$

A first nonlinear optimization enables the estimation of R_2* and PDFF by considering a model with fixed C_k coefficients. The R_2* can then be replaced in the equation above and, by means of two other subsequent optimizations, *ndb* and *nmidb* can be estimated to retrieve the lipid composition.

In the previous lines, we mentioned that the frequency shift related to the B_0 field inhomogeneities was a superposition of undesired effects and an inherent physical property of tissues, magnetic susceptibility. Thus, the maps of field inhomogeneity reconstructed with the method described above provide access to such information.

Some research groups have shown that it is possible to decompose the field related to the B_0 inhomogeneities into two contributions: an external field composed of low spatial frequencies that combines the macroscopic aspects, such as the effects of the shim coils or other undesired effects, and an internal field with high frequencies that results from the effects of internal susceptibility of the tissues (Schweser et al. 2017). To separate the two contributions, several approaches have been proposed. Among these, we can cite the methods based on filtering techniques such as those based on homodyne high-pass filtering of the complex image (Abduljalil et al. 2003), on a polynomial correction of the phase images; or methods using parametric models, in particular those employing spherical harmonics (SHARP (Schweser et al. 2011) method, followed by V-SHARP (Wu et Liu 2011) and RESHARP (Sun et Wilman 2014)) and the projection onto a dipole field (PDF method (Liu et al. 2011)) that exploits the principle of orthogonality between perturbations contributing to the internal and external field. The PDF and RESHARP methods are the most used ones.

To estimate the magnetic susceptibility of tissues, an analytical expression of the internal field B_{int} induced by a distribution of susceptibility χ has been introduced by integrating Maxwell's equations (Salomir et al. 2003; de Rochefort et al. 2010). By considering Maxwell's magnetostatic equations with a Lorentz-sphere correction term, we obtain:

$$\mathrm{B_{int}}(\mathbf{r}) = \mathrm{B_0} \int_{\mathrm{r} \neq \mathrm{r}'} \chi_{\mathrm{int}}(\vec{\mathrm{r}}) \frac{3\cos^2(\theta_{\mathrm{rr}'}) - 1}{4\pi|\mathbf{r}' - \mathbf{r}|^3} \mathrm{d}^3\mathrm{r}' \qquad [10.9]$$

where $\boldsymbol{r}$ is the position vector, θ is the angle between the position vector and the $\overrightarrow{B_0}$ field and B_0 is the value of the applied static field.

Overall, the internal field B_{int} can be considered as a linear system whose transfer function h(θ) is the equation of the magnetic field emitted by a unitary dipole, with the susceptibility distribution χ_{int} given as an input. Thus, we obtain:

$$\mathrm{B_{int}} = \mathrm{B_0}\left(\chi_{\mathrm{int}} \otimes \mathrm{h}(\theta)\right) \qquad [10.10]$$

In the frequency domain (or k-space), we have:

$$\mathrm{F(B_{int})} = \mathrm{B_0}\ \mathrm{F}(\chi_{\mathrm{int}}) \times \mathrm{H(k)} \qquad [10.11]$$

F represents the Fourier transform and H(k) is the dipolar kernel in k-space:

$$\mathrm{H(k)} = \left(\frac{1}{3} - \frac{\mathrm{k_z^2}}{\mathrm{k^2}}\right) \qquad [10.12]$$

Thus, calculating χ_{int} consists of inverting the equation above in k-space or performing a deconvolution in the image domain. However, this inversion leads to an ill-posed problem since the kernel can become equal to zero when $k^2 = 3\ k_z^2$, which represents a conical region in k-space observed from the three spatial dimensions and a spin orientation θ with respect to the B_0 field equal to the magic angle (54.7°). In such cases, the consequences are amplified noise, and artifacts in the reconstructed image (streaking artifact).

Several methods have been proposed to tackle this problem. Among the first ones, there were methods with thresholding of the transfer function and those based on Wiener deconvolution. Other approaches using regularizations have shown good performance in terms of stability and artifact suppression. de Rochefort et al. (2010) have introduced additional regularization terms based on spatial a priori data extracted from magnitude images to penalize the contours, together with boundary conditions and signal-to-noise conditions.

10.2.3. *Clinical and preclinical applications*

We have described that the artifacts of the gradient echo scans can be exploited to simultaneously retrieve quantitative parameters for tissue characterization. The latter has several clinical applications, which mainly include hepatic diseases related to metabolism disorders and obesity. In fact, such patients have a high risk of developing nonalcoholic fatty liver diseases (NAFLD). These diseases are often asymptomatic and can evolve into severe conditions where steatosis (presence of intrahepatic fat) is accompanied by inflammation or fibrosis, the so-called steatohepatitis. If left untreated, these patients can develop cirrhosis or hepatocellular carcinomas. The methods described here could be an alternative to hepatic biopsies for monitoring such patients. Besides PDFF, which is capable of precisely measuring the amount of intrahepatic fat, Xie et al. (2013) have shown that magnetic susceptibility could enable the evaluation of fibrosis because the macromolecules that compose it increase the diamagnetism of the tissues. In chronic hepatic diseases, this is particularly important given that fibrosis is the main prognosis factor and influences the therapeutic strategy. Leporq et al. (2017) have shown that the simultaneous measurement of adiposity, lipid composition and magnetic susceptibility can provide a complete and quick analysis of the liver in a single breath-hold to distinguish simple steatoses from steatohepatitis in patients with NAFLD.

Research works have exploited these techniques to evaluate bone health in osteoporosis. In the context of femoral bone marrow, while simple adiposity measurements via PDFF appear limited due to age-related confounding factors, considerable differences in lipid compositions, especially an increase of saturated fatty acids fraction, have been reported in postmenopausal patients compared to premenopausal ones (Martel et al. 2018). On the other hand, different lipid profiles have been observed within a population of postmenopausal women between primary osteoporosis and secondary osteoporosis in response to glucocorticoid treatment (Martel et al. 2019). Moreover, it has been shown that magnetic susceptibility measurements enable the evaluation of trabecular density in the calcaneum (Diefenbach et al. 2019). Finally, simultaneity could provide an overview of bone health for monitoring osteoporosis via the evaluation of lipid metabolism and trabecular density.

Proof-of-concept investigations in healthy volunteers have also shown the value of simultaneous measurements of lipid composition and adiposity in nutrition studies for multi-organ monitoring of the therapeutic fasting effect (Viallon et al. 2019) or in monitoring an overfeeding protocol (Nemeth et al. 2019).

We have seen that, by exploiting the information obtained from scans that sample the echo time dimension (or acquisitions sensitive to chemical shifts), relevant multiparametric information can be extracted. In the following, we cover other approaches capable of extracting multiparametric information from gradient echo acquisitions.

10.3. Multiparametric MRI using steady-state acquisitions in repeated fast sequences

10.3.1. *Steady state in a stationary sequence without transverse effects*

In general, gradient echo sequences consist of quickly repeating (at every *TR*) (Brown et al. 2014) a radiofrequency pulse with an angle α, eventually accompanied by a slice-selection gradient. Between two consecutive pulses, a series of gradients partially cover the k-space. We have mentioned before that the apparent transverse relaxation modulates the contrast of this type of sequence through the echo time *TE*. It is also well known that the flip angle α and *TR* both affect longitudinal magnetization. Indeed, if the transverse magnetization is considered negligible between two repetitions, the signal obtained after some identical repetitions, at the "Ernst's" equilibrium for the transverse magnetization, can be simply described as:

$$M_t = M_0 E_2^* \sin\alpha \frac{(1 - E_1)}{1 - E_1 \cos\alpha} \quad [10.13]$$

with $E_1 = \exp(-R_1\, TR)$ and $E_2^* = \exp(-R_2^* TE)$, where R_1 and R_2* are the inverse relaxation rates of T_1 and T_2^*, respectively. For this equilibrium, several important flip angles can be defined (Buxton et al. 1987):

– the Ernst angle, which maximizes the signal for a given tissue:

$$\cos\alpha_{Ernst} = E_1 \quad [10.14]$$

– the Buxton angle that maximizes the contrast (e.g. the sensitivity to T_1 variations when a contrast agent is injected):

$$\cos\alpha_{Buxton} = \frac{1 - 2E_1}{E_1 - 2} \quad [10.15]$$

This simple description of the NMR signal is based on the hypothesis of effective suppression of transverse magnetization between repetitions.

The first mechanism is the apparent transverse relaxation which is a combination of the intrinsic irreversible transverse relaxation T_2 and the local dephasing effects, which are more or less reversible. The decay via transverse relaxation between two TR ($E_2 = \exp(-R_2\, TR)$, with R_2 being the inverse transverse relaxation rate of T_2)

is however weak for fast repetitions (T_2 is of the order of 100–1,000 ms and TR is around 10 ms).

Diffusion is another irreversible phenomenon occurring in these sequences. To consider its effects, we should describe a sequence design element of the so-called spoiling gradients (Brown et al. 2014), which will be called here the residual gradients. These gradients are consistently applied in the so-called "unbalanced" sequences. When inserted after the imaging gradients, the spoiling gradients cause a dephasing along the same given direction between two RF pulses. As a result, the average transverse magnetization in a voxel is zero before applying the next RF pulse. Since these gradients have a dephasing role, they cause signal attenuation due to diffusion. To characterize this effect, we can simply express the distance a over which a dephasing of 2π is produced and introduce the value of diffusion attenuation between two TR:

$$E_d = \exp -bD = \exp -\left(\frac{2\pi}{a}\right)^2 TR \times D \qquad [10.16]$$

with D as the free-water diffusion coefficient and $b = \left(\frac{2\pi}{a}\right)^2 TR$ as the sequence's sensitivity to diffusion. Typically, the residual distance is smaller than the voxel size, which is of the order of millimeters in clinical routine, TR is of the order of 10 ms and D is close to the free-water diffusion coefficient of 2×10^{-9} m^2.s^{-1}. We can observe that diffusion is negligible in the residual gradient between two repetitions ($E_d \sim 0.9992$ with the values above).

Therefore, in practice, we can seldom obtain sufficient destruction of transverse magnetization in fast sequences, either via transverse relaxation, or via diffusion, and hence this common approximation has to be reconsidered. The dephasing produced by the residual gradients must be taken into account to rigorously describe the obtained contrast.

10.3.2. *Transverse effects considerations for describing steady states*

The existence of non-negligible transverse magnetization implies a dependency on the history of phase coherence that results, on the one hand, from the gradients, and, on the other hand, from the radiofrequency pulses (since the pulses can have different phases at each repetition).

The residual gradient is applied along a fixed direction; here, we suppose that its spatial coordinate is x. Then, the magnetization can be conveniently expressed as two polynomes in the Z variable:

$$M_l\ (x) = \sum_{k=-\infty}^{k=+\infty} m_{l,k}\, Z^{-k} \quad [10.17]$$

$$M_t\ (x) = \sum_{k=-\infty}^{k=+\infty} m_{t,k}\, Z^{-k} \quad [10.18]$$

M_l represents the longitudinal magnetization, and M_t is the transverse magnetization. By defining $Z = \exp -2i\pi x/a$, this formulation represents a discrete Fourier series, which corresponds to the formalism of configuration states and extended phase graphs (Hennig 1991), which are also used for designing radiofrequency pulses (Pauly et al. 1991). Instead of being described by two coefficients, the magnetization is now expressed via vectors of coefficients corresponding to the longitudinal and transverse components, respectively, for each voxel of an image. Indeed, since the dephasing is the same between two TR, the magnetization can be represented as such a discrete series.

This formalism is convenient because it enables relatively simple modeling and manipulation of the events that affect the magnetization via applied gradients, relaxation and diffusion (Freed et al. 2001; Weigel 2015). Indeed:

– residual gradients shift the indexes k of the series that describes the transverse magnetization;

– relaxation attenuates all of the coefficients, notably except for the coefficient $k = 0$ of the longitudinal magnetization that relaxes toward thermal equilibrium;

– diffusion is taken into account by filtering the series (e.g. by a Gaussian filter in the case of free diffusion) (Kaiser et al. 1974);

– flip angles "mix" the coefficients between longitudinal and transverse series.

The latter mixing effect that results from the radiofrequency pulses is more difficult to comprehend. Indeed, up to now, we have considered pulses producing flip angles with respect to the axis of the B_0 field, but without specifying the rotation axis in the transverse plane. However, repeated sequences employ periodic phase cycling. This feature is often called radiofrequency spoiling (Zur et al. 1991) and is performed by incrementing the phase by $\Delta\varphi$. Hence, at the rth repetition, the phase of the radiofrequency pulse is increased by the value $r.\Delta\varphi$, yielding a quadratic evolution of the phase. After a certain number of repetitions with pulses of the same amplitude but with a quadratically changing phase, a dynamic steady state is achieved. The measured transverse magnetization is still demodulated with the same phase as the radiofrequency pulse and it can be shown that the demodulated order $k = 0$ is stationary. Apart from specific variations (Hardy et al. 1996; Heule et al. 2014), the order $k = 0$ of the transverse component is typically the effectively measured one (the residual gradient is applied after readout). The other orders, with an average value of zero, have a negligible effect on the measurement, although they are still present and store a part of magnetization that contributes to the order $k = 0$ after some repetitions. The formation of this coherence corresponds to stimulated echos. In summary, the order $k = 0$ corresponds to a superposition of several terms that are more or less combined in phase, depending on the chosen increment.

Figure 10.3 shows some examples of the effects of different parameters of the residual gradient, flip angle and phase increment on the order k = 0, illustrating how the signal can be modulated using these sequence parameters.

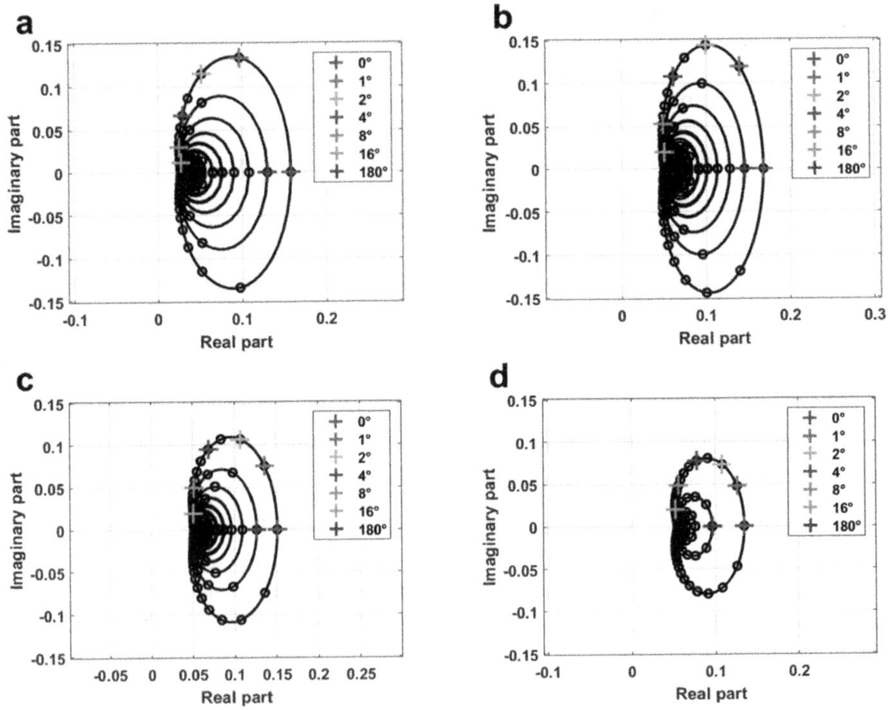

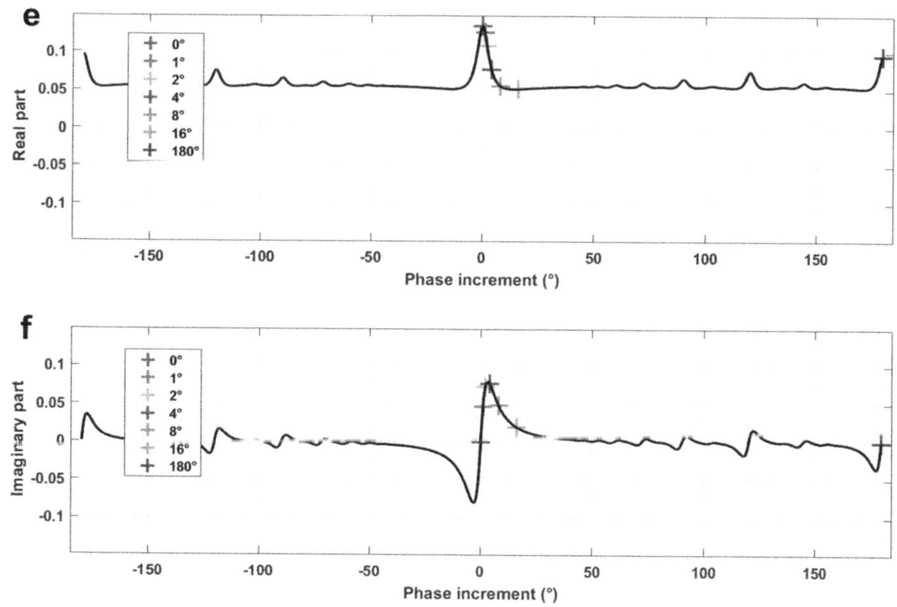

Figure 10.3. *(a) Complex-plane representation of the real and imaginary parts of the NMR signal at dynamic steady-state for the order k = 0 simulated for a flip angle of 25°, TR of 12 ms, and a diffusion coefficient D of 2 × 10^{-9} $m^2 \cdot s^{-1}$ with phase increment varying between – 180° and 180°. (b) Complex-plane representation of the real and imaginary parts of the NMR signal at dynamic steady state for the order k = 0 simulated for a flip angle of 25°, TR of 12 ms and a diffusion coefficient D of 2 × 10^{-9} $m^2.s^{-1}$ with phase increment varying between – 180° and 180°. For a color version of this figure, see www.iste.co.uk/ratiney-beuf/challenges.zip*

COMMENT ON FIGURE 10.3.– *Black circles represent each phase increment: (a) for T_1 = 1,500 ms and T_2 = 800 ms, with a characteristic distance of 1.25 mm; b) for T_1 = 800 ms and T_2 = 500 ms and a characteristic distance of 1.25 mm; c) for T_1 = 800 ms and T_2 = 250 ms and a characteristic distance of 1.25 mm; d) for T_1 = 800 ms and T_2 = 250 ms and a characteristic distance of 0.3125 mm. The (e) and (f) plots represent the real and imaginary parts of the signal, respectively, for case (d) as a function of phase increment. The colored crosses represent the signal for specific phase increment values (0°, 1°, 2°, 4°, 8° and 180°). These plots show the considerable effect of the parameters T_1 and T_2 on the signal at equilibrium, but also the effect of diffusion weighting, which depends on the residual gradient. It should be noted that the obtained equilibrium can be very different, in particular depending on the two parameters, the residual gradient and phase increment. In addition, the phase with which the stimulated echos combine produces* *an equilibrium signal with an additional phase that adds up to the effects related to chemical shifts and susceptibility described in section 10.2. Figure 10.4 illustrates this phase stemming from the combination of stimulated echos (de Rochefort et al. 2016).*

This phenomenon has not been extensively exploited so far, but has significant implications due to the fact that the basic sequences of MRI manufacturers have different settings for these sequence parameters (direction and amplitude of the residual gradient, as well as phase increments) that are not usually accessible to the user and are rarely stored in the scan's metadata. As a result, this limits the possibility of quantifying and reproducing contrasts obtained on different systems, which does not allow for properly controlled experimental conditions.

In conclusion, the approaches seeking to extract physical parameters (for relaxometry) from fast acquisitions of this kind often neglect the transverse effects, which is mostly an unjustified approximation considering the value of the applied residual gradient. The phase increment leads to variabilities in the measured signal that are seldom taken into account. These two elements can modulate the signal depending on diffusion and relaxation times, thereby providing the opportunity to optimize the contrast and quantify the underlying physical parameters by means of fast sequences.

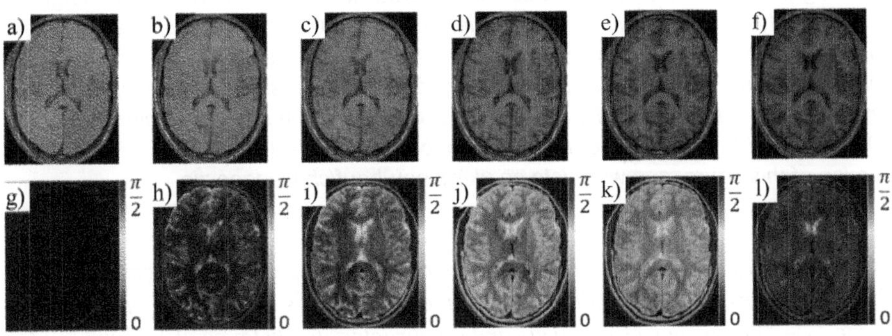

Figure 10.4. *Brain slice acquired at the center of a 3D volume for several fast gradient echo scans with a residual gradient along the readout at 1.5 T with the following parameters: acquired voxel size 1.25 x 1.25 x 2.5 mm³, TR = 12 ms, flip angle 25°, a = 0.3125 mm, and phase increments of (a, g) 0°, (b, h) 1°, (c, i) 2°, (d, j) 4°, (e, k) 8°, (f, l) 16°. For a color version of this figure, see www.iste.co.uk/ratiney-beuf/challenges.zip*

COMMENT ON FIGURE 10.4.– *The first line (a, b, c, d, e, f) corresponds to signal amplitude, while the second line (g, h, i, j, k, l) to the phase once TE dephasing effects, identical for all of the scans, have been removed. Clear changes in amplitude and phase depending on the tissue are visible, illustrating the strong effect of phase cycling on the NMR signal.*

10.3.3. Uses in multiparametric quantitative imaging

In section 10.3.2, we have seen how the magnetization can be modeled by means of two polynomials describing the longitudinal and transverse components, respectively, for each voxel. We have seen that the order $k = 0$ is generally the one that contributes the most to the image signal. Here, we consider a case where several measurements have been performed using a steady-state sequence with a fixed flip angle, always of order $k = 0$, but with different acquisition parameters (such as the residual gradient and the phase increment). For simplicity, the reconstruction problem is expressed voxel by voxel and we consider that the dynamic equilibrium state at each point of the image can be written as a function of derived variables E_1, E_2, E_d, and α, the effective flip angle in the considered voxel that has to be quantified. The complex signal corresponding to the n-th measurement is expressed as:

$$S_{0,n} = M_0\ E_2^*\exp i\varphi_0 \times m_{t,0}(E_1\ , E_2\ , E_d\ , \alpha, f_n, a_n, \Delta\varphi_n) = M_e\ \times m_n \qquad [10.19]$$

where M_0 is the magnetization at thermal equilibrium, E_2^* and φ_0 are terms that take into account the apparent relaxation and dephasing at echo time (as previously described). The term $m_{t,0}$ corresponds to the model: it depends on the parameters that have to be quantified, which are the same for all of the acquisitions $(E_1\ , E_2\ , E_d\ , \alpha)$, and on acquisition parameters that vary from one scan to another $(f_n, a_n, \Delta\varphi_n)$. The parameter f_n is introduced to account for the different flip angles between the acquisitions, whose absolute value αf_n is not known, but its relative variation is well controlled. Thus, from a series of N measurements $S_{0,n}$, the data can be fitted to the model to determine $M_e = M_0\ E_2^*\exp i\varphi_0$, and the combination of $E_1\ , E_2\ , E_d\ , \alpha$ that is the most relevant considering the measurements, diffusion and the effective flip angle, that is, performing parametric quantitative relaxometry imaging.

This approach can be expressed in generic terms as a least-squares minimization:

$$\min_{M_e, E_1\ , E_2\ , E_d\ , \alpha} \sum_{n=1}^{n=N} \left\|S_{0,n} - M_e\ \times m_n\right\|^2 \qquad [10.20]$$

Such a problem can be solved using iterative algorithms, such as the Gauss–Newton algorithm (Leroi et al. 2018, 2020; de Rochefort 2018a), for example. The latter implies calculating the Jacobian matrix, which is defined as:

$$J_n = \begin{bmatrix} real(m_n) & real\left(\frac{\partial m_n}{\partial R1}\right) & real\left(\frac{\partial m_n}{\partial R2}\right) & real\left(\frac{\partial m_n}{\partial D}\right) & real\left(\frac{\partial m_n}{\partial \alpha}\right) \\ imag(m_n) & imag\left(\frac{\partial m_n}{\partial R1}\right) & imag\left(\frac{\partial m_n}{\partial R2}\right) & imag\left(\frac{\partial m_n}{\partial D}\right) & imag\left(\frac{\partial m_n}{\partial \alpha}\right) \end{bmatrix} \quad [10.21]$$

$$J = \begin{bmatrix} J_1 \\ \vdots \\ J_N \end{bmatrix} \quad [10.22]$$

The "optimal" series of measurements can then be defined using protocol optimization approaches. For this purpose, the Fisher information matrix is employed:

$$FIM = \frac{|M_e|^2}{\sigma^2} J^H J \quad [10.23]$$

In this expression, the real and imaginary parts are separated, and it is hypothesized that each measurement includes Gaussian noise with a mean of zero and a constant variance σ^2. The error σ_i of an unbiased estimator θ_i (M_e, R_1, R_2, D or α) is then constrained by the Cramér–Rao lower bound:

$$\sigma_i \geq CRLB_i = \sqrt{(FIM^{-1})_{ii}} \quad [10.24]$$

Therefore, an optimization criterion can be defined, for example, minimization of the sum of relative errors of the corrected parameters:

$$CF = \sum_{i=1}^{i=N_{par}} \frac{{\sigma_i}^2}{{\theta_i}^2} \quad [10.25]$$

At this point, we need to tackle a pure problem of minimization in a large space (the space of experimental possibilities of combinations of flip angles, phase increments, gradients and, eventually, TR) to which we can apply stochastic optimization algorithms to obtain a satisfying solution (Valabregue and de Rochefort 2016; Leroi et al. 2018, 2020) (see Figure 10.5 for an illustration of this principle).

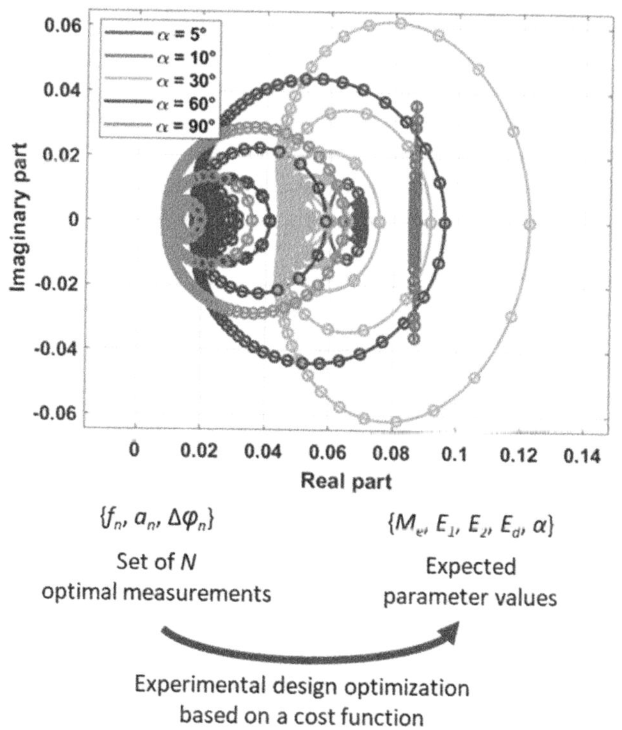

Figure 10.5. *Principle of protocol optimization. For a color version of this figure, see www.iste.co.uk/ratiney-beuf/challenges.zip*

COMMENT ON FIGURE 10.5.– *Among all of the possibilities available in terms of sequence parameters (different angles parametrized by f_n, characteristic distances parametrized by a_n, and phase increment $\Delta\varphi_n$), the goal is to find a set of N points (represented as black circles) that minimizes a cost function for a set of expected values of signal amplitude, relaxation time, diffusion coefficient and effective flip angle. Once this optimization is performed, we obtain a set of N measurements to be performed, from which corrections can be made to determine the sought physical parameters R_1, R_2, apparent diffusion coefficient and α.*

10.3.4. *Clinical and preclinical applications*

Mapping quantitative parameters such as R_1, R_2, and apparent diffusion coefficients on different systems responds to the need of comparing populations among them in an absolute and reproducible way, or to follow up the evolution of these parameters in the same patient over time regarding a physiopathological process.

A limitation of such quantifications lies in the diversity of quantification techniques, with some requiring long acquisition times and sometimes high specific absorption rates (SAR). The variability of sequence implementations with some approximations that are not always justified and of different correction techniques is also a source of bias. To reduce the scan time and the SAR, fast sequences with low flip angles can be used, but they need to take into account the residual gradients and phase increment as well as include appropriate modeling.

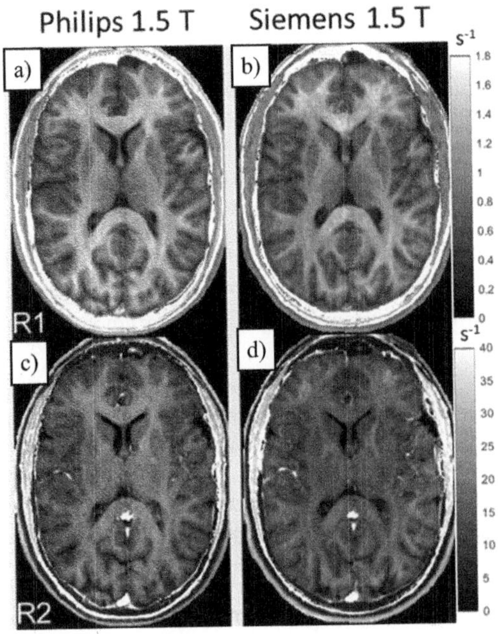

Figure 10.6. *Slice of a 3D volume of the brain after correction with 13 different optimized contrasts providing similar parametric maps of R_1 and R_2 in the same subject at 1.5 T for two different manufacturers: (a and b) maps of R_1 and (c and d) maps of R_2*

To illustrate how these biases are reduced, let us consider two applications. In the first one (Figure 10.6), scans are performed on two systems from different manufacturers for fast three-dimensional relaxometry of the brain in the same subject (de Rochefort et al. 2017).

In the second one (Figure 10.7), the goal is to correct the inhomogeneities of a surface coil used in transmit/receive mode on a mouse to obtain images with uniform contrast without flip angle variation effects (Guillot et al. 2017; de Rochefort et al. 2018b).

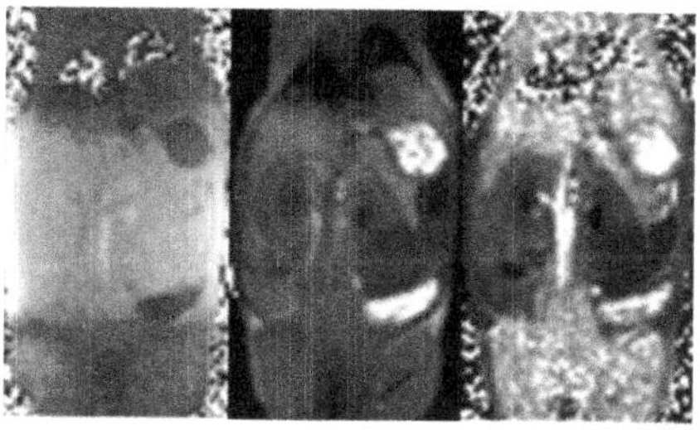

a) b) c)

Figure 10.7. *Slice of a 3D volume from whole-body imaging of a mouse at 1.5 T with a surface coil. Since the sensitivity profile of the coil is the same for transmission and reception (a, correction result), it is possible to reconstruct a T_1-weighted map that is insensitive to transmit and receive inhomogeneities (b), as well as a parametric map of R2 (c). In these images, the different regions in the kidneys (cortex and medulla) can be distinguished, together with a tumor from a xenograft in the left kidney (on the right as per radiology convention)*

10.3.5. *Conclusion*

We have seen that the so-called "spoiled" MRI sequences that involve repeated excitations with a residual gradient and periodic phase cycling have to take into account the evolution of transverse magnetization in clinical imaging situations. They lead to a complex dynamic steady state that can be exploited to generate phase contrast that is related, for example, to the relaxation times and diffusion and to perform multiparametric imaging. Protocol optimization methods can help determine the acquisition parameters required for the accurate quantification of this bias. Proof-of-concept works aim to reduce the variability between different imaging systems and the dependence on the inhomogeneities of the excitation radiofrequency field.

10.4. MRI fingerprinting

10.4.1. *Concept*

Initially introduced by Ma et al. (2013), the MR fingerprinting (MRF) method is an alternative to quantitative MRI methods based on analytical models of the NMR signal. Instead of using theoretical considerations on the signal's evolution around an equilibrium state and correcting an equation to fit the data, the underlying idea of the MRF method is that a theoretical knowledge of the nuclear magnetization's evolution is not required to generate an MRI sequence as long as its temporal behavior can be simulated in silico. Thus, the MRF technique includes a new approach for obtaining parametric MRI maps, consisting of the following steps, described in Figure 10.8:

– Step 0: design of an MRF acquisition pattern, that is, an MRI sequence sensitive to several biomarkers (e.g. T_1 and T_2) and composed of a series of scans with parameters that vary over time (*TR*, *TE*, flip angles, etc.). This acquisition pattern can be optimized for a given application or simply generated randomly.

– Step 1: execute the MRF pattern on an MRI scanner to acquire a sequence of MRI images of the investigated object. In this way, a temporal signal is obtained for each pixel, called the "measured fingerprint".

– Step 2: simulate the MRF pattern thousands of times by considering virtual voxels with properties spanning a range of (e.g. T_1 = 100, 120... 3,000 ms, T_2 = 40, 50... 2,000 ms). This produces a database of "simulated fingerprints", called the "dictionary".

– Step 3: for each acquired fingerprint (for each image pixel), search for the simulated fingerprint in the dictionary that is the closest to the measured fingerprint. If the distance between the two signals is small, the parameters used during the simulation can be assigned to this pixel (matching).

– Step 4: repeat step 3 for each pixel of the acquired image to reconstruct the parametric maps of all of the parameters used during the simulation (maps of T_1, T_2, etc.).

Not only the MRF concept provides simultaneous access to several NMR parameters, but it also quantifies them. Thanks to steps 2 and 5 and to the dictionary search, the initial images can be strongly under-sampled, thereby providing considerable time gains during the scans. Acquiring all of the data with a single MRF scan also reduces the duration of MRI protocols by avoiding dead times between sequences and all of the processes of optimization and achievement of pseudo-equilibrium states. Finally, the influence of acquisition system imperfections (coils, magnet) and patient movements can be reduced, either by taking them into account in the simulations and thus by increasing the dictionary size, or by guiding the matching step with the help of complementary measurements (e.g. separate acquisitions of B_0 or B_1 maps).

10.4.2. *Different types of measurements*

From the beginning, the MRF method has shown extremely encouraging results for mapping T_1, T_2 and proton density M_0 in healthy human volunteers (Ma et al. 2013). An inversion recovery bSSFP sequence and two patterns of acquisitions (random or sinusoidal variations of the repetition time and flip angle over 1,000 points) were tested at first. Each image was acquired by means of a spiral trajectory with a variable density that rotated at each image. This approach creates noise incoherence in the images and thus aids the matching step. Overall, acquiring an MRF slice (1,000 images) takes 12.3 s with this implementation. The measurements were compared to results obtained via traditional relaxometry methods based on spin-echo acquisitions and DESPOT1 and DESPOT2 methods (Deoni et al. 2005) with correlation coefficients greater than 0.92 in all of the cases. The efficiency of MRF (calculated as precision per unit time) was also 1.85 times greater than in the DESPOT method which was at that time considered to be the most efficient method. Following this work, several types of basic sequences (FISP, GRE, SE, etc.), acquisition patterns (random, partially linear, partially sinusoidal, etc.) and k-space filling trajectories (Cartesian, EPI, radial) have been proposed for MRF (Jiang et al. 2015; Buonincontri and Sawiak 2016).

The original implementation of the MRF method has shown the capability of this approach to simultaneously and efficiently generate parametric maps representing transverse and longitudinal relaxation times. However, it is clear that the concept underlying this method can provide much more information on tissues. Conventional magnetization preparation modules, such as diffusion ones, can be included in the design of some fingerprints. Applying diffusion gradients with random amplitudes gives access to the apparent diffusion coefficient (Jiang et al. 2013). ASL-type sequences that alternate control and labeling acquisitions with durations that vary from one image to another are capable of measuring parameters of cerebral microperfusion related to blood flow (Su et al. 2016). Adding bipolar gradients (with variable amplitudes) to a bSSFP MRF sequence also enables the quantification of blood flow in large vessels (Flassbeck et al. 2019). By varying the echo time or performing quadratic phase cycling in a bSSFP sequence, quantitative T_2^* information is obtained (Rieger et al. 2017; Wang et al. 2019, Khajehim et al. 2021). Finally, using different types of multiband RF pulses, magnetization transfer information can be retrieved (West et al. 2021). A comprehensive review of the MRF methods in 2019 listed about 15 different applications, typically with several versions of acquisition patterns (Poorman et al. 2020).

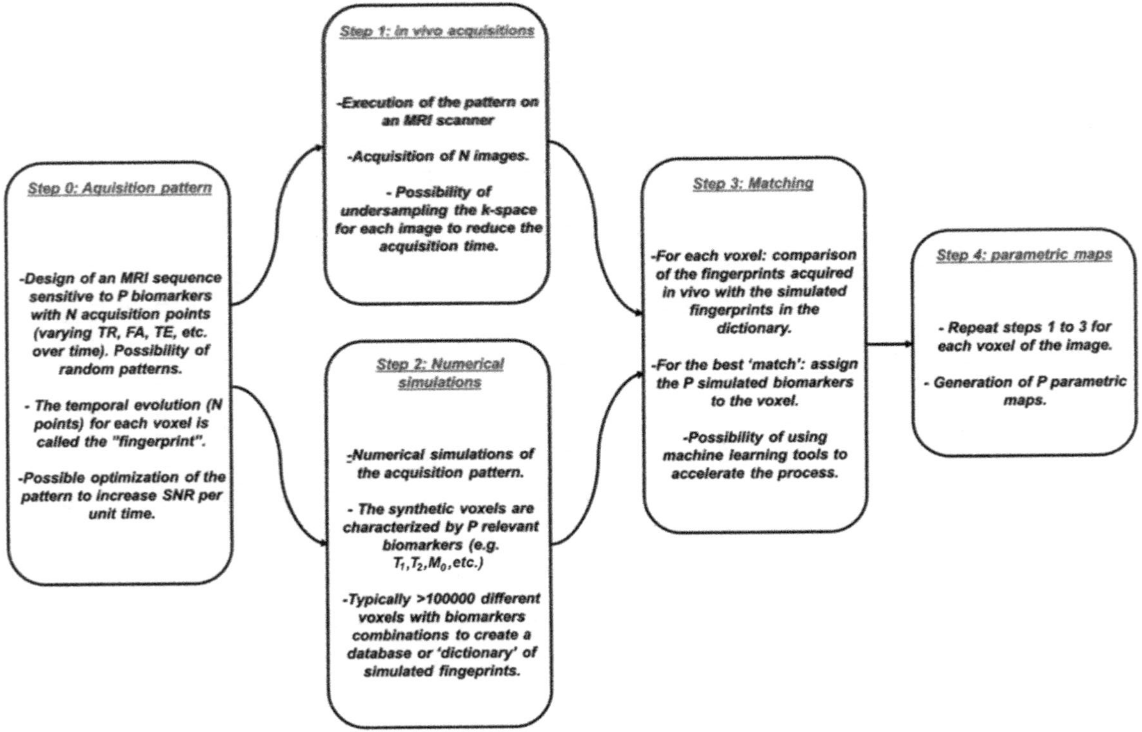

Figure 10.8. *Diagram of the MRF principle*

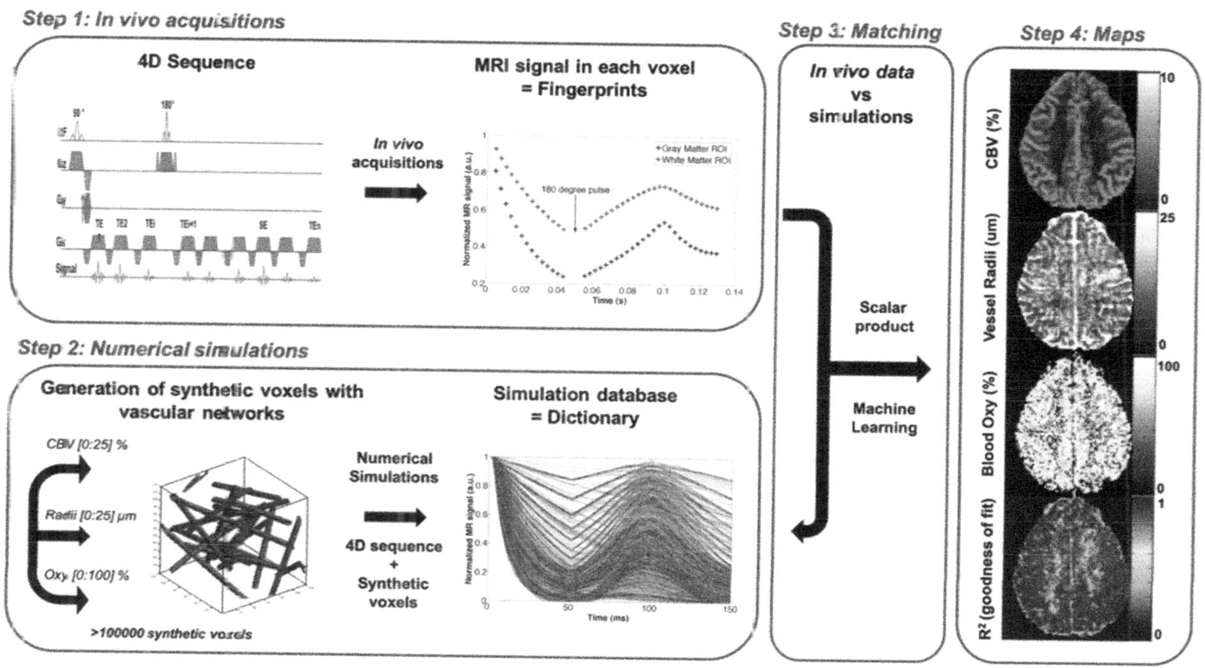

Figure 10.9. *Acquisition of vascular parameters of a human brain with the vascular MRF method. Contrary to the original MRF method, the acquisitions are performed with Cartesian trajectories and several echo times. The simulations are performed for synthetic voxels containing vascular structures with varying features (cerebral blood volume fraction (CBV), vessel size (Radia), and oxoygenation (Oxy)). For a color version of this figure, see www.iste.co.uk/ratiney-beuf/challenges.zip*

In addition, the MRF method makes the most sense when we have to investigate phenomena that are hard to describe with simple equations but can nevertheless be simulated. For example, if simulations employ virtual voxels containing internal geometrical structures (e.g. blood vessels), after calculating the distribution of the magnetic field and taking into account the effects of water molecules' diffusion and relaxation, it is possible to produce maps representing different features of the cerebral microvascular network (geometrical structure or blood oxygenation) (Christen et al. 2014; Lemasson et al. 2016). Such approaches provide results that are superior compared to classical perfusion MRI since the MRF approach enables the use of very rich biophysical models that include specific pathological situations while conventional analyses employ models with many simplifying hypotheses. Other microscopic features (cells, myelin fibers, etc.) could also be investigated with the same approach, in particular by leveraging the properties of water diffusion.

10.4.3. *Technical developments*

Although the MRF method theoretically enables quantitative multidimensional measurements, creating advanced MRF protocols for simultaneously measuring more than three parameters faces some technical difficulties. The large number of parameters to be measured and thus a large number of dictionary dimensions immediately lead to considerable acquisition and reconstruction times. Moreover, correcting acquisition artifacts (B_1, B_0, motion) adds more complexity to the task. To enable advanced MRF protocols, methods optimizing the acquisition steps and the reconstruction have to be devised.

10.4.3.1. *K-space data acquisition*

In MRF scans, several thousands of images have to be acquired to generate fingerprints. Therefore, spending the least time possible in acquiring each of them is crucial. To reduce the acquisition time as much as possible, several approaches have been proposed: (1) k-space undersampling (compressed sensing and metric learning (Wang et al. 2016)); and (2) optimization of temporal information of the fingerprints (sliding windows (Liao et al. 2017)). To further reduce scan times, the MRF approach can be combined with multi-channel coils and parallel excitations (multiband) that enable the simultaneous acquisition of several slices (Ye et al. 2017).

10.4.3.2. *Dictionary search*

When a large number of parameters has to be determined for a scan, the dictionary size can become too large (several terabytes) and the search (matching) is time consuming (several hours/days/brains). Several approaches that are capable of fast information search in databases can be used: (1) a method based on fast group matching (Cauley et al. 2015) that exploits the correlations within the dictionary to create groups of elements; (2) an approach based on singular value decomposition (SVD) which compresses the dictionary in the time domain (McGivney et al. 2014); and (3) an approach based on the k-d tree used to reorganize the elements and aid the search. Deep learning methods have also been introduced with extremely encouraging results. A fully connected neural network called DRONE (Cohen et al. 2018), trained to directly relate a temporal fingerprint to a set of parameters (e.g. T_1 and T_2) or, in other words, to learn the dictionary, has allowed reconstruction acceleration factors of the order of 300–5,000 compared to direct matching. Other research works aim to reduce not only the reconstruction time but also the number of simulations required to create dictionaries (Boux et al. 2018).

10.4.3.3. *Design of acquisition patterns*

In the MRF method, all of the acquisition parameters and the number of their repetition (or temporal length of the fingerprints) can be chosen in a random way. Thus, there is a great number of possibilities regarding the design of fingerprints ($\sim 1{,}000^{1000}$). Until now, this aspect has not been fully exploited and the acquisition patterns are chosen in a pseudo-empirical way. The introduction of automatic procedures based on numerical optimization and calculation of metrics such as the Cramér–Rao bound is gradually taking place (Sommer et al. 2017; Lee et al. 2019; Zhao et al. 2019) and such approaches could determine the fingerprint with the highest signal-to-noise ratio per unit time for a given application. For example, a procedure based on gradient descent (also used in machine learning tools) and models based on Bloch equations or EPG formalism can optimize the patterns of TR and flip angles in a few minutes with a reduction of the Cramér–Rao bound of about 60% compared to the pattern that was initially proposed by Ma et al. (2013) and Lee et al. (2019).

10.4.3.4. *Artifact corrections*

In the first MRF study, it was suggested (although not proven) that the method could be robust to involuntary patient motion during the acquisition. A subsequent investigation has explored the influence of the movements on MRF scans and determined which types of motion can be corrected (Ma et al. 2013). A method called MORPH has been also proposed for a retrospective correction of motion artifacts (Mehta et al. 2018). An iterative algorithm performs a standard matching step, identifies the images affected by motion artifacts during the scan using several metrics (e.g. root mean square error (RMSE)), estimates motion with a co-registration step, corrects the data and performs a new matching step. With this approach, satisfying results were obtained even when more than 54% of images were corrupted by motion. To correct for the artifacts caused by inhomogeneities in B_0 and B_1 fields, several approaches can be considered:

1) Introducing these parameters as new simulation dimensions to create parametric maps of B_0 and B_1 directly after the matching step. In this case, it is even possible to change the acquisition patterns to make them more sensitive to artifacts (Buonincontri and Sawiak 2016).

2) Employing independent scans to obtain B_0 and B_1 maps and constrain the dictionary search (Ma et al. 2017). Moreover, the slice selection profile can be included in the simulations to improve the results (Hong et al. 2017; Ma et al. 2017).

10.4.4. *Applications and perspectives*

MRF represents an astounding playground for method development. Using combinations of the different presented methods, MRF data (T_1, T_2 and M_0 maps) can be acquired in 3D for the entire human brain (with 1 mm^3 spatial resolution) in 7.5 minutes (Liao et al. 2017) with a possible acceleration of two or three times in the case of multiband acquisitions (Ye et al. 2017). Data reconstruction takes only a few seconds when neural networks are used. 3D MRF relaxometry measurements are quite reproducible and repeatable in a human brain at 1.5 teslas and 3 teslas (variation coefficient <10% in test/retests on eight MRI scanners (Buonincontri et al. 2019)). Several clinical applications investigating the brain (healthy tissues and cerebral tumors), breast, heart, cartilage, eyes or prostate have already shown promising results (Poorman et al. 2020). However, the MRF method may exhibit its power only when the original acquisition patterns that combine equilibrium and pseud-equilibrium states, and random acquisitions efficiently covering the entire Bloch sphere for all of the parameters are automatically generated. With protocols optimized through machine learning tools, it could even be possible to create multiparametric sequences that would replace entire MRI examinations.

10.5. Conclusion

In this chapter, we have presented various methods that use the signal of gradient echo MRI acquisitions to simultaneously extract several useful parameters. These metrics all have the common aspect of representing from a macroscopic point of view a parameter that characterizes tissues at a microscopic scale and they constitute the raw material for biomarkers. Besides the choice of acquisition sequences, we have covered several existing reconstruction approaches (physical models, comparison of signals with a dictionary generated in silico) for quantifying the information extracted from the MR signal. However, several validation and standardization steps, not tackled here, are still required to make multiparametric quantitative MRI a tool for clinical routine. Outside imaging biomarkers research, these methods, intrinsically less dependent on the scan protocols and imaging systems, can also play an important role in generating high-quality data. A remaining open question concerns the determination of the excitation sequences that enable the quantification of multiple parameters in the shortest time possible, as well as the development of correction methods or machine learning analyses to obtain representation models capable of handling the generated multidimensional data and making them interpretable. Artificial intelligence approaches will probably provide innovative tools for these purposes.

10.6. References

Abduljalil, A.M., Schmalbrock, P., Novak, V., Chakeres, D.W. (2003). Enhanced gray and white matter contrast of phase susceptibility-weighted images in ultra-high-field magnetic resonance imaging. *Journal of Magnetic Resonance Imaging*, 18(3), 284–290.

Boux, F., Forbes, F., Arbel, J., Barbier, E.L. (2018). Dictionary-free MR fingerprinting parameter estimation via inverse regression. In *Joint Annual Meeting ISMRM-ESMRMB 2018*, 1–2, Paris [Online]. Available at: https://hal.archives-ouvertes.fr/hal-01941630 [Accessed October 28 2019].

Brown, R.W., Cheng, Y.-C.N., Mark Haacke, E., Thompson, M.R., Venkatesan, R. (eds) (2014). Fast imaging in the steady state. In *Magnetic Resonance Imaging*. John Wiley & Sons, New York.

Buonincontri, G. and Sawiak, S.J. (2016). MR fingerprinting with simultaneous B1 estimation. *Magnetic Resonance in Medicine*, 76(4), 1127–1135.

Buonincontri, G., Biagi, L., Retico, A., Cecchi, P., Cosottini, M., Gallagher, F.A., Gómez, P.A., Graves, M.J., McLean, M.A., Riemer, F. et al. (2019). Multi-site repeatability and reproducibility of MR fingerprinting of the healthy brain at 1.5 and 3.0 T. *NeuroImage*, 195, 362–372.

Buxton, R.B., Edelman, R.R., Rosen, B.R., Wismer, G.L., Brady, T.J. (1987). Contrast in rapid MR imaging: T1- and T2-weighted imaging. *Journal of Computer Assisted Tomography*, 11(1), 7–16.

Bydder, M., Girard, O., Hamilton, G. (2011). Mapping the double bonds in triglycerides. *Magnetic Resonance Imaging*, 29(8), 1041–1046.

Cauley, S.F., Setsompop K., Ma, D., Jiang, Y., Ye, H., Adalsteinsson, E., Griswold, M.A., Wald, L.L. (2015). Fast group matching for MR fingerprinting reconstruction. *Magnetic Resonance in Medicine*, 74(2), 523–528.

Christen, T., Pannetier, N.A., Ni, W.W., Qiu, D., Moseley, M.E., Schuff, N., Zaharchuk, G. (2014). MR vascular fingerprinting: A new approach to compute cerebral blood volume, mean vessel radius, and oxygenation maps in the human brain. *NeuroImage*, 89, 262–270.

Cohen, O., Zhu, B., Rosen, M.S. (2018). MR fingerprinting Deep RecOnstruction NEtwork (DRONE). *Magnetic Resonance in Medicine*, 80(3), 885–894.

Deoni, S.C.L., Peters, T.M., Rutt, B.K. (2005). High-resolution T_1 and T_2 mapping of the brain in a clinically acceptable time with DESPOT1 and DESPOT2. *Magnetic Resonance in Medicine*, 53(1), 237–241.

Diefenbach, M.N., Meineke, J., Ruschke, S., Baum, T., Gersing, A., Karampinos, D.C. (2019). On the sensitivity of quantitative susceptibility mapping for measuring trabecular bone density. *Magnetic Resonance in Medicine*, 81(3), 1739–1754.

Dixon, W.T. (1984). Simple proton spectroscopic imaging. *Radiology*, 153(1), 189–194.

Flassbeck, S., Schmidt, S., Bachert, P., Ladd, M.E., Schmitter, S. (2019). Flow MR fingerprinting. *Magnetic Resonance in Medicine*, 81(4), 2536–2550.

Freed, D.E., Scheven, U.M., Zielinski, L.J., Sen, P.N., Hürlimann, M.D. (2001). Steady-state free precession experiments and exact treatment of diffusion in a uniform gradient. *The Journal of Chemical Physics*, 115(9), 4249–4258.

Guillot, G., Jourdain, L., Chanet, N., Dubuisson, R.-M., Poirier-Quinot, M., de Rochefort, L. (2017). R1, R2 and B1 mapping with an inhomogeneous T/R coil by QuICS. Meeting guide, ESMRMB, 34th Annual Scientific Meeting, 793.

Hamilton, G., Yokoo, T., Bydder, M., Cruite, I., Schroeder, M.E., Sirlin, C.B., Middleton, M.S. (2011). In vivo characterization of the liver fat ^{1}H MR spectrum. *NMR in Biomedicine*, 24(7), 784–790.

Hardy, P.A., Recht, M.P., Piraino, D., Thomasson, D. (1996). Optimization of a dual echo in the steady state (DESS) free-precession sequence for imaging cartilage. *Journal of Magnetic Resonance Imaging*, 6(2), 329–335.

Hennig, J. (1991). Echoes – How to generate, recognize, use or avoid them in MR-imaging sequences. Part I: Fundamental and not so fundamental properties of spin echoes. *Concepts in Magnetic Resonance*, 3(3), 125–143.

Hernando, D., Kellman, P., Haldar, J.P., Liang, Z.-P. (2010). Robust water/fat separation in the presence of large field inhomogeneities using a graph cut algorithm. *Magnetic Resonance in Medicine*, 63(1), 79–90.

Heule, R., Ganter, C., Bieri, O. (2014). Triple echo steady-state (TESS) relaxometry. *Magnetic Resonance in Medicine*, 71(1), 230–237.

Hines, C.D.G., Yu, H., Shimakawa, A., McKenzie, C.A., Brittain, J.H., Reeder, S.B. (2009). T_1 independent, T_2* corrected MRI with accurate spectral modeling for quantification of fat: Validation in a fat-water-SPIO phantom. *Journal of Magnetic Resonance Imaging*, 30(5), 1215–1222.

Hong, T., Han, D., Kim, M.-O., Kim, D.-H. (2017). RF slice profile effects in magnetic resonance fingerprinting. *Magnetic Resonance Imaging*, 41, 73–79.

Horng, D.E., Hernando, D., Hines, C.D.G., Reeder, S.B. (2013). Comparison of R_2* correction methods for accurate fat quantification in fatty liver. *Journal of Magnetic Resonance Imaging*, 37(2), 414–422.

Jiang, Y., Hamilton, J.I., Lo, W.-C., Wright, K.L., Ma, D., Coristine, A.J., Seiberlich, N., Gulani, V., Griswold, M.A.. (2013). Simultaneous T_1, T_2, diffusion and proton density quantification with MR fingerprinting. In *Proceedings of the 22th Annual Meeting of ISMRM*, London.

Jiang, Y., Ma, D., Seiberlich, N., Gulani, V., Griswold, M.A. (2015). MR fingerprinting using fast imaging with steady state precession (FISP) with spiral readout. *Magnetic Resonance in Medicine*, 74(6), 1621–1631.

Kaiser, R., Bartholdi, E., Ernst, R.R. (1974). Diffusion and field-gradient effects in NMR Fourier spectroscopy. *The Journal of Chemical Physics*, 60(8), 2966–2979.

Khajehim, M., Christen, T., Tam, F., Graham, S.J. (2021). Streamlined magnetic resonance fingerprinting: Fast whole-brain coverage with deep-learning based parameter estimation. *NeuroImage*, 238, 118237.

Lee, P.K., Watkins, L.E., Anderson, T.I., Buonincontri, G., Hargreaves, B.A. (2019). Flexible and efficient optimization of quantitative sequences using automatic differentiation of Bloch simulations. *Magnetic Resonance in Medicine*, 82(4), 1438–1451.

Lemasson, B., Pannetier, N., Coquery, N., Boisserand, L.S.B., Collomb, N., Schuff, N., Moseley, M., Zaharchuk, G., Barbier, E.L., Christen, T. (2016). MR vascular fingerprinting in stroke and brain tumors models. *Scientific Reports*, 6, 37071.

Leporq, B., Ratiney, H., Pilleul, F., Beuf, O. (2013). Liver fat volume fraction quantification with fat and water T_1 and T_2* estimation and accounting for NMR multiple components in patients with chronic liver disease at 1.5 and 3.0 T. *European Radiology*, 23(8), 2175–2186.

Leporq, B., Lambert, S.A., Maxime Ronot, M., Vilgrain, V., Van Beers, B.E. (2014). Quantification of the triglyceride fatty acid composition with 3.0 T MRI. *NMR in Biomedicine*, 27(10), 1211–1221.

Leporq, B., Lambert, S.A., Ronot, M., Vilgrain, V., Van Beers B.E. (2017). Simultaneous MR quantification of hepatic fat content, fatty acid composition, transverse relaxation time and magnetic susceptibility for the diagnosis of non-alcoholic steatohepatitis. *NMR Biomed*, 30(10). doi: 10.1002/nbm.3766.

Leroi, L., Coste, A., de Rochefort, L., Santin, M.D., Valabregue, R., Mauconduit, F., Giacomini, E., Luong, M., Chazel, E., Valette, J. et al. (2018). Simultaneous multi-parametric mapping of total sodium concentration, T_1, T_2 and ADC at 7 T using a multi-contrast unbalanced SSFP. *Magnetic Resonance Imaging*, 53, 156–163.

Leroi, L., Gras, V., Boulant, N., Ripart, M., Poirion, E., Santin, M.D., Valabregue, R., Mauconduit, F., Hertz-Pannier, L., Le Bihan, D. et al. (2020). Simultaneous proton density, T_1, T_2, and flip-angle mapping of the brain at 7 T using multiparametric 3D SSFP imaging and parallel-transmission universal pulses. *Magnetic Resonance in Medicine*, 84(6), 3286–3299.

Li, W., Wu, B., Liu, C. (2011). Quantitative susceptibility mapping of human brain reflects spatial variation in tissue composition. *NeuroImage*, 55(4), 1645–1656.

Liao, C., Bilgic, B., Manhard, M.K., Zhao, B., Cao, X., Zhong, J., Wald, L.L., Setsompop, K. (2017). 3D MR fingerprinting with accelerated stack-of-spirals and hybrid sliding-window and GRAPPA reconstruction. *NeuroImage*, 162, 13–22.

Liu, C.Y., McKenzie, C.A., Yu, H., Brittain, J.H., Reeder, S.B. (2007). Fat quantification with IDEAL gradient echo imaging: Correction of bias from T(1) and noise. *Magnetic Resonance in Medicine*, 58(2), 354–364.

Liu, T., Khalidov, I., de Rochefort, L., Spincemaille, P., Liu, J., Tsiouris, A.J., Wang, Y. (2011). A novel background field removal method for MRI using projection onto dipole fields (PDF). *NMR in Biomedicine*, 24(9), 1129–1136.

Ma, D., Gulani, V., Seiberlich, N., Liu, K., Sunshine, J.L., Duerk, J.L., Griswold, M.A. (2013). Magnetic resonance fingerprinting. *Nature*, 495(7440), 187–192.

Ma, D., Coppo, S., Chen, Y., McGivney, D.F., Jiang, Y., Pahwa, S., Gulani, V., Griswold, M.A. (2017). Slice profile and B_1 corrections in 2D magnetic resonance fingerprinting. *Magnetic Resonance in Medicine*, 78(5), 1781–1789.

Martel, D., Leporq, B., Bruno, M., Regatte, R.R., Honig, S., Chang, G. (2018). Chemical shift-encoded MRI for assessment of bone marrow adipose tissue fat composition: Pilot study in premenopausal versus postmenopausal women. *Magnetic Resonance Imaging*, 53, 148–155.

Martel, D., Leporq, B., Saxena, A., Belmont, H.M., Turyan, G., Honig, S., Regatte, R.R., Chang, G. (2019). 3T chemical shift-encoded MRI: Detection of altered proximal femur marrow adipose tissue composition in glucocorticoid users and validation with magnetic resonance spectroscopy. *Journal of Magnetic Resonance Imaging*, 50(2), 490–496.

McGivney, D.F., Pierre, E., Ma, D., Jiang, Y., Saybasili, H., Gulani, V., Griswold, M.A. (2014). SVD compression for magnetic resonance fingerprinting in the time domain. *IEEE Transactions on Medical Imaging*, 33(12), 2311–2322.

Mehta, B.B., Ma, D., Pierre, E.Y., Jiang, Y., Coppo, S., Griswold, M.A. (2018). Image reconstruction algorithm for motion insensitive MR Fingerprinting (MRF): MORF. *Magnetic Resonance in Medicine*, 80(6), 2485–2500.

Nemeth, A., Segrestin, B., Leporq, B., Seyssel, K., Faraz, K., Sauvinet, V., Disse, E., Valette, P.-J., Laville, M., Ratiney, H., Beuf, O. (2019). 3D chemical shift-encoded MRI for volume and composition quantification of abdominal adipose tissue during an overfeeding protocol in healthy volunteers. *Journal of Magnetic Resonance Imaging*, 49(6), 1587–1599.

O'Regan, D.P., Callaghan, M.F., Wylezinska-Arridge, M., Fitzpatrick, J., Naoumova, R.P., Hajnal, J.V., Schmitz, S.A. (2008). Liver fat content and T_2*: Simultaneous measurement by using breath-hold multiecho MR imaging at 3.0 T – Feasibility. *Radiology*, 247(2), 550–557.

Pauly, J., Le Roux, P., Nishimura, D., Macovski, A. (1991). Parameter relations for the Shinnar-Le Roux selective excitation pulse design algorithm [NMR imaging]. *IEEE Transactions on Medical Imaging*, 10(1), 53–65.

Peterson, P. and Månsson, S. (2013). Simultaneous quantification of fat content and fatty acid composition using MR imaging. *Magnetic Resonance in Medicine*, 69(3), 688–697.

Poorman, M.E., Martin, M.N., Ma, D., McGivney, D.F., Gulani, V., Griswold, M.A., Keenan, E.K. (2020). Magnetic resonance fingerprinting. Part 1: Potential uses, current challenges, and recommendations. *Journal of Magnetic Resonance Imaging*, 51(3), 675–692.

Reeder, S.B., Pineda, R.P., Wen, Z., Shimakawa, A., Yu, H., Brittain, J.H., Gold, G.E., Beaulieu, C.H., Pelc, N.J. (2005). Iterative decomposition of water and fat with echo asymmetry and least-squares estimation (IDEAL): Application with fast spin-echo imaging. *Magnetic Resonance in Medicine*, 54(3), 636–644.

Reeder, S.B., McKenzie, C.A., Pineda, A.R., Yu, H., Shimakawa, A., Brau, A.C., Hargreaves, B.A., Gold, G.E., Brittain, J.H. (2007). Water-fat separation with IDEAL gradient-echo imaging. *Journal of Magnetic Resonance Imaging*, 25(3), 644–652.

Rieger, B., Zimmer, F., Zapp, J., Weingärtner, S., Schad. L.R. (2017). Magnetic resonance fingerprinting using echo-planar imaging: Joint quantification of T_1 and T_2* relaxation times. *Magnetic Resonance in Medicine*, 78(5), 1724–1733.

de Rochefort, L. (2018a). Method and device for imaging by magnetic resonance. *Espacenet* [Online]. Available at: https://worldwide.espacenet.com/publicationDetails/biblio?FT=D&date=20180727&DB=EPODOC&locale=fr_EP&CC=FR&NR=3036189B1&KC=B1&ND=5.

de Rochefort, L. (2018b). Spatially-resolved relaxometric mapping with an inhomogeneous transmit-receive coil designed for mouse in a fast-field cycling magnetic resonance imaging insert. In *Conference on NMR Relaxometry and Related Methods*, Turin.

de Rochefort, L., Liu, T., Kressler, B., Liu, J., Spincemaille, P., Lebon, V., Wu, J., Wang. Y. (2010). Quantitative susceptibility map reconstruction from MR phase data using Bayesian regularization: Validation and application to brain imaging. *Magnetic Resonance in Medicine*, 63(1), 194–206.

de Rochefort, L., Guillot, G., Dubuisson, R.-M., Valabrègue, R. (2016). In vivo feasibility of multi-parametric mapping based on fast steady-state sequences. In *24th Scientific Meeting of the International Society for Magnetic Resonance in Medicine (ISMRM 2016)*, Singapore.

de Rochefort, L., Leroi, L., Valabregue, R., Girard, O., Duhamel, G., Santin, M., Loureiro de Sousa, P., Lamy, J., Mauconduit, F., Dubuisson, R.-M. et al. (2017). Multi-parametric maps from multi-contrasts steady-state sequences on multiple manufacturers and fields. Meeting guide, ESMRMB, 34th Annual Scientific Meeting, 456 [Online]. Available at: https://hal.archives-ouvertes.fr/hal-02553615.

Salomir, R., de Senneville, B.D., Moonen, C.T. (2003). A fast calculation method for magnetic field inhomogeneity due to an arbitrary distribution of bulk susceptibility. *Concepts in Magnetic Resonance*, 19B(1), 26–34.

Schweser, F., Deistung, A., Lehr, B.W., Reichenbach, J.R. (2011). Quantitative imaging of intrinsic magnetic tissue properties using MRI signal phase: An approach to in vivo brain iron metabolism? *NeuroImage*, 54(4), 2789–2807.

Schweser, F., Robinson, SD., de Rochefort, L., Li, W., Bredies K. (2017). An illustrated comparison of processing methods for phase MRI and QSM: Removal of background field contributions from sources outside the region of interest. *NMR Biomed*, 30(4). doi: 10.1002/nbm.3604

Sommer, K., Amthor, T., Doneva, M., Koken, P., Meineke, J., Börnert, P. (2017). Towards predicting the encoding capability of MR fingerprinting sequences. *Magnetic Resonance Imaging*, 41, 7–14.

Su, P., Mao D., Liu, P., Li, Y., Pinho, M.C., Welch, B.G., Lu, H. (2016). Multiparametric estimation of brain hemodynamics with MR fingerprinting ASL. *Magnetic Resonance in Medicine*, 78(5), 1812–1823.

Sun, H. and Wilman, A.H. (2014). Background field removal using spherical mean value filtering and Tikhonov regularization. *Magnetic Resonance in Medicine*, 71(3), 1151–1157.

Valabregue, R. and de Rochefort, L. (2016). Fisher information matrix for optimizing the acquisition parameters in multi-parametric mapping based on fast steady-state sequences. In *24th Scientific Meeting of the International Society for Magnetic Resonance in Medicine (ISMRM 2016)*, Singapore [Online]. Available at: https://hal.archives-ouvertes.fr/hal-02532390/.

Viallon, M., Leporq, B., Drinda, S., Wilhelmi de Toledo, F., Galusca, B., Ratiney, H., Croisille, P. (2019). Chemical-shift-encoded magnetic resonance imaging and spectroscopy to reveal immediate and long-term multi-organs composition changes of a 14-days periodic fasting intervention: A technological and case report. *Frontiers in Nutrition*, 6, 5.

Wang, Z., Li, H., Zhang, Q., Yuan, J., Wang, X. (2016). Magnetic resonance fingerprinting with compressed sensing and distance metric learning. *Neurocomputing*, 174, 560–570.

Wang, C.Y., Coppo, S., Mehta B.B., Seiberlich, N., Yu, X., Alan Griswold, M.A (2019). Magnetic resonance fingerprinting with quadratic RF phase for measurement of T_2* simultaneously with δ_f, T_1, and T_2. *Magnetic Resonance in Medicine*, 81(3), 1849–1862.

Weigel, M. (2015). Extended phase graphs: Dephasing, RF pulses, and echoes – Pure and simple. *Journal of Magnetic Resonance Imaging*, 41(2), 266–295.

West, D.J., Cruz, G., Teixeira, R.P.A.G., Schneider, T., Tournier, J.-D., Hajnal. J.V., Prieto, C., Malik, S.J. (2021). An MR fingerprinting approach for quantitative inhomogeneous magnetization transfer imaging. *Magnetic Resonance in Medicine*, 28984, 87(1), 220–235.

Xie, L., Sparks, M.A., Li, W., Qi, Y., Liu, C., Coffman, T.M., Johnson, G.A. (2013). Quantitative susceptibility mapping of kidney inflammation and fibrosis in type 1 angiotensin receptor-deficient mice. *NMR in Biomedicine*, 26(12), 1853–1863.

Ye, H., Cauley, S.F., Gagoski, B., Bilgic, B., Ma, D., Jiang, Y., Du, Y.P., Griswold, M.A., Wald, L.L., Setsompop, K. (2017). Simultaneous multislice magnetic resonance fingerprinting (SMS-MRF) with direct-spiral slice-GRAPPA (ds-SG) reconstruction. *Magnetic Resonance in Medicine*, 77(5), 1966–1974.

Zhao, B., Haldar, P.H., Liao, C., Ma, D., Jiang, Y., Griswold, M.A., Setsompop, K., Wald, L.L. (2019). Optimal experiment design for magnetic resonance fingerprinting: Cramér-Rao bound meets spin dynamics. *IEEE Transactions on Medical Imaging*, 38(3), 844–861.

Zur, Y., Wood, M.L., Neuringer, L.J. (1991). Spoiling of transverse magnetization in steady-state sequences. *Magnetic Resonance in Medicine*, 21(2), 251–263.

11

Interventional MRI

Bruno QUESSON[1,2] and Valéry OZENNE[1]
[1] *CRMSB, CNRS, Université de Bordeaux, France*
[2] *IHU Liryc, Université de Bordeaux, France*

11.1. Introduction to interventional MRI

The goal of interventional MRI is to provide visual real-time feedback to the personnel performing therapeutical interventions (puncture, surgery, thermal ablation, radiotherapy, etc.) via a medical therapeutic device (MTD). It is employed in several medical fields (neurology, oncology, urology, cardiology, etc.). Many imaging modalities (X-rays, ultrasounds, pre-operative optical imaging and MRI) can be exploited, with the choice dependent on several aspects (targeted application, access to instrumentation, type of information sought in the images, equipment cost and compatibility with the MTD).

Regardless of the application and imaging modality, the procedures typically include the steps listed below.

11.1.1. *Intervention planning*

In this pre-interventional phase, the goal is to define the main steps of the intervention that include (i) delimiting the location to be reached and/or the region to be treated via the MTD and critical adjacent tissues to be preserved; (ii) the choice of the access path: percutaneous, vascular or non-invasive; and (iii) the choice of the MTD and its interventional mode. For this purpose, a map of the subject's anatomy

For a color version of all the figures in this chapter, see www.iste.co.uk/ratiney-beuf/challenges.zip.

The Challenges of MRI,
coordinated by Hélène RATINEY and Olivier BEUF. © ISTE Ltd 2024.

(ideally in 3D) that covers the entire region penetrated by the MTD is usually obtained before the treatment. This map can be an anatomical image, a 3D model (e.g. a 3D mesh) or a functional representation (e.g. a 3D map of the electrical cardiac activity). Such pieces of information can be acquired several days before the intervention or at the very beginning of the interventional session if the imaging device makes it possible.

11.1.2. *Pre-operatory imaging*

This phase requires real-time imaging to interactively guide the intervention by combining live images with data obtained during the planning phase. This sets a minimum image acquisition rate for a smooth and, ideally, latency-free display of relevant information to the person performing the intervention. At first, the MTD is typically moved (ballistically) toward the area to be treated, and then the intervention is performed. Ideally, these steps are guided via real-time imaging. However, if this is impossible (e.g. if the device cannot be operated during image acquisition), intermittent imaging is performed, for example, by iteratively re-positioning the therapeutic device at the target area.

11.1.3. *Post-operative follow-up imaging*

Once the therapeutic intervention has been performed, one or several imaging modalities can be used to evaluate the treatment effect. Such post-operative imaging can be performed immediately after the intervention and/or several weeks later, if necessary.

Table 11.1 lists the different imaging modalities for each intervention step.

	X-ray scan	Fluoroscopy	Ultrasound	MRI
Planning	++	–	–	++
MTD positioning	++	++	++	++
Real-time imaging	–	+	Depending on the application	
Post-treatment imaging	++	–	+	++

Table 11.1. *Comparison of the performance of different imaging modalities: ++: excellent; +: acceptable; –: poor*

MRI presents undeniable advantages for several procedural steps. However, the issues of costs and instrumentation accessibility have so far hindered the clinical development of interventional MRI in favor of other imaging modalities such as ultrasound and X-ray scans or fluoroscopy. On the other hand, a certain number of technical barriers related to the acquisition and image reconstruction techniques, hardware of medical devices that are used in highly magnetic environments, and numerical computation capabilities have also challenged the growth of this discipline. Nevertheless, all these obstacles are getting tackled, paving the way for interventional MRI applications with significant potential.

Figure 11.1 provides a schematic representation of an MTD guided via MRI.

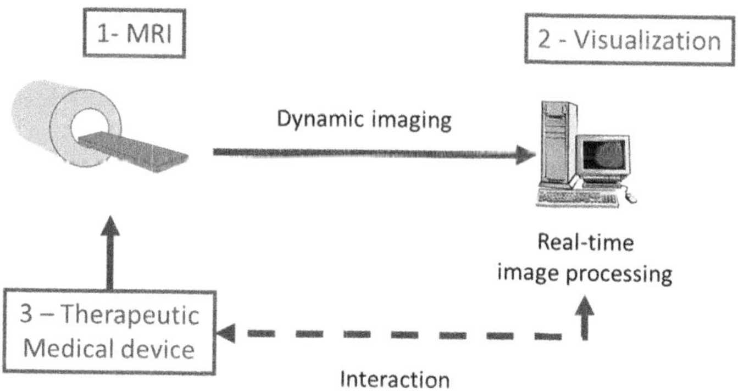

Figure 11.1. *Schematic representation of an interventional MRI device. (1) MRI provides images during the therapeutic procedure. (2) These images are analyzed and visualized in real time via software that eventually interacts with the MTD (3) to optimize the therapy*

Before continuing, the notion of real-time imaging has to be defined.

It would not make any sense to provide absolute values of imaging rate in seconds or minutes. In fact, the rate strongly depends on the application and type of information that has to be obtained. The notion of real-time imaging has to be put in perspective with the characteristic time of the biological phenomenon that has to be investigated, the specific constraints related to the foreseen treatment and the targeted organ. To illustrate this point, let us consider the example of thermal radiofrequency therapies that are commonly used to treat liver tumors (via percutaneous access) and cardiac arrhythmias (via vascular access). Although the MTD technology is similar in the two applications, the constraints are very different. The treatment duration is in the order of 10–15 min for the liver and about 1 min for the atrium. Hence, while it is acceptable to update the images every 10 s for the liver, such a rate is not sufficient in the heart. On the other hand, the dimensions of thermal lesions induced in the liver are in the order of several centimeters and a few millimeters in the heart. As a result, the spatial image resolution has to be much higher for the imaging of cardiac arrhythmias than for liver tumor treatments. Furthermore, motion (only respiratory versus respiratory and cardiac) that occurs in these two organs also leads to different constraints regarding the MRI acquisition sequences.

Therefore, the concept of real-time imaging has to take into account all the hardware and physiological constraints to provide relevant information to the operator.

11.2. Technical considerations in interventional MRI

This section focuses on real-time imaging compared to planning and post-interventional imaging that make use of conventional diagnostic imaging techniques.

11.2.1. *Choice of the MRI acquisition sequence*

Interventional MRI involves more significant technical constraints than diagnostic imaging because useful information has to be immediately available during the therapeutic intervention. For this purpose, the same image acquisition has to be repeated to analyze and visualize the evolution of contrasts over time in the reconstructed images. Several fast MRI sequences exist, and their choice depends on the requirements in terms of spatial resolution, volume coverage, acquisition rate and radiofrequency energy deposited during the scan in the sample or around an implanted medical device (risk of tissue heating; see the SAR notion in section 2.6.1). A trade-off among acquisition parameters thus has to be met in order to guarantee sufficient signal-to-noise ratio (SNR) while providing suitable contrasts for visualizing the relevant phenomenon.

For all such reasons, fast gradient echo sequences, such as FLASH (Markl and Leupold 2012) or True-FISP (Bieri and Scheffler 2013), represent the preferred choice. If the scans have to be accelerated, some variations can be employed, such as echo planar imaging (EPI) (Mansfield 1984) as a multishot EPI (ms-EPI) or single-shot EPI (ss-EPI). These techniques acquire several lines (ms-EPI) or all the lines (ss-EPI) of the k-space following an RF pulse. Therefore, the acquisition time is shorter compared to FLASH, since the number of pulses is reduced to record all the k-space lines, with the highest acceleration factor provided by ss-EPI where all the lines are acquired after a single pulse. However, this choice entails longer echo times, which can decrease the SNR in organs with short T_2*. On the other hand, artifacts can occur, including in particular geometric distortions and magnetic susceptibility artifacts around medical devices positioned inside the organs during the treatment.

11.2.2. *Image reconstruction*

An additional intrinsic constraint in interventional MRI is the reconstruction of images at a rate at least as fast as the acquisition rate. Indeed, if the image reconstruction process leads to delays with respect to the scans, there will be lags between the acquisition and display of useful information for the personnel performing the intervention. Today's computational performance is capable of providing reconstructed images in real time at rates of at least 10 images/s, which is sufficient for many applications. Among the usually available algorithms on the clinical scanners, parallel imaging techniques (e.g. SENSE, GRAPPA and ASSET) can reduce the number of acquired lines (by a factor of 2 or 3) in the k-space and reconstruct good-quality images in real time by means of simultaneous measurements of an undersampled k-space using multi-element receive coils positioned around the patient.

This acceleration can be exploited in several ways, for example, to increase the number of slices for a fixed scan time, reduce the number of lines acquired at each *TR*, reduce the echo time (decreasing the T_2* weighting) or decrease possible susceptibility artifacts or geometric distortions. Another approach consists of simultaneously exciting several slices (simultaneous multi-slices techniques) to gather a composite signal resulting from a mixture of all the slices, and then extracting each slice via a reconstruction algorithm that uses the spatial sensitivities of the different receive coils. This approach can be combined with a FLASH, ms-EPI, or ss-EPI sequence, among others, or include k-space undersampling to benefit from the advantages of parallel imaging and fast sequences.

Nevertheless, it should be reminded that the final quality of the images and the eventual artifacts induced by the combination of these acceleration and parallel imaging techniques have to be taken into account.

11.2.3. *Image analysis and display*

Once the images are reconstructed, they should be processed to extract useful information and deliver it to the operator or MTD to guide the treatment. This typically requires a real-time transfer of reconstructed MRI images to a separate console that performs this operation via specifically developed software for the target application. The provided images can be visualized inside or outside the MRI room depending on the application, for example, when the operator performs the intervention by means of interactive imaging (e.g. insertion of a device into the tumor). The image analysis software should not introduce any latency, especially if high amounts of data are generated at each second.

11.2.4. *Motion management*

Physiological motion, in particular cardiac and respiratory movements, is quite constraining for MRI. Typically, synchronizing the acquisition of a part of k-space with the respiratory and/or cardiac phase can tackle motion, although at the price of lower temporal resolution, an essential aspect in real-time MRI. On the other hand, using breath holds is difficult to envision. Employing acquisition sequences that are faster than the duration of the considered motion (typically 6 s for the respiratory cycle and 1 s for the cardiac cycle) is thus a viable solution (see section 11.2.1). In this way, the displacement during the acquisition of a given k-space is minimized, although it may be necessary to correct the displacement between subsequent scans for the same k-space plane. The most straightforward way is to use some physiological synchronization (respiratory/cardiac sensor, navigator echo). Another approach consists of correcting the motion that is directly visible on the images of the same slice over time by means of image co-registration. For this purpose, an estimated vector field representing the voxel displacement between an image obtained during the treatment and a reference image has to be calculated. This displacement is then applied to the present image to make it correspond as much as possible to the reference image. The process is then repeated for each newly acquired image. Several algorithms based on rigid and/or deformable transformations have been introduced for different target applications. Such functionalities are particularly important when the analysis of the intensity variation in a pixel during treatment has to be displayed. Another approach to remove motion effects consists of using 3D positioning systems integrated with the MTD (when these are available) and synchronizing the image acquisition with the images of the position of such a system. For example, several existing technologies exploit electromagnetic triangulation systems or MRI measurements from projections along three orthogonal directions by means of small MRI detectors integrated into the MTD.

Knowing the instantaneous position in 3D of the organ or medical device also enables the automatic repositioning of a slice at each scan. This dynamic monitoring makes it possible to choose the image refresh rate without necessarily depending on the characteristic time of the physiological motion. However, this requires greater interaction with the MR system by implementing a dynamic feedback loop that analyzes this position in real time to instantaneously reposition the MRI slices over the target region.

11.3. Interventional MRI hardware

Interventional MRI involves an MTD and must provide real-time images during an intervention to optimize the use of the device or to guide its operation via the images obtained during the treatment. The variety of possible MTDs includes, for example, single-use consumables, such as a puncture probes, intracardiac catheters or thermoablation systems (radiofrequency needles, microwaves, laser or cryotherapy). These devices are first positioned at the target tissues percutaneously or via vascular pathways (intracardiac catheters) and then used to perform the therapeutic action. Other MTDs are extracorporeal, such as high-intensity focused ultrasound (HIFU), magnetic hyperthermia devices or linear accelerators for radiotherapy.

11.3.1. *Intracorporeal medical devices*

11.3.1.1. *Access and operation of the MTD*

Current clinical MRIs generally consist of a cylinder with an internal diameter of about 70 cm, with 80 cm reached in some new-generation MRI scanners. On the other hand, the length of MRI scanners tends to become shorter, approaching the length of X-ray scanners in which interventional procedures are often performed. However, the available space around a patient remains relatively limited, which makes the positioning of the MTDs via percutaneous access complicated with only MRI guidance. Therefore, the design of MTDs must be adapted to these accessibility constraints. Additionally, the MTD positioning procedure can be performed via alternative imaging modalities, such as ultrasound, by bringing this modality system close to the MRI bed. It should be noted that several MRI manufacturers provide mobile beds, which enable patient preparation and MTD positioning to be done outside the MRI room. Another alternative consists of using interactive imaging for the positioning, but this remains impractical for the operator.

11.3.1.2. *MRI compatibility and electromagnetic interference*

MRI compatibility with the MTD is an indispensable prerequisite. A suitable choice of materials composing the MTD can prevent it from being attracted to the

MRI magnet. Moreover, the MTD's magnetic susceptibility should preferably be as close as possible to that of the human tissues to avoid perturbing the spatial homogeneity of the magnetic field B_0 in the vicinity of the device. In the negative case, the MRI image will exhibit a loss of signal intensity near the MTD, with the size of the affected area dependent on the employed acquisition sequence (see section 11.2.1), with a more prominent effect in gradient echo sequence, in particular in their accelerated versions such as ms-EPI and ss-EPI. Furthermore, this artifact is more intense when B_0 and TE increase and the bandwidth per pixel decreases. Laser fiber and cryotherapy devices have excellent compatibility with MRI, while radiofrequency and microwave systems typically produce stronger artifacts in MRI images.

If the MTD emits electromagnetic waves (especially for cardiac ablation radiofrequency catheters, percutaneous radiofrequency needles, or microwaves), it is of critical importance to avoid any electromagnetic interference that could cause artifacts in the MRI images, making them useless. Although these devices operate at frequencies far from those of the clinical MRI systems (around 500 kHz for radiofrequency systems and 1 GHz for microwave systems), the emitted power is in the order of hundreds of watts, which can produce parasitic signals with sufficient intensity at the MRI frequency if the signal emitted by the MTD is not mono-frequential. Since the MRI signal is very low (in the order of microwatts), the parasitic signal produced by the MTD generator and detected by the receiving MRI coils can be larger than the MRI signal. To tackle this problem, a filtering system has to be implemented within the transmitting hardware that links the energy source to the MTD positioned inside the target organ, in particular when the source is located outside the Faraday cage of the MRI scanner. This filtering system can also prevent the transmission of an electrical signal generated by the radiofrequency pulses of the MRI scanner that could be sensed by the electrical cables of the MTD and perturb the operation of the energy source. Several approaches have been introduced to electrically isolate the MTD and the MRI scanner, for example, using passive filters (low-pass or band-stop LC type) or impedance transformers distributed along the transmission line of the MTD.

11.3.1.3. *Risk of heating in conducting parts of the MTD*

The radiofrequency pulses emitted by the MRI sequence can induce currents in conductive parts of the MTD. A consequence of this is an increased risk of generating hot spots in the tissues in contact with the MTD's tip. The heating can quickly lead to necroses and irreversible coagulation. The inclusion of stop-band filters tuned to the MRI frequency and distributed along the transmission line at intervals smaller than the wavelength of the MR signal can reduce this effect.

Another solution consists of modifying the characteristic impedance of the MTD during the transmission of the radiofrequency pulse by MRI coils (Ozen et al. 2019), which implies an appropriate design of the MTD. Other research groups have proposed using multi-element MRI transmit coils. This approach optimizes the currents in each transmit coil to minimize the currents induced in the MTD (Godinez et al. 2020), and the current in the latter can be measured by an inductive system without requiring specific modifications of the MTD.

11.3.2. *Extracorporeal therapeutic medical devices*

HIFU and magnetic hyperthermia devices are non-invasive and operate inside the MRI bore. Their considerations regarding access, MRI compatibility and electromagnetic interference risks are analogous to percutaneous MTDs. However, the risks of artifacts in the target region are almost non-existent, which offers more possibilities in the choice of acquisition sequences. The combination of MRI with a radiotherapy device (MR-Linac) is a relatively recent technology. It has the advantage of an MTD located outside the MRI bore, with a modification of the magnet to let the radiotherapy beam pass through it. For the three MTDs mentioned above, one of the challenges is to manage the relative displacement of a moving target (respiratory or cardiac activity) with respect to the local area where the energy is delivered by the MTD. A dynamic feedback system must be devised to control the energy deposition in real time such that this energy is always oriented toward the target and avoids damaging adjacent healthy tissues.

11.4. MR-Linac

This device combines a linear accelerator for radiotherapy with an MRI. It is a completely non-invasive MTD since the radiotherapy emitter is located outside the MRI magnet's bore. The treatment is performed by radiotherapists and the most used image-guiding modality is X-rays.

Radiotherapy treatment is subdivided into various sessions distributed over several days. This means that the target area has to be precisely repositioned with respect to the radiotherapy emitter for each session in order to optimize the delivered dose and avoid damage to adjacent healthy tissues. On the other hand, the geometry of the region to be treated can evolve during the treatment, which ideally requires adaptive approaches.

The advantages of combining MRI and linear accelerators are as follows:

– being able to make use of the rich contrasts provided by MRI to accurately visualize the treatment target (planning phase) and the surrounding tissues to be preserved;

– suppression of the image co-registration step when planning is performed using images obtained on another system (X-ray or MRI scanner), which can be a source of therapeutical imprecisions or limitations in the delivered dose for avoiding damage to healthy tissues;

– the ability to follow the tumor displacement (breathing) during the treatment via fast imaging to synchronize the emission of the radiotherapy beam with the target motion – since the MRI can acquire images of any plane, it is also possible to visualize the displacement of the target by acquiring images of a coronal or sagittal plane;

– the ability to scan the patient as much as necessary via a non-ionizing modality in 2D and 3D;

– the ability to visualize the evolution of 3D tumor geometry during the treatment to adjust the radiation dose with respect to the initial planning (adaptive treatment);

– ability to use MRI images acquired at the end of each treatment session to extract markers for therapy prognosis, in particular via diffusion MRI.

Today, two clinical systems are available, one employing low-field MRI (0.35 T, MRIdian) and the other using a high magnetic field (1.5 T, Unity Elekta). The low-field system consists of an MRI with two main coils that surround the radiotherapy device. The main acquisition sequences enable the co-registration of the target at each session. During the treatment, cine imaging (True-FISP sequence) can be performed to control the emission/arrest of the radiotherapy beam. The system working at 1.5 T is more recent and includes a Philips scanner that is quite similar to conventional diagnostic scanners, with an aperture for the radiotherapy beam near its center. The advantage of working at 1.5 T lies in images with a higher quality (gain in SNR) or higher spatial resolution and in all the imaging methods available on diagnostic clinical scanners. On the downside, combining high-field MRI with a radiotherapy system involves considerable technological challenges (risk of radiofrequency interference between the waves emitted by the two devices, requiring mutual shielding via dedicated Faraday cages, minimization of radiotherapy overdose effects due to the generation of secondary electrons at some tissue interfaces – the so-called electron return effect).

These two systems are used in clinics and aim to provide adaptive radiotherapy for personalized treatment with better control of the radiation dose (higher dose in the target region and lower dose in the organs at risk).

11.5. MRI thermometry for guided thermal therapies

11.5.1. *Principle of MRI thermometry*

Several physical parameters affecting the contrast of MRI images are sensitive to temperature (Quesson et al. 2000). They include longitudinal (T_1) and transverse (T_2) relaxation times, magnetization (M_0) and the resonant frequency of water protons (ν_0). Based on the latter, the proton resonance frequency shift (PRFS) technique has become the standard for acquiring images of temperature distribution inside the organs whenever a thermotherapy MTD (radiofrequency, microwaves, laser, HIFU) is used. The variation of ν_0 is almost linear over the range of temperatures in liquid water and depends very little on the investigated organ. The variation of ν_0 with temperature (the PRF constant called σ in the following) is about 0.01 ppm/°C, which corresponds to a variation of 0.63 Hz/°C for a scanner operating at 1.5 T (ν_0 = 63 MHz). Thus, the phase φ of the MRI signal varies as a function of temperature according to the following equation:

$$\varphi(x,y,z,t) = \omega(x,y,z,t).T_E$$

$$\varphi(x,y,z,t) = \omega_{REF}(x,y,z).T_E + \gamma.B_0.\sigma.(T(x,y,z,t) - T_0(x,y,z)).T_E$$

$$\varphi(x,y,z,t) = \varphi_{REF}(x,y,z) + \gamma.B_0.\sigma.\Delta T(x,y,z,t).T_E$$

It leads to:

$$\Delta T(x,y,z,t) = \frac{\varphi(x,y,z,t) - \varphi_{REF}(x,y,z,t)}{\gamma.B_0.\sigma.T_E} = k.\Delta\varphi(x,y,z,t) \qquad [11.1]$$

where φ_{REF} is the phase measured at the initial temperature (37 °C) and $\Delta T(x,y,z,t)$ is the temperature variation with respect to the initial physiological temperature T_0. By subtracting the phase of two consecutive images obtained via a gradient echo sequence pixel by pixel, the temperature variation can be calculated for each pixel of the image, as illustrated in Figure 11.2.

Thermometry is rather useful because, from the temperature maps obtained during the treatment, an image of the cumulative thermal dose can be calculated. In order to be able to compare different thermotherapy treatment protocols, an

Arrhenius law model has been proposed by Sapareto and Dewey (1984) with the following formula for the cumulative equivalent minutes at 43°C (*CEM43*):

$$CEM43(t) = \int_0^t R^{T(t)-43} dt \qquad [11.2]$$

where *R* is the ratio of the exposure duration yielding the same fraction of cell death. Although *R* can vary depending on the cells, a fixed value of 2 is typically used for R in clinical thermal ablations during which the temperature around the MTD can reach or exceed 100°C. The factor of 2 chosen for the *R* parameter indicates that the exposure duration is halved to obtain the same CEM43 for each additional degree.

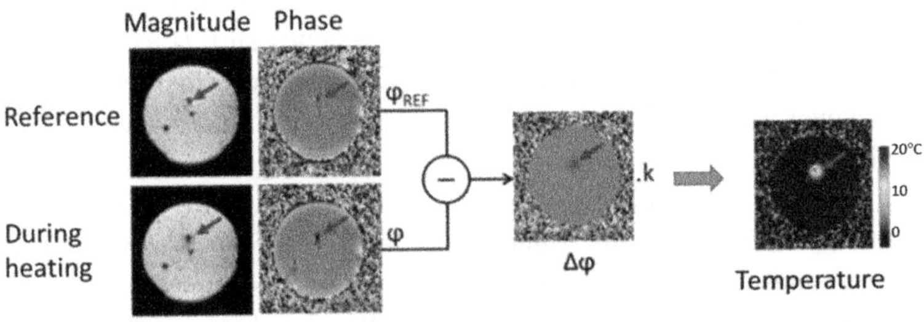

Figure 11.2. *Example of MRI thermometry using the PRFS method in an agar gel sample during radiofrequency heating. The phase image φ obtained during the heating is subtracted from the reference image φREF measured before the heating. The temperature image with a color scale is obtained by multiplying the phase difference image by a factor k, which is then overlaid onto the magnitude image*

This index permits converting an exposure duration at a given temperature into an equivalent duration at the reference temperature of 43°C for the same biological effect (e.g. the lethal thermal dose that corresponds to an exposure of 240 min at 43°C). Consequently, exposure at 51°C for 1 min or at 55°C for 3 s will provide the same cumulative equivalent lethal dose.

MRI thermometry enables the calculation and real-time display of instantaneous temperature maps and cumulative dose maps. Such information helps visualize the evolution of the thermal treatment induced by a thermoablation MTD and thus to evaluate whether the treatment is complete or not inside a target region and the eventual risks of damage to surrounding healthy tissue.

The equation for calculating CEM43 is nonlinear and, therefore, requires a rather high accuracy from thermometry (ideally, in the order of 1°C or less) to avoid overestimation of the thermal dose that is effectively deposited locally.

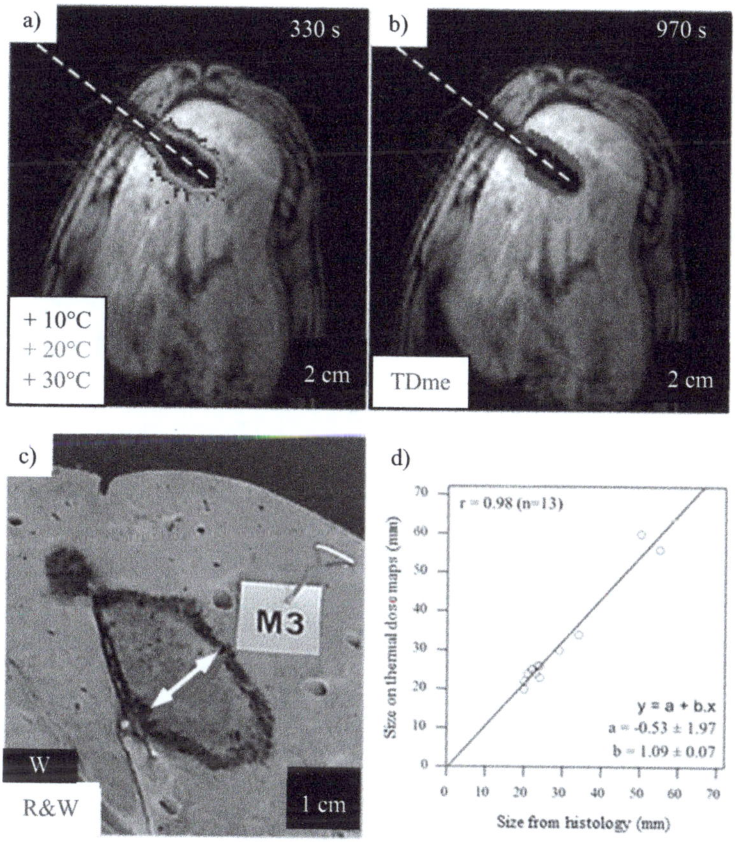

Figure 11.3. *Example of preclinical liver thermal ablation via percutaneous radiofrequency needle guided via MRI thermometry*

COMMENT ON FIGURE 11.3.– *(a) Instantaneous image of the temperature obtained during the application of radiofrequency energy showing the isolevels at +10°C, +20°C and +30°C above physiological temperature. The susceptibility artifact produced by the needle extends over 10 mm, and the white dashed line represents the actual size of the needle. (b) Image of the cumulative thermal dose (CEM43). The pixels in red have reached or exceeded the lethal value of 240 min. (c) Macroscopic slice of the lesion induced in an explanted liver. The transverse size of the coagulation necrosis is represented by the white arrow and the total area (including the peripheral transition area) is represented by the red arrow. (d) Correlation between the transverse dimensions of the lesions measured in the explants (red arrow) and those obtained from thermal dosimetry maps (image b). Illustrations adapted from Seror et al. (2008).*

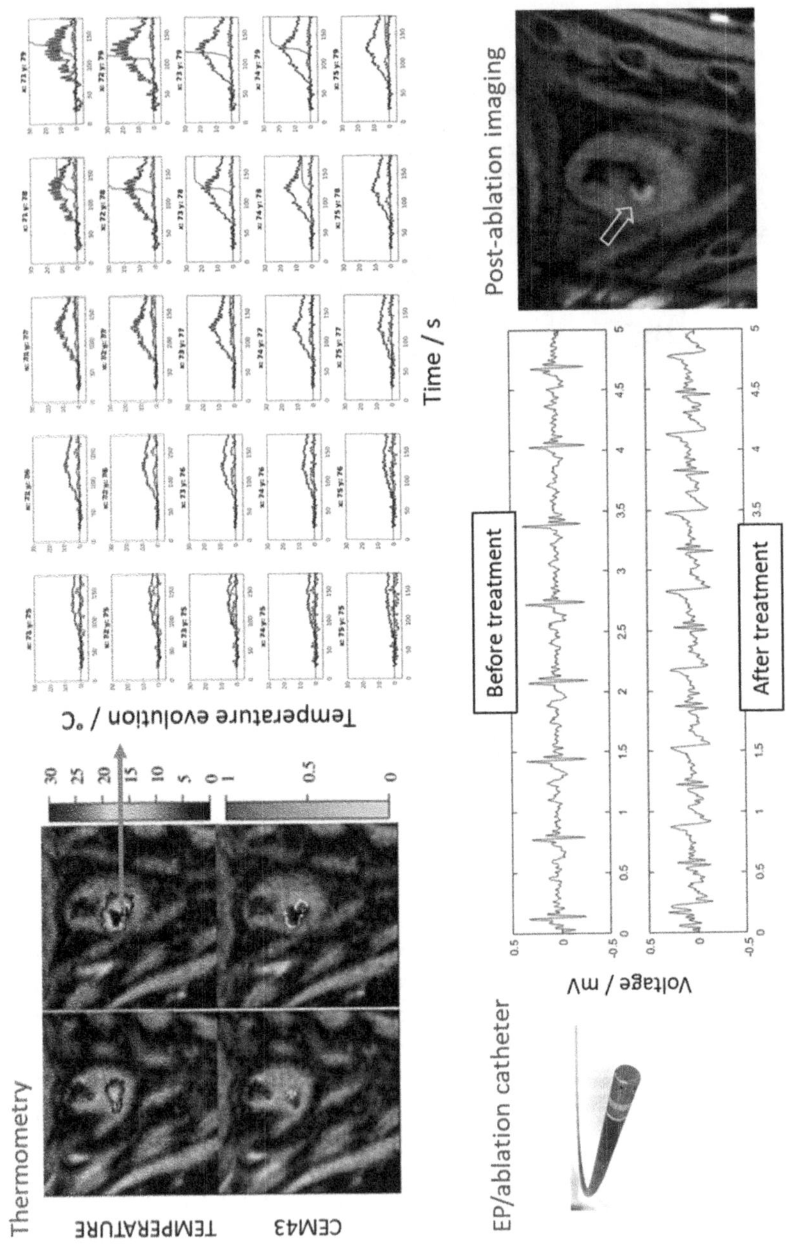

Figure 11.4. *Example of cardiac treatment via radiofrequency catheter in the left ventricle guided by MRI thermometry*

COMMENT ON FIGURE 11.4.– *An electrophysiology and radiofrequency ablation (EP/ablation) catheter is positioned in contact with the myocardium via vascular pathways; thereafter, radiofrequency energy is delivered to the tissue to introduce coagulation necrosis with a simultaneous recording of electrophysiological signals by contact. MRI thermometry (5 slices/heartbeat) provides the visualization of the temperature and CEM43 during the treatment. The top right plot shows temperature curves in several heated pixels (blue curves) and non-heated pixels (black) as well as the evolution of CEM43 (red). The recording of the EP contact signals shows a decrease in signal amplitude corresponding to the regions where tissues were damaged (CEM43 greater than or equal to the lethal value – red pixels in CEM43 images). Post-ablation imaging (3D inversion recovery sequence without contrast agent) confirms the lesion (hypersignal, yellow arrow), which enables the repositioning of the catheter for performing more RF ablation if necessary. See Ozenne et al. (2017) for details on the sequence.*

The above illustrations show examples of the treatment of a liver tumor via a radiofrequency needle (Figure 11.3) and a thermal lesion induced in a heart via an intracardiac catheter (Figure 11.4). In these images, the size of the susceptibility artifact in the liver is much larger than in the heart. This can be explained by an optimized design of the intracardiac catheter.

Thermometry associated with thermal therapy MTDs represents a considerable advantage compared to the imaging techniques in MR-Linac systems as the therapeutic effect can be quantified during the heat deposition and not via imaging obtained after the treatment.

11.5.2. *Practical implementation, advantages and limitations of MRI thermometry*

The PRFS method is only valid for the water signal. Therefore, the lipid signal has to be suppressed using conventional techniques (inversion-recovery, selective excitation of water using binomial pulses, selective fat excitation with a dephasing gradient before the water excitation, etc.). If the targeted organ has a high lipid content (e.g. breast), the resulting image will have few pixels with detectable signal, which requires appropriate image processing to extract temperature information.

An important aspect is related to the uncertainty of the measured temperature, which is directly proportional to the uncertainty of the MRI signal's phase measurement. It has been shown that the optimal accuracy is obtained when the TE of the sequence is equal to the T_2* of the considered tissue. However, in practice, a TE shorter than T_2* can be used to exploit the higher SNR and decrease the phase uncertainty. An SNR of about 10 calculated on the magnitude image is usually sufficient for obtaining a temperature uncertainty in the order of 1°C.

The literature has shown that clinical scanners (1.5 T and 3 T) can provide temperature images with a spatial resolution in the order of a millimeter, an uncertainty of 1°C, and a refresh rate in the order of seconds for a volumetric coverage of about 1–2 cm in most of the organs yielding usable MRI signal. The PRFS method is, however, more complicated to implement in bones, lungs and the digestive system.

Several imaging sequences have been introduced, from standard 2D gradient echo sequence (FLASH) or its accelerated variations (echo shifting (de Zwart et al. 1996), ms-EPI (Celicanin et al. 2014) and ss-EPI (Ozenne et al. 2019)) combined with parallel imaging and multiband excitations, up to more advanced 3D versions (Svedin et al. 2018; Odeen and Parker 2019) with sophisticated reconstruction. It should be noted that using fast gradient echo sequences introduces geometrical distortions, although these can be corrected. The interested reader can refer to analogous techniques developed for functional MRI imaging of the brain.

Regardless of the employed sequence, a crucial requirement is that the generated data flow is processed in real time. For motionless organs (e.g. the brain), the processing pipeline is relatively simple. On the other hand, in moving organs (abdomen, thorax), the phase variations related to spatial changes in magnetic susceptibility can exceed those due to the local temperature changes. Synchronizing the scans with breathing is, for example, a simple solution for tackling this problem, although at the expense of temporal resolution for thermometry. To remove this limitation, a continuous acquisition can be performed with the aid of alignment and phase correction algorithms. One of the approaches is based on creating a set of reference images (atlas) acquired in different organ positions. During the intervention, each new image is compared to the most similar image in the atlas to subtract the phase contributions related to motion and keep only the contribution related to temperature variation. The so obtained temperature image is then co-registered with a unique reference image to be able to extract the temporal evolution of temperature in each pixel. Several implementations have been proposed with the goal of accelerating the image processing steps and improving temperature accuracy (Toupin et al. 2017). Examples of processing pipelines are presented in many scientific papers (de Senneville et al. 2010, 2011, 2021; Roujol et al. 2012; Ozenne et al. 2017). Another approach consists of extracting the contribution of the phase related to motion by analyzing the spatial variations of the phase in each new image by means of a mathematical model. During the intervention, using model knowledge, spatial variations are estimated on new images and then subtracted. This technique leads to the hypothesis that the phase around the heated area is accurately defined, which is sometimes difficult to ensure in practice. PRFS-based thermometry is well suited for treatments inducing high temperature rises. In contrast, in cryotherapy, the shortening of T_2* during the creation of ice around the implanted MTD makes this imaging technique ineffective. Other approaches based on ultrashort echo time (UTE) techniques have been proposed but they remain at the research stage. We invite the reader to refer to a recent review (Lutz and Bernard 2020).

In conclusion, MRI thermometry can be considered to be quite mature from a technical point of view and it successfully guides several MTDs in clinical use.

11.6. High-intensity focused ultrasound

11.6.1. *General principles*

HIFU focus mechanical ultrasound waves emitted from the surface of a transducer (typically, a portion of a sphere) outside the body toward tissues located deep inside the body. The size of the focal spot depends on the geometry of the emitter (focal distance "f" and aperture "D") as well as on the wavelength (λ) of the produced waves, as indicated in Figure 11.5.

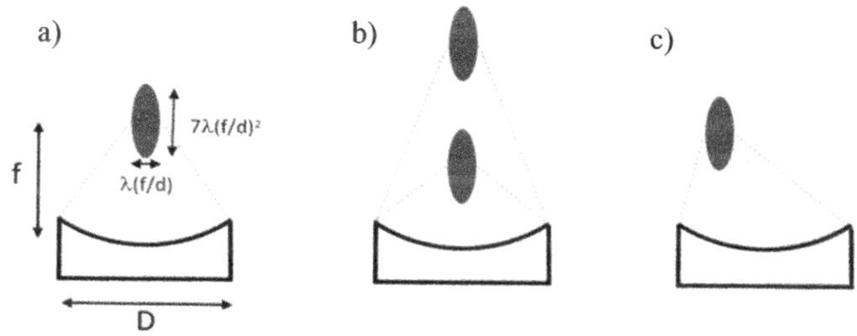

Figure 11.5. *Schematic representation of a HIFU transducer with aperture D and focal distance f*

COMMENT ON FIGURE 11.5.– *The dimensions of the focal spot are indicated in (a) as a function of the ultrasound wavelength, aperture and focal distance of the transducer. For example, for a transducer operating at 1 MHz (λ ~ 1 mm) with f ~ D, the size of the focal spot is 1 × 7 mm. If the transducer has many elements that can be activated via electrical signals with individually controllable phases, then the focus can be oriented closer or farther along the beam axis (b) or to a side (c).*

HIFU can be employed in several operation modes. Depending on the emitted ultrasound wave intensity and its duration, different biological effects can be induced (heating, stable or inertial cavitation, lithotripsy, histotripsy). Using continuous emission at relatively low intensity, deep tissues can be heated with a local temperature increase, similar to percutaneous MTDs. MRI thermometry (see section 11.5) can monitor the local temperature increase until the target level. Using fast multislice imaging by means of ss-EPI type of sequences, the local induced heating can be visualized in the target area as well as along the trajectory of the focal cone, as illustrated in Figure 11.6.

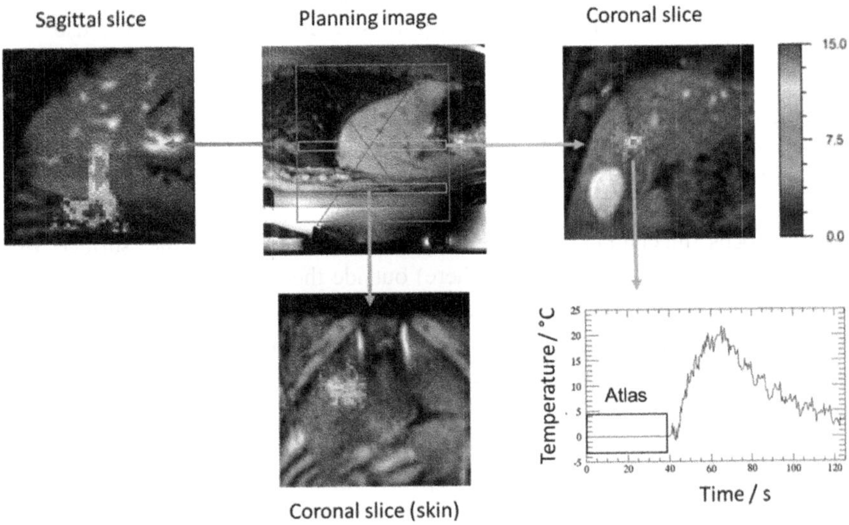

Figure 11.6. *HIFU in the liver guided by MRI thermometry*

COMMENT ON FIGURE 11.6.– *The planning image provides the visualization of the HIFU cone (red lines) and enables the positioning of thermometry slices: a coronal slice (orange box) and a sagittal slice (blue slice) centered at the focal point, as well as a slice at the skin (green box). Each slice is acquired in 80 ms thanks to a single shot EPI sequence. The temporal evolution of the temperature measured at the focal point is represented in the plot. Thanks to the first phase images, the artifacts in temperature curves related to breathing could be corrected. An increase of 20°C in 20 s is observed at the focal point.*

In pulsed mode, tissue displacement in the order of micrometers can be induced (acoustic radiation force) and detected by means of diffusion-weighted MRI sequences with at least two gradients, the first inducing a spin dephasing that is compensated by the second gradient. This technique includes a set of MRI sequences and is referred to as acoustic radiation force imaging (ARFI). Ultrasound pulse emission is synchronized with a gradient lobe in the MRI sequence. In the region where displacements are induced, the dephasing of the MRI signal is not counterbalanced by the second magnetic field gradient with opposite polarity. As a result, the phase image exhibits contrast that is related to the displacement induced by the acoustic radiation force, as illustrated in Figure 11.7.

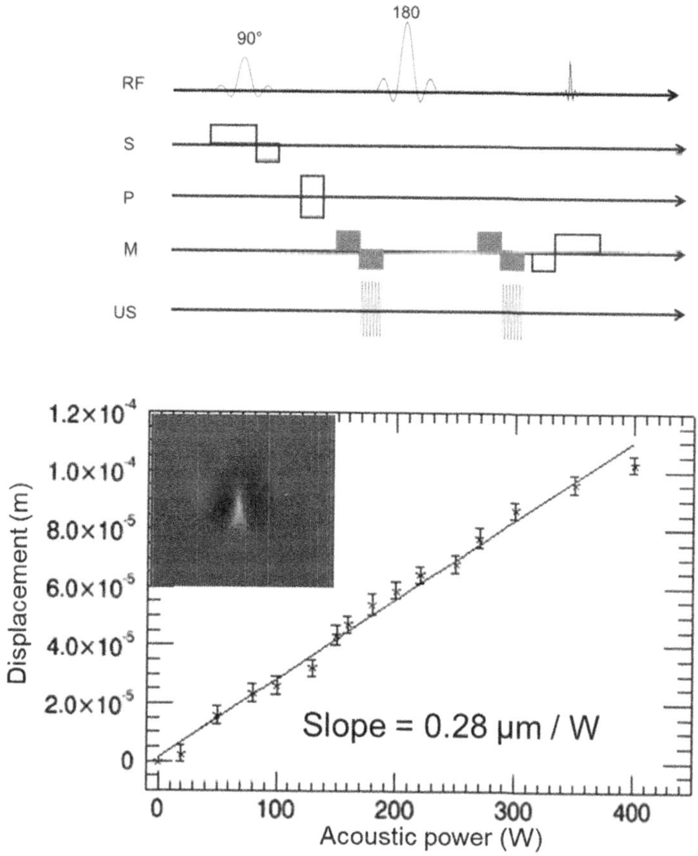

Figure 11.7. *ARFI technique for visualizing the displacement induced by an ultrasound pulse*

COMMENT ON FIGURE 11.7.– *The chronogram presents a spin echo sequence in which two bipolar gradients (orange) have been added on both sides of the refocusing 180° pulse. Ultrasound pulses are synchronized with each negative lobe of the gradient. Once reconstructed, the phase image is converted into a displacement image by integrating the duration and amplitude of the gradients, enabling the area displaced by the ultrasounds to be accurately localized in the image. The curve below shows the measurement of displacement at the focal point by repeating the MRI ARFI measurement using varying acoustic power emitted by the HIFU transducer. A linear fit yields a slope of* $0.28\mu m/W_{acoustic}$ *in this case.*

Several implementations of MRI-ARFI sequences have been introduced using gradient echo (Mougenot et al. 2016) or spin echo sequences (Marsac et al. 2012). Using pulsed focused ultrasound guided via MRI-ARFI can, for example, accurately target the area of ultrasound beam application in the brain to open the brain–blood barrier or to optimize the ultrasound beam to counterbalance the distortions and intensity attenuations in a heterogeneous or a strongly damping medium, such as the skull. Another application of the MRI-ARFI method is the control of acoustic intensity required to locally modify the propagation of the ultrasound beam to reach the focal spot. The result is an increased absorption, which leads to greater and more spatially distributed heating and avoids damaging deep tissues and interfaces between tissues with large differences in acoustic impedance (Zderic et al. 2008).

Displacement and temperature can be encoded simultaneously in the phase of the MRI image (Auboiroux et al. 2012; Bour et al. 2017; de Bever et al. 2018). Depending on the polarity of the magnetic field gradients, these contributions can be added or subtracted in the phase of the MRI signal. Relatively simple image processing (sum and difference between consecutive images) is capable of reconstructing a temperature image (and thus thermal dose maps) and a displacement image.

11.6.2. *Application domains*

The therapeutic potential of focused ultrasound with MRI guidance is highly promising in many biomedical domains. A large number of clinical therapeutic devices exist and most of them can be guided via non-MRI methods. Nevertheless, using MRI offers the advantage of multiplane imaging with a large variety of contrasts, in addition to the possibility of monitoring the thermal and mechanical effects of focused ultrasound in real time. The main clinical application domains for MRI-guided HIFU are the treatment of uterine fibroids, essential tremors and bone metastases.

Other oncologic applications are being developed with advanced proofs of concept and first clinical results on the treatment of breast or prostate cancer, for example. The website of the Fus Foundation (www.fusfoundation.org) provides an exhaustive review of the technogical advancements and preclinical and clinical applications of this technology.

11.7. Perspectives of interventional MRI

Interventional MRI is a growing domain with high application potential. One of the current limitations consists of the accessibility (especially in France) and the cost of MRI equipment. However, the latter is mitigated with the recent market availability of dedicated interventional MRI systems with a large diameter (up to 80 cm) providing the benefits of strong magnetic field gradients and a lower main magnetic field ($B_0 < 1$ T) with reduced acquisition and operating costs. Several fast acquisition sequences are provided by the main MRI manufacturers with real-time image reconstruction capabilities thanks to the wide spread of processors capable of high-performance parallelized calculations. On the other hand, fast communication interfaces allow for the export of reconstructed images to external consoles that interface with the MTDs. Another important feature regards the user interaction with an external console for MRI use enabling the selection of sequences and controlling their execution. For example, the slices can be repositioned during the sequence scan depending on a signal that is external to MRI. Thus, MRI becomes a component of the MTD, changing its initially intended use as a radiological diagnostic device. This modification is not exempt from complications from the regulatory point of view and affects the choice of MRI manufacturers regarding the provided sequences.

Interventional MRI should benefit from the advent of artificial intelligence techniques. For example, their application can include automatic organ segmentation, acceleration of image reconstruction, artifact correction and automatic re-positioning of slices for a percutaneous device.

An important aspect is related to hardware considerations. These include dedicated MRI receive coils that must provide sufficient access for inserting a percutaneous MTD or that do not affect the therapeutic capabilities of the MTD (HIFU, MR-Linac), the development of motorized positioning accessories (e.g. mechanical systems with piezoelectrical motors for HIFU), or optimized MTDs that minimize magnetic susceptibility artifacts, heating risks and electromagnetic interference with MRI. Many technical solutions already exist for each of these challenges.

Acquiring MRI images simultaneously with MTD operation paves the way for the development of robotic systems. The power delivered by a thermal ablation system can be controlled to achieve local heating with accuracy in the order of 1°C by means of a feedback loop employing tissue temperature measured via thermometry to continuously adjust the delivered ultrasound power (Salomir et al. 2000; Sebeke et al. 2019) and perform a 3D treatment adapted to the target. In this way, for example, local chemical therapeutical treatments (active principle encapsulated into a thermosensitive nanoparticle) can be delivered by means of moderate temperature increase (Cheng et al. 2020), while reducing the secondary effects compared to conventional treatments (in particular, cardiotoxicity) or a relevant gene can be activated via a thermosensitive promoter (Deckers et al. 2009).

Many technological barriers have been overcome, allowing for the MRI advantages to be combined with different innovative therapeutic solutions (puncture, radiotherapy, thermal ablation, etc.). The goals are to (i) provide the practitioners with a better way to control the therapy in real time while reducing any secondary effects and (ii) increase the number of patients eligible for image-guided therapies without having to compromise between safety and treatment efficacy. Finally, accurate 3D guidance in real time offered by MRI, in addition to the diagnostic performance pre- and post-intervention that it provides in many clinical domains, represents significant value.

11.8. References

Auboiroux, V., Viallon, M., Roland, J., Hyacinthe, J.N., Petrusca, L., Morel, D.R., Goget, T., Terraz, S., Gross, P., Becker, C.D. et al. (2012). ARFI-prepared MRgHIFU in liver: Simultaneous mapping of ARFI-displacement and temperature elevation, using a fast GRE-EPI sequence. *Magn. Reson. Med.*, 68(3), 932–946.

de Bever, J.T., Odeen, H., Hofstetter, L.W., Parker, D.L. (2018). Simultaneous MR thermometry and acoustic radiation force imaging using interleaved acquisition. *Magn. Reson. Med.*, 79(3), 1515–1524.

Bieri, O. and Scheffler, K. (2013). Fundamentals of balanced steady state free precession MRI. *J. Magn. Reson. Imaging*, 38(1), 2–11.

Bour, P., Marquet, F., Ozenne, V., Toupin, S., Dumont, E., Aubry, J.F., Lepetit-Coiffe, M., Quesson, B. (2017). Real-time monitoring of tissue displacement and temperature changes during MR-guided high intensity focused ultrasound. *Magn. Reson. Med.*, 78(5), 1911–1921.

Celicanin, Z., Auboiroux, V., Bieri, O., Petrusca, L., Santini, F., Viallon, M., Scheffler, K., Salomir, R. (2014). Real-time method for motion-compensated MR thermometry and MRgHIFU treatment in abdominal organs. *Magn. Reson. Med.*, 72(4), 1087–1095.

Cheng, B., Bing, C., Staruch, R.M., Shaikh, S., Wodzak Staruch, M., Szczepanski, D., Williams, N.S., Laetsch, T.W., Chopra, R. (2020). The effect of injected dose on localized tumor accumulation and cardiac uptake of doxorubicin in a Vx2 rabbit tumor model using MR-HIFU mild hyperthermia and thermosensitive liposomes. *Int. J. Hyperthermia*, 37(1), 1052–1059.

Deckers, R., Quesson, B., Arsaut, J., Eimer, S., Couillaud, F., Moonen, C.T. (2009). Image-guided, noninvasive, spatiotemporal control of gene expression. *Proc. Natl. Acad. Sci. USA*, 106(4), 1175–1180.

Godinez, F., Scott, G., Padormo, F., Hajnal, J.V., Malik, S.J. (2020). Safe guidewire visualization using the modes of a PTx transmit array MR system. *Magn. Reson. Med.*, 83(6), 2343–2355.

Lutz, N.W. and Bernard, M. (2020). Contactless thermometry by MRI and MRS: Advanced methods for thermotherapy and biomaterials. *iScience*, 23(10), 101561.

Mansfield, P. (1984). Real-time echo-planar imaging by NMR. *Br. Med. Bull.*, 40(2), 187–190.

Markl, M. and Leupold, J. (2012). Gradient echo imaging. *J. Magn. Reson. Imaging*, 35(6), 1274–1289.

Marsac, L., Chauvet, D., Larrat, B., Pernot, M., Robert, B., Fink, M., Boch, A.L., Aubry, J.F., Tanter, M. (2012). MR-guided adaptive focusing of therapeutic ultrasound beams in the human head. *Med. Phys.*, 39(2), 1141–1149.

Mougenot, C., Waspe, A., Looi, T., Drake, J.M. (2016). Variable ultrasound trigger delay for improved magnetic resonance acoustic radiation force imaging. *Phys. Med. Biol.*, 61(2), 712–727.

Odeen, H. and Parker, D.L. (2019). Improved MR thermometry for laser interstitial thermotherapy. *Lasers Surg. Med.*, 51(3), 286–300.

Ozen, A.C., Lottner, T., Bock, M. (2019). Safety of active catheters in MRI: Termination impedance versus RF-induced heating. *Magn. Reson. Med.*, 81(2), 1412–1423.

Ozenne, V., Toupin, S., Bour, P., de Senneville, B.D., Lepetit-Coiffe, M., Boissenin, M., Benois-Pineau, J., Hansen, M.S., Inati, S.J., Govari, A. et al. (2017). Improved cardiac magnetic resonance thermometry and dosimetry for monitoring lesion formation during catheter ablation. *Magn. Reson. Med.*, 77(2), 673–683.

Ozenne, V., Bour, P., de Senneville, B.D., Toupin, S., Vaussy, A., Lepetit-Coiffe, M., Jais, P., Cochet, H., Quesson, B. (2019). Assessment of left ventricle magnetic resonance temperature stability in patients in the presence of arrhythmias. *NMR Biomed.*, 32(11), e4160.

Quesson, B., de Zwart, J.A., Moonen, C.T. (2000). Magnetic resonance temperature imaging for guidance of thermotherapy. *J. Magn. Reson. Imaging*, 12(4), 525–533.

Roujol, S., Benois-Pineau, J., de Senneville, B.D., Ries, M., Quesson, B., Moonen, C.T. (2012). Robust real-time-constrained estimation of respiratory motion for interventional MRI on mobile organs. *IEEE Trans. Inf. Technol. Biomed.*, 16(3), 365–374.

Salomir, R., Vimeux, F.C., de Zwart, J.A., Grenier, N., Moonen, C.T. (2000). Hyperthermia by MR-guided focused ultrasound: Accurate temperature control based on fast MRI and a physical model of local energy deposition and heat conduction. *Magn. Reson. Med.*, 43(3), 342–347.

Sapareto, S.A. and Dewey, W.C. (1984). Thermal dose determination in cancer therapy. *Int. J. Radiat. Oncol. Biol. Phys.*, 10(6), 787–800.

Sebeke, L., Deenen, D.A., Maljaars, E., Heijman, E., de Jager, B., Heemels, W., Grull, H. (2019). Model predictive control for MR-HIFU-mediated, uniform hyperthermia. *Int. J. Hyperthermia*, 36(1), 1040–1050.

de Senneville, B.D., Roujol, S., Moonen, C.T., Ries, M. (2010). Motion correction in MR thermometry of abdominal organs: A comparison of the referenceless vs. the multi-baseline approach. *Magn. Reson. Med.*, 64(5), 1373–1381.

de Senneville, B.D., Ries, M., Maclair, G., Moonen, C.T. (2011). MR-guided thermotherapy of abdominal organs using a robust PCA-based motion descriptor. *IEEE Trans. Med. Imaging*, 30(11), 1987–1995.

de Senneville, B.D., Coupe, P., Ries, M., Facq, L., Moonen, C.T. (2021). Deep correction of breathing-related artifacts in real-time MR-thermometry. *Comput. Med. Imaging Graph*, 87, 101834.

Seror, O., Lepetit-Coiffe, M., Le Bail, B., de Senneville, B.D., Trillaud, H., Moonen, C.T., Quesson, B. (2008). Real time monitoring of radiofrequency ablation based on MR thermometry and thermal dose in the pig liver in vivo. *Eur. Radiol.*, 18(2), 408–416.

Svedin, B.T., Payne, A., Bolster Jr., B.D., Parker, D.L. (2018). Multiecho pseudo-golden angle stack of stars thermometry with high spatial and temporal resolution using k-space weighted image contrast. *Magn. Reson. Med.*, 79(3), 1407–1419.

Toupin, S., de Senneville, B.D., Ozenne, V., Bour, P., Lepetit-Coiffe, M., Boissenin, M., Jais, P., Quesson, B. (2017). Combination of principal component analysis and optical-flow motion compensation for improved cardiac MR thermometry. *Phys. Med. Biol.*, 62(4), 1208–1224.

Zderic, V., Foley, J., Luo, W., Vaezy, S. (2008). Prevention of post-focal thermal damage by formation of bubbles at the focus during high intensity focused ultrasound therapy. *Med. Phys.*, 35(10), 4292–4299.

de Zwart, J.A., Van Gelderen, P., Kelly, D.J., Moonen, C.T. (1996). Fast magnetic-resonance temperature imaging. *J. Magn. Reson. B*, 112(1), 86–90.

12

Ultra-high Field Imaging

Virginie CALLOT[1,2] and Alexandre VIGNAUD[3]

[1] CRMBM, CNRS, Université Aix-Marseille, France

[2] CEMEREM, AP-HM, Hôpital de la Timone, Marseille, France

[3] NeuroSpin, CEA, Gif-Sur-Yvette, France

At the time of the writing, and although there are no strict conventions, the "ultra-high field" term used in this chapter dedicated to human investigations refers to a magnetic field strength greater than, or equal to, 7 teslas[1].

12.1. Historical overview

Since its introduction in clinical routine in the mid-1980s, magnetic resonance imaging (MRI) has gained importance in radiology diagnostis, becoming a reference tool in various clinical applications. Since the first research works in this domain, this trend has been accompanied by a regular increase in the strength of the static magnetic field (B_0) systems. From the instruments used in proof-of-concept demonstrations in the 1970s (Lauterbur 1973), to the scanners currently used in clinical research, the magnetic field strength has increased by two orders of magnitude (Figure 12.1).

1 The systems dedicated to small-animal imaging used in preclinical research will not be covered in this chapter. For these applications, ultra-high field systems typically refer to field strengths greater than 9.4 T or 11.75 T.

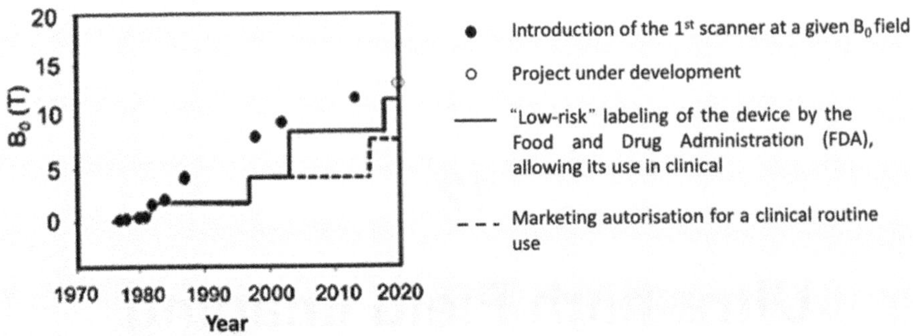

Figure 12.1. *Evolution of the MRI's static magnetic field strength (B_0 in tesla) over time. Figure adapted from Rooney et al. (2007)*

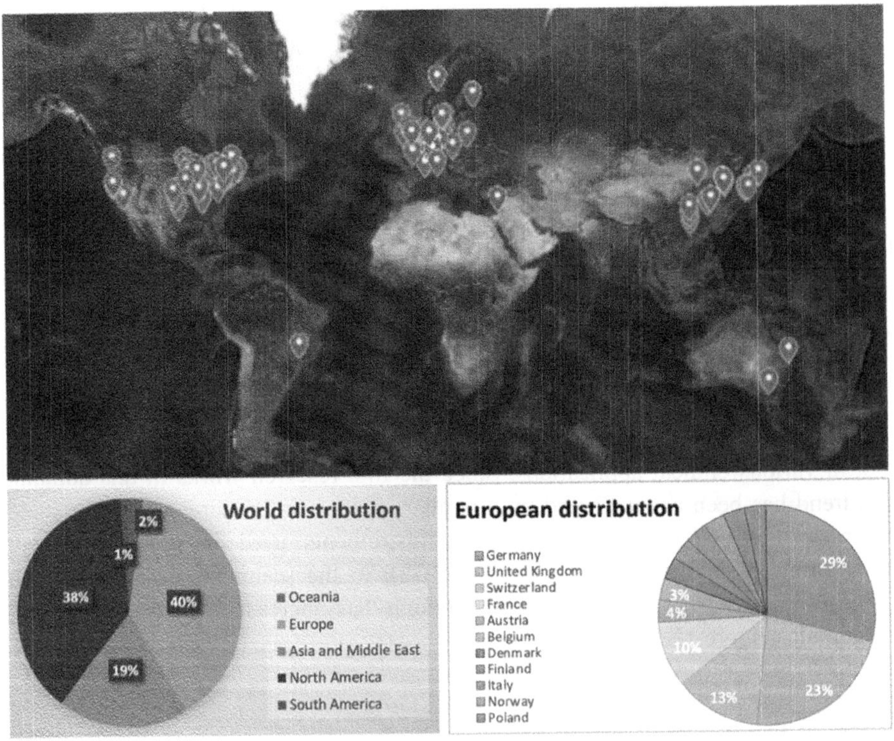

Figure 12.2. *Geographic distribution of ultra-high field systems installed worldwide (spring 2021). In France, three systems are currently installed (Saclay, Marseille, Poitiers). For a color version of this figure, see www.iste.co.uk/ratiney-beuf/challenges.zip*

While in vivo ultra-high-field imaging was initially demonstrated in 1998 in a brain on an 8 T scanner (Robitaille et al. 1998), 7 T field strength has become the field of reference in this domain (Uğurbil 2018), with the first operating device developed in the early 2000s (Vaughan et al. 2001) in Minneapolis. Twenty years later, these devices have become well established in the clinical research landscape with more than 90 systems installed over the world in 2021 (Figure 12.2). Since 2017, these scanners have been certified for clinical exams in the brain, including sodium imaging, and for musculoskeletal applications (exclusively in the knee).

12.2. Quest toward higher field MR systems – why?

Although widely used and undergoing continuous improvement thanks to several technological advancements (gradient system, RF coils, parallel imaging, etc.) over the last two decades, anatomical MRI at standard fields (1.5 and 3 T) often remains constrained to spatial resolutions in the range of a millimeter. At such field strengths, quantitative MRI, exotic nuclei MRI (also known as X-nuclei) and spectroscopy can also suffer from low sensitivity (in the sense of "available signal" for detection). To overcome these limitations, visualize human body structures in more detail, and improve the detection of physiological variations, ultra-high field systems thus represent a promising solution (just as 3 T or 4 T systems appeared as a better alternative to 1.5 T scanners in the 1990s) providing much better signal-to-noise ratio (SNR), contrast due to susceptibility effects and spectral resolution, as will be described in the following.

12.2.1. *Advantages and benefits of ultra-high field systems*

12.2.1.1. *Signal-to-noise ratio and sensitivity*

SNR is one of the most important parameters in MRI because its increase can be exploited to improve spatial (Figure 12.3) or temporal resolution. For fixed temporal and spatial resolutions, it provides better sensitivity, which is particularly beneficial for quantitative imaging.

According to theory, the SNR variation is supralinear as a function of the main magnetic field strength (Ocali and Atalar 1998). This has recently been confirmed by experimental measurements. Considering all of the parameters influencing the measurements for a range of B_0 between 1.5 and 9.4 T, the SNR was found to increase as $B_0^{1.65}$ (Pohmann et al. 2016). Thus, the expected gain in SNR when using 7 T instead of 3 T, assuming the same RF coil design, is approximately a factor of 3.1 (see Figure 12.4).

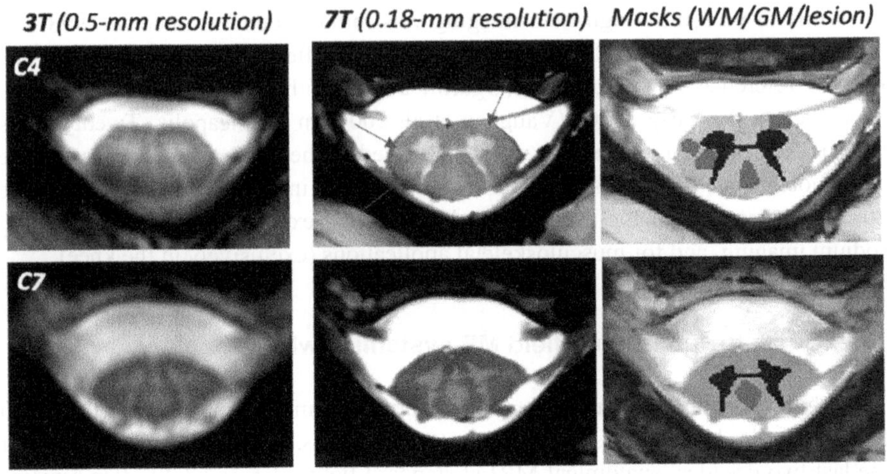

Figure 12.3. *Imaging of the spinal cord in the context of multiple sclerosis: the contours of the white matter (WM), gray matter (GM) and lesion become much more prominent at the higher field; some undetected lesions at 3 T become visible at 7 T (red arrows) with a direct impact on the diagnosis and patient treatment. Images from CRMBM-CEMEREM (V. Callot). For a color version of this figure, see www.iste.co.uk/ratiney-beuf/challenges.zip*

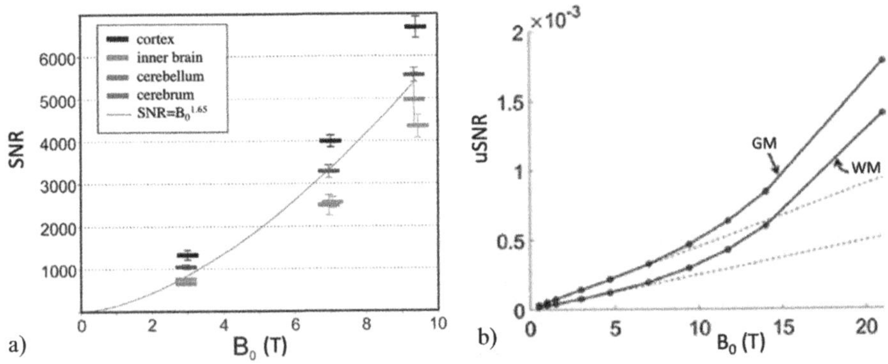

Figure 12.4. *SNR variation as a function of the magnetic field B_0. For a color version of this figure, see www.iste.co.uk/ratiney-beuf/challenges.zip*

COMMENT ON FIGURE 12.4.– *(a) SNR variation as a function of magnetic field B_0. Modified from Pohmann et al. (2016), with the authors' permission. (b) Simulated variation of the ultimate SNR (a.u.) in gray matter (GM) and white matter (WM) as a function of the magnetic field. The dashed lines represent the linear extrapolation* *of uSNR at lower fields. Modified from Guérin et al. (2017), with the authors' permission. The notion of ultimate SNR refers to the maximum theoretically possible SNR, regardless of the coil geometry (Ocali and Atalar 1998).*

SNR is even more important in parallel imaging with SENSE- or GRAPPA-based reconstructions, which have been widely adopted to reduce the scan time at the price of decreased SNR (compared to conventional Cartesian-based MRI with a receive coil array). This reduction is dependent on the acceleration factor R and the geometry factor "g" related to coil geometry according to the formula $SNR_R = SNR_0/(g.R^{1/2})$ (Pruessmann et al. 2001). However, for a given coil design, it has been shown that, when B_0 increases, g has less influence on the result, thereby increasing the advantage of parallel imaging at ultra-high field (Wiesinger et al. 2004).

Finally, while MRI usually detects hydrogen nuclei (^1H), other nuclei (X) with a nonzero nuclear spin can also be used. Due to the concentration of the isotope in the human body and its gyromagnetic value, the observable signal is typically very low at conventional magnetic fields employed in clinics, leaving little room for alternative approaches. At 7 T, the SNR gain partially compensates for this weakness, thereby opening new perspectives for X-nuclei imaging and spectroscopy (see Chapter 9). The best candidates are in the order of decreasing available signal: ^{23}Na sodium, which can be used as a marker of tissue viability and the investigation of inflammatory and (neuro-)degenerative processes (Thulborn 2018), particularly through the measurement of the total sodium concentration (Burstein and Springer 2019); ^{31}P phosphorus for investigating the energy metabolism and pH measurement (Liu et al. 2017); and ^{13}C carbon. Lower-abundance ^{39}K potassium and ^{17}O oxygen remain hardly detectable at 7 T. Finally, it should be noted that the low-sensitivity nuclei that are naturally absent in the human body can also be considered for 7 T imaging. This is the case of ^7Li lithium used in psychiatry to evaluate the efficacy of some treatments (Stout et al. 2020).

12.2.1.2. *Contrasts (BOLD/T_2*, T_1, etc.)*

Besides the SNR and sensitivity, the contrast-to-noise ratio (CNR), measured from the difference in signal between two tissues, is also very important. High CNR can be useful for medical diagnosis in detecting small pathological anomalies or simply for the identification and delimitation of tissues from their intrinsic properties (T_1, T_2, T_2*). At 7 T, T_2* and T_1 contrasts can be particularly useful.

For a variation of the magnetic field (B) in a sample according to $B = \mu_0.(1+\chi).B_0$, with μ_0 as the vacuum permeability and χ as the magnetic susceptibility of the sample, the magnetic field non-uniformities at the interface between two tissues with different magnetic susceptibility properties ($\Delta\chi = \chi_2 - \chi_1$)

are given by $\Delta B \propto \Delta\chi.B_0$. Therefore, increasing the magnetic field leads to linearly increased sensitivity to magnetic field inhomogeneities at the interface between compartments with different magnetic susceptibility. These variations of the local magnetic field, created at microscopic and mesoscopic scales (contributions to T_2) as well as at a macroscopic scale ($\gamma.\Delta B_0$), perturb the transverse relaxation, leading to the so-called T_2* that satisfies the equation $1/T_2^* = 1/T_2 + \gamma.\Delta B_0$ (van der Kolk et al. 2013). These perturbations imply greater sensitivity of T_2*-weighted sequences, such as gradient echo ones, at 7 T compared to conventional fields.

	Relaxation time	1.5 T	3 T	7 T
Blood (venous)	T_2* (ms)	42–70	20–29	7–13
	T_1 (ms)	1,250	1,650	2,100
Gray matter (brain)	T_2* (ms)	65–84	42–66	33–36
	T_2 (ms)	80	71	47
	T_1 (ms)	1,200	1,300	2,100
White matter (brain)	T_2* (ms)	66	48–53	27–35
	T_2 (ms)	84	72	47
	T_1 (ms)	650	840	1,220
Cerebrospinal fluid	T_1 (ms)	4,100	4,310	4,420

Table 12.1. *Examples of relaxation values (T_2*, T_2, T_1) as a function of the magnetic field. Adopted from Rooney et al. (2007); Koopmans et al. (2008); Cox and Gowland (2010); and Zhang et al. (2013)*

This sensitivity offers new perspectives, in particular for functional imaging (fMRI). fMRI is based on the variations of blood flow and volume, as well as deoxyhemoglobin concentration, during neuronal activation, which cause changes in magnetic susceptibility and, as a consequence, in signal (blood oxygenation level dependent (BOLD) effect (see Chapter 5)). Combined with a possible improvement of spatial resolution, ultra-high field fMRI (Yacoub and Wald 2018) becomes more sensitive and enables us to, for example, distinguish the activation within subcortical layers (Figure 12.5).

It should be noted that increasing the strength of the magnetic field causes additional distortions but also greater sensitivity to physiological noise (see section 12.2.2). As a result, the parameters of a functional imaging sequence should be selected to maintain the temporal SNR (tSNR) within the thermal noise regime (Triantafyllou et al. 2011) to fully benefit from the increased field.

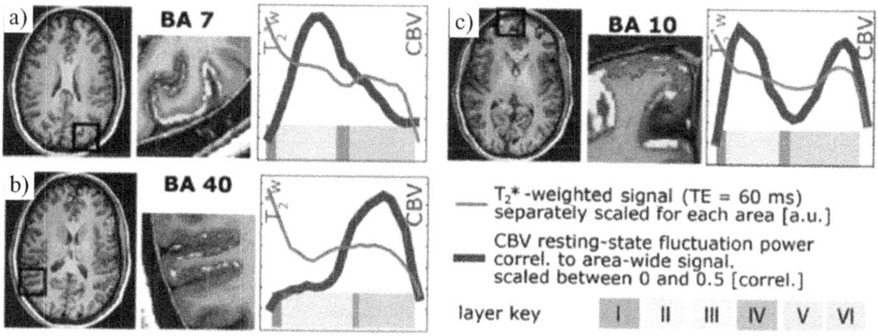

Figure 12.5. *Functional maps of different cortical regions, highlighting layout-specific activity features. (a) Large signal activity in superficial layers for BA7 (Brodmann area), (b) activity mainly in the deeper layers (BA40), (c) activity on the surface and in the deep layers for BA10. Modified from Finn et al. (2020), with authors' permission. For a color version of this figure, see www.iste.co.uk/ratiney-beuf/challenges.zip*

The literature suggests that an advantage exists in using T_2 weighting rather than T_2* weighting at ultra-high magnetic fields. Indeed, T_2 weighting improves the specificity of the BOLD signal by strengthening the contribution of capillaries compared to the large vessels inside a voxel (Uludağ et al. 2009). However, in practice, T_2 weighting is rarely used because it requires spin-echo sequences that deposit a considerable amount of energy in the tissues, which limits their applications to small volumes of interest.

Susceptibility weighting imaging (SWI) (Haacke et al. 2004) and quantitative susceptibility mapping (QSM) (de Rochefort et al. 2010) methods also greatly benefit from higher magnetic fields. The most spectacular applications include vascular network imaging (venography) (Koopmans et al. 2008) (see Figure 12.6), imaging of deep brain structures (subthalamic nuclei, basal ganglia, etc.) (Abosch et al. 2010), or the visualization of the central vein in the context of multiple sclerosis (MS), as described in section 12.4.

Finally, some applications also benefit from the variation of the longitudinal relaxation time (T_1) with the magnetic field. In biological tissues, the value of T_1 increases with the field strength (Rooney et al. 2007; Rodgers et al. 2013). In its generalized form, the variation of T_1 is expressed as T_1 (s) ~ A.ν_0 ^{B}, with ν_0 as the resonance frequency (Hz) and A and B two tissue-dependent constants (Bottomley et al. 1987).

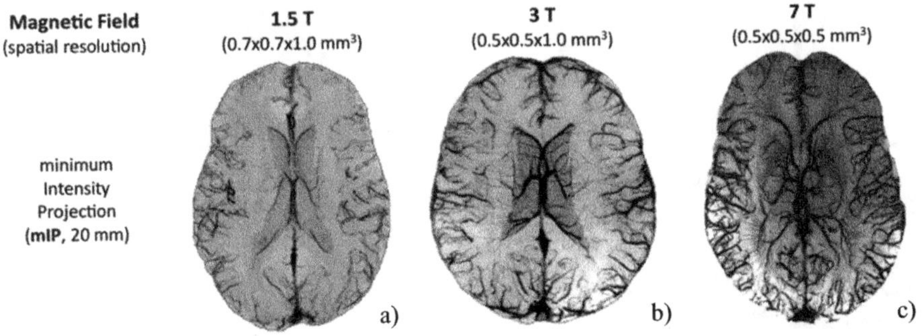

Figure 12.6. *SWI imaging (mIP) acquired at different magnetic fields. (a) 1.5 T, (b) 3 T and (c) 7 T. The contrast and spatial resolution (voxel size) achieved at 7 T are particularly useful for detailed visualization of the venous network and its possible anomalies. From Monti et al. (2017), with the authors' permission*

At first glance, this increase could be perceived as a disadvantage. For instance, in neuroradiology, distinguishing between gray and white matter can become more difficult on conventional T_1-weighted images. However, this increase can be exploited for vascular imaging with contrast injection (Hagberg and Scheffler 2013) and without contrast agents (time of flight (ToF)) (Kang et al. 2010). In fact, the relaxation times of the blood and contrast agents, such as gadolinium, are less affected by the increase in B_0 than the adjacent tissues (Zhang et al. 2013). Thanks to a better SNR, spatial resolution and efficacy in suppressing the background signal (von Morze et al. 2007), the difference between the blood (injected or not) and static tissues is amplified, providing a better demarcation of the arterial network and eventual extravasation toward surrounding tissues.

A longer T_1 is also advantageous for applications with longitudinal magnetization preparation before the image acquisition; an example consists of cardiac tagging (used for investigating myocardial contractions), whose efficacy is improved over several cardiac cycles thanks to the longer T_1 values at 7 T (Rodgers et al. 2013).

12.2.1.3. *Spectral broadening (MRS, CEST, etc.)*

The domains of metabolic imaging and magnetic resonance spectroscopy (MRS) benefit from increased magnetic fields as well. Both for single voxel applications (single voxel spectroscopy (SVS)) or for spectroscopic imaging (chemical shift imaging (CSI)), the increased SNR in MRS can be exploited to reduce the voxel size and, hence, the partial volume effects in order to make the acquired metabolic spectrum more specific to the investigated tissues (e.g. discrimination of neurochemical profiles within the thalamic nuclei (Donadieu et al. 2016)).

More importantly, the spectral resolution between two species ($\Delta\omega$) increases linearly with B_0 (according to $\Delta\omega = \gamma\cdot(\sigma_2 - \sigma_1)\cdot B_0$, with σ being the chemical shift of each of these two species), thus highlighting the contribution of proton populations that could not be previously distinguished, thereby improving both the sensitivity and specificity of the technique. To fully benefit from these advantages, a good uniformity of B_0 and B_1^+ is required, together with the implementation of specific acquisition and post-processing strategies (adiabatic pulses, frequency stabilization, etc.) (Henning 2018).

Chemical exchange saturation transfer (CEST) (Ward et al. 2000; Kogan et al 2013), which enables the indirect detection of metabolites or molecules containing protons that can be exchanged via magnetization transfer from the pool of bound protons to the pool of free protons, can also benefit from a higher magnetic field. In the human body, these metabolites include the amide protons (APT), glycosaminoglycans (gag), glycogen, glutamate (Glu), etc., which can be notably used to investigate tumors (APT-CEST) or the cartilage (gag-CEST), for example. Once again, higher SNR provides better sensitivity (Singh et al. 2012) and improved frequency separation is advantageous due to the possibility of distinguishing components that were so far hardly discernible from the water peak (e.g. hydroxyl protons, which have a chemical shift between 0.5 and 1.5 ppm). It should be noted that at 7 T, all of these CEST applications remain still largely challenged by the problems related to the non-uniformities of the static and radiofrequency fields.

12.2.2. *Disadvantages and challenges*

Despite several advantages listed above, which have been predicted by the theory for a long time, the introduction of 7 T scanners for clinical use had not taken place until very recently. The cost/benefit ratio could have been a reasonable justification for this late appearance, but this was rather due to the need to first solve problems linked to heterogeneity of the static B_0 and radiofrequency B_1^+ fields, as well as the specific absorption rate (SAR) associated with the latter.

12.2.2.1. *B_0 inhomogeneity*

The scanners are manufactured to provide certain hardware specifications of constant uniformity of the static magnetic field B_0 inside the MRI bore over a diameter of spherical volume (DSV), regardless of the system's field (see Chapter 1).

Introducing an object or a patient inside the bore causes local field inhomogeneities (Schenck 1996) that increase linearly with B_0.

This heterogeneity, in particular at the interfaces between media with different magnetic susceptibilities χ, can be partially corrected using shim coils installed in the gradient insert. However, even if significant improvements can be obtained locally, these non-uniformities cannot be always compensated; this is the case of bone/tissue interfaces in the spine, air/tissue in the nasal cavity or near the lungs, or in the presence of metallic implants. Depending on the type of sequences, these effects can translate into artifacts, distortions, and signal loss in the images, especially in non-Cartesian imaging sequences, EPI sequences used in functional and diffusion imaging, or in spectroscopy.

This problem can be addressed using more B_0 shim coils (third spherical harmonic orders), gradient coil inserts dedicated to the organ to be scanned (Stockmann and Wald 2018), or dynamic shim strategies for multislice acquisitions with a controlled current in the shim coils for each imaging slice (Sengupta et al. 2011).

It should be noted that the variations of the B_0 field due to breathing (variation of the lung volume and intrinsic susceptibility effects) can also be problematic at 7 T, in particular for EPI- or gradient echo-based imaging and spectroscopy. This phenomenon, called "dynamic variation of the B_0 field", can induce a significant and penalizing signal attenuation. When imaging the spinal cord for instance, B_0 variations in the order of 70 Hz have been reported during the breathing cycle, associated with a signal loss between 40 and 120% (Vannesjo et al. 2019). In the brain, these fluctuations are lower, in the order of 10 Hz, but they are still present (Vannesjo et al. 2015).

12.2.2.2. *Feasibility of ultra-high resolution imaging*

Increasing the spatial resolution provided by 7 T is hindered by higher sensitivity to the patient's motion (physiological or involuntary). Physiological movements are related to the cardiac rhythm, cerebrospinal fluid pulsations, as well as breathing, which cause dynamic variations of B_0 non-uniformities in addition to organ displacement. Synchronizing the MRI acquisition with the respiratory or cardiac cycle (via pressure or pulse sensors or ECG electrodes) remains necessary for cardiac, medullar or abdominal applications as conventionally performed at lower fields. Physiological data can also be recorded, such that they can be filtered or their influence uncorrelated during image post-processing (Lévy et al. 2021). It should be noted that the signal quality of the electrocardiogram at 7 T can be considerably perturbed inside the magnet by the magnetohydrodynamic effects of blood flow (Stäb et al. 2016).

Motion can also be related to patient compliance (Marrakchi-Kacem et al. 2016). For brain applications, dedicated devices have been developed to ensure the reliability and reproducibility of investigations with very high spatial resolution. These devices employ motion control systems based on optical cameras (Stucht et al. 2015; Mattern et al. 2018) or magnetic field cameras (Haeberlin et al. 2015) and involve a feedback loop that modifies in real-time the gradients applied by the imaging sequence to take into account the changes in the patient's position. Furthermore, the information can be also used a posteriori to correct the motion effects during post-processing. Regardless of the approach, these methods are currently limited to research settings.

12.2.2.3. B_1^+ *non-uniformity*

In terms of SNR and CNR, the benefit of MRI at 7 T mentioned in section 12.2.1 is neutralized by the inhomogeneous propagation of the radiofrequency field in the human body at this frequency. Maxwell equations governed by the electromagnetism laws show that when the resonance frequency is increased, the wavelength of the RF fields inside the tissues decreases down to the size of the body region to be scanned (between 10 and 15 cm, see Figure 12.7(a)), potentially with destructive interferences (Collins and Wang 2011) or dielectric artifacts (Hoult and Phil 2000) with conventional excitation approaches, depending on the coil geometry, scanned region and its relative permittivity ε_r and electrical conductivity σ. In practice, this translates into a modification of the B_1^+ field within the tissues (nonuniform flip angle over the image, see Figures 12.7(f) and (g)), and consequently into spatial heterogeneities of the signal (signal loss artifacts) (see Figures 12.7(d) and (e)).

For scanners approved for clinical use, with currently authorized medical scans only in the brain and knee, radiofrequency heterogeneity in these anatomical regions remains overall limited and permits good diagnostic interpretation. Nevertheless, some precautions have to be taken in the frontotemporal regions and during quantitative imaging. To minimize these problems, other approaches are required: passive approaches based on dielectric pads, or active ones, based on imaging with parallel transmission (see section 12.5).

The non-uniformities of B_1^+ field are also a limitation for all of the imaging sequences that exploit global inversions or saturations of the magnetization.

In quantitative imaging, such as CEST or T_1 relaxometry, the B_1^+ heterogeneities have to be corrected to remove quantification biases (Kogan et al. 2013). Some sequences, such as the T_1-MP2RAGE (Marques et al. 2010), can be adapted to be relatively immune to B_1^+ variations thanks to the type of employed RF pulses and a smart adjustment of the acquisition parameters (RF angles, inversion times, etc.).

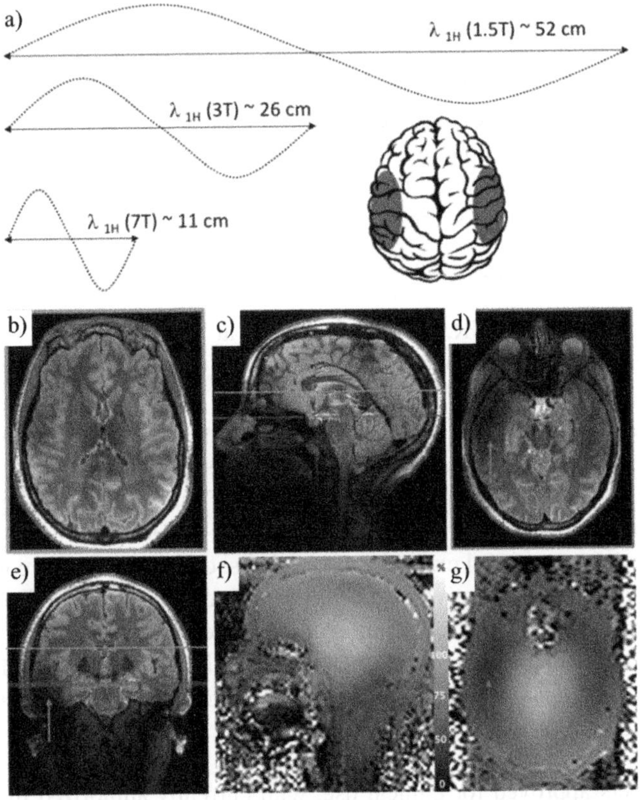

Figure 12.7. *Illustration of the radiofrequency wavelength in water at different magnetic fields (a) (Schick 2005). Anatomical brain imaging (b–e) and B_1^+ mapping (f and g). The green arrow points at a less uniform signal area in the temporal region. The variations of B_1^+ are around –25% in the frontal region (e) and about 50% in the temporal region (f, green arrow). Images provided by CRMBM-CEMEREM (Marseille). For a color version of this figure, see www.iste.co.uk/ratiney-beuf/challenges.zip*

Fat saturation techniques and other specific suppression techniques or spatially selective water excitation methods, such as the ones employed in spectroscopy, can also suffer from B_1^+ heterogeneity, which makes them inefficient over the entire volume of interest. Arterial spin labeling (ASL) techniques are also heavily penalized (Teeuwisse et al. 2010). Since RF emission is usually optimized for the slice plane, the labeling in a region far away from the imaging plane is less effective and suboptimal. Whenever possible, the use of adiabatic pulses that produce RF pulses with relatively low sensitivity to B_1^+ variations is recommended and can provide considerable improvements (Zimmer et al. 2016).

12.2.2.4. *Specific absorption rate*

One of the main risks of MRI is related to the heating of biological tissues during a scan (see Chapter 2). Within the range of frequencies of operation of modern MRI scanners, a non-negligible amount of energy of the RF excitation is absorbed by the body, causing heating that can cause severe damage if it is too intense. In a first approximation, this part of energy increases following B_0^2 for a given flip angle inside the volume (Hoult and Phil 2000). The SAR is the parameter used to quantify the energy dissipated per unit time in the patient (W/kg). SAR can be measured in several ways: SAR_{global} is the average SAR over the patient's body mass in the scanner and SAR_{local} is calculated per unit 10 g of tissue. SAR_{local} describes the energy deposited locally in the tissue that is capable of affecting it without necessarily being dangerous from a global point of view. SAR values are calculated and monitored by the manufacturers when the scanner is employed in single-channel transmission mode and are limited by regulations (3.2/10 W/kg for SAR_{global}/SAR_{local} in the head in normal mode, 2 W/kg for the body, etc.) (International Standard (IEC) 2010) in the same way for any field, which in practice makes high-field imaging more constrained, with a global increase by a factor of ~5 from 3 to 7 T.

The penalties related to energy deposition occur particularly in sequences employing several RF pulses with a large flip angle, such as turbo spin echo sequences. Usually, in such sequences, the number of slices that can be acquired has to be reduced or the repetition time has to be increased. Magnetization transfer sequences require high peak power and are also strongly penalized. These effects can be reduced using parallel transmission (pTx) and specific RF pulse design approaches (see section 12.5).

12.3. Quest toward higher fields – how?

12.3.1. *Technical constraints*

To fully reach the theoretically expected gain in terms of SNR, spatial resolution and image quality, improved performances in terms of power and slew rate of gradients, second and third-order shims, and RF systems, had to be achieved, optimizing each component to reduce coupling between gradient and shim coils, Foucault currents, acoustic vibrations or peripheral nerve stimulations (Winkler et al. 2018). Ultra-high field systems thus become more sophisticated, larger (see Table 12.2), and more expensive.

A major technical and physical constraint in ultra-high field MRI is the need for an RF coil adapted to the organ to be scanned. Indeed, the transmitted wavelength in human tissues decreases from ~ 55 cm at 1.5 T to 13 cm at 7 T, leading to destructive interferences of the MRI signal and limited penetration depth. As a result, whole-body coils that are usually integrated inside the bore and commonly used for RF excitation in scanners at 1.5 or 3 T are inadequate and inefficient at 7 T. Coil manufacturers have thus focused on the development of systems for 7 T imaging working in transmit/receive mode and adapted as much as possible to each organ of interest. While the number and efficiency of the coils are still low (Kraff and Quick 2019), in particular for applications outside the brain, the development of new coil technologies (dipoles, striplines, ceramic ones, etc.) is a very active domain, promising a wider deployment of ultra-high fields.

	1.5 T	3 T	7 T	10.5 T	11.7 T
Length (cm)	125–170	160–180	270–300	410	500
Bore diameter (cm)	60–70	60–70	60	60	60
Strength (mT/m) / Slew Rate (T/m/s)	40–45/200	40–80/200	70–80/200	70/200	70/200
Weight (t)	3–6	5–10	25	110	134

Table 12.2. *Some hardware features of standard scanners at 1.5, 3 T, 7 T, 10.5 T (CMRR, Minnesota)(*) and 11.7 T (Quettier et al. 2020) (Neurospin, Saclay). All scanners employ horizontal cylindrical bores with active shielding, except for (*) with passive shielding*

12.3.2. *Physiological constraints, contraindications and safety*

A long-standing and recurrent question related to MRI investigations at 7 T and its introduction in clinical practice concerned its potential "danger" and the precautions to be taken for the currently available devices.

Perception feedbacks collected from carefully monitored and instructed subjects during one or several repeated scans at 7 T have not shown any negative health effects (van Osch and Webb 2014). Some effects, such as light (< 40% of the subjects) to moderate dizziness (20%), metallic-taste feeling (5%), nausea (2%) and light flashes (magnetophosphenes) (1%), can occur when entering/exiting the bore or when moving within the magnet's fringe field (Rauschenberg et al. 2014), but these effects are temporary, well known and physiologically characterized (Schenck 2000). Minor magnetohydrodynamic effects on the cardiovascular system (increased arterial pressure or cardiac rhythm) have also been reported, but they have a low probability of occurring at fields below 8 T according to the World Health Organisation (Internationale Arbeitsorganisation, International Commission on Non-Ionizing Radiation Protection and Weltgesundheitsorganisation 2006). Moreover, all of these effects are nowadays greatly attenuated by active shielding systems in MRIs, slow motions of the scanner table when entering the bore, and slow movements around the table during the patient's positioning. With the new-generation systems, scans are very well tolerated by patients

Regarding exclusion criteria and the possibility to scan a patient with an implant, whether it is a passive (cardiac stent, dental implant, osteosynthesis materials) or active one (pacemaker, neurostimulation electrodes, etc.), the indications and precautions to be taken into account have evolved during the last decade (Hoff et al. 2019; Fagan et al. 2021) and they now approve the patient's exam in some conditions (material composition, conditional classification at 3 T, localization of the implant with respect to the coil, etc.). These indications should further evolve with the deployment of 7 T in clinics and better knowledge of material compatibility. However, many advances remain to be pursued in this domain and great caution must be used in case of doubts.

To conclude, SAR is regulated as for lower fields and thus does not represent a greater risk. Peripheral nerve stimulations (PNS) are induced by the variations of the encoding gradients and therefore are only affected by their technical characteristics. The acoustic noise produced by the gradient switching increases with the B_0 field for a given magnet and gradient design (Laplace forces (Price et al. 2001)), hence proper acoustic protection remains necessary and sufficient. Increased vigilance is also compulsory regarding the risks of external magnetic metallic objects (keys, rolling chairs, etc.) being attracted to the center of the magnet (so-called "projectile" risks).

12.4. Main applications and novel opportunities

Ultra-high field imaging systems have enabled a significant step forward in our ability to visualize and study the body organs and their impaired functioning. 7 T MRI is of course inappropriate for all diagnostic cases, but it has become unavoidable for some applications in the brain and knee, for which, as we have seen previously, the latest generations of 7 T MRI scanners have received regulatory approval (CE/FDA) in the European Union and the United States. Some application examples are illustrated below.

In the brain, the five main applications for which 7 T MRI has already been a game-changer are (van der Kolk et al. 2013; Trattnig et al. 2018): cerebrovascular diseases (microbleeding, aneurysms); cerebral tumors; epilepsy; MS; and degenerative diseases such as Parkinson's disease.

12.4.1. *Cerebrovascular diseases*

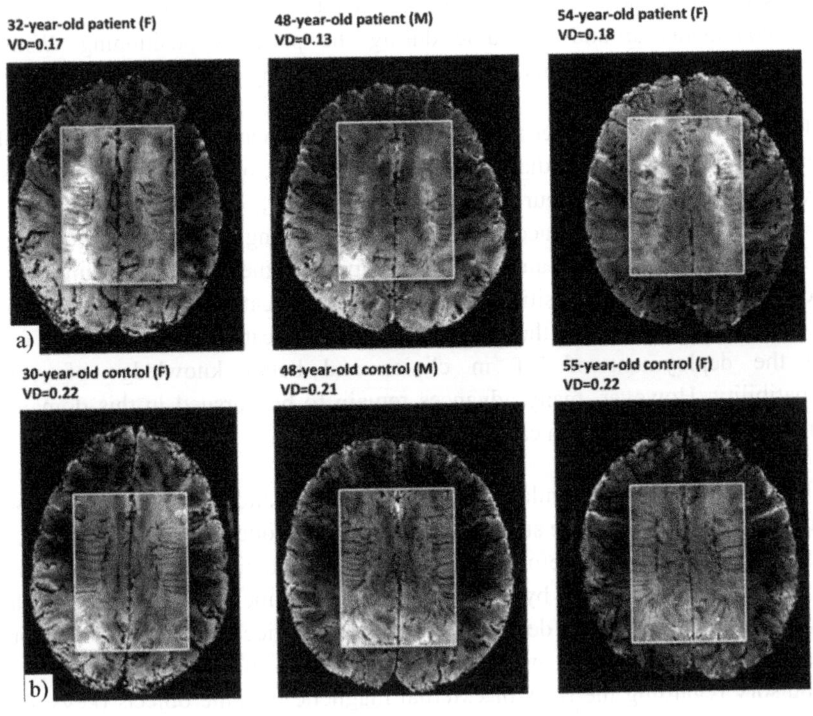

Figure 12.8. *Illustration of vein density reduction in the CADASIL disease (a) compared to healthy volunteers paired by age and gender (b). Minimum intensity projection. VD represents the average vein density. Lower densities are observed in patients, in particular in the hyperintense signal areas in the white matter (yellow rectangle). Images modified from De Guio et al. (2014), with the authors' permission. For a color version of this figure, see www.iste.co.uk/ratiney-beuf/challenges.zip*

Thanks to the increased spatial resolution (reaching 0.2 mm isotropic voxels), magnetic resonance angiography at 7 T has been revolutionary in revealing ramifications of the vascular network that were until now invisible on conventional scanners (e.g. lenticulostriate arteries that feed deep brain structures or perforating arteries of the cerebral trunk). 7 T angiography offers new opportunities (Park et al. 2018) in the context of early detection of cerebrovascular diseases (aneurysms, etc.), investigation of vascular mechanisms in small-vessel diseases (e.g. Cerebral Autosomal Dominant Arteriopathy with Subcortical Infarcts and Leukoencephalopathy (CADASIL)) (see Figure 12.8) or for functional angiography.

Thanks to an increased contrast in T_2*-weighted imaging, microbleeding is also more detectable. Compared to 3 T scanners, this technique detects the microbleeding of atypical small venous vessels, providing complementary information that can be useful to better understand vascular ischemic or traumatic pathologies (Moenninghoff et al. 2015).

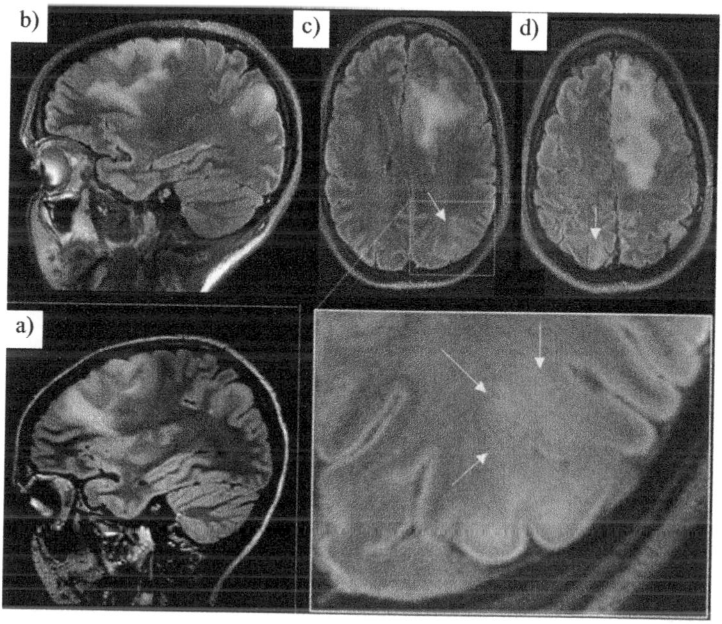

Figure 12.9. *Imaging performed after the first epileptic seizure. 3 T imaging provided an initial diagnosis of a left frontal infiltrating lesion (a) without detectable lesions. Additional imaging at 7 T (b) revealed two more lesions (c, d) in the left (c) and right parietal junction, leading to the final diagnosis of an anaplastic glioma with a therapeutic incidence of the multifocal nature. Images kindly provided by Prof. R. Guillevin (CHU Poitiers). For a color version of this figure, see www.iste.co.uk/ratiney-beuf/challenges.zip*

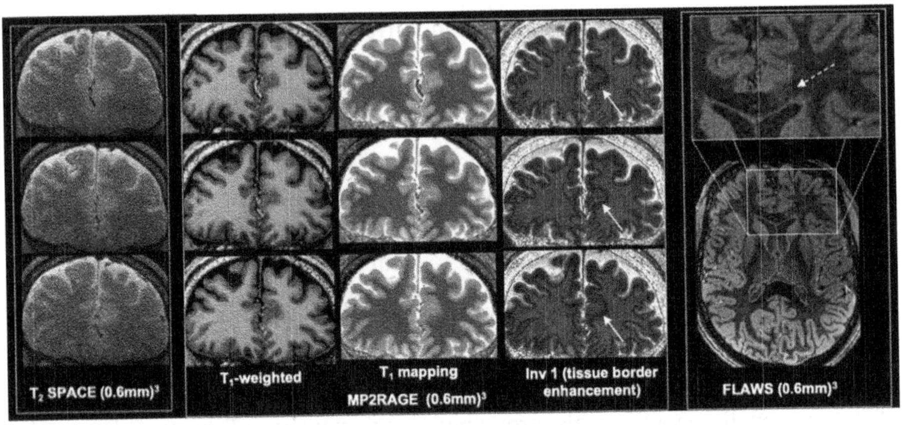

Figure 12.10. *Structural MRI at 7 T of a patient with focal cortical dysplasia (FCD) type II, not diagnosed at 3 T*

COMMENT ON FIGURE 12.10.– *Dysplasia located in the anterior part of the left cingular gyrus is visible with the three high-resolution 3D sequences (T_2 SPACE, MP2RAGE and FLAWS). The first inversion time (inv1) of the MP2RAGE sequence was chosen to highlight the interface between the gray and the white matter (void signal indicated by the white arrow). Remarkably and importantly for the patient's treatment, the "transmantle sign", that is, a hypersignal between the dysplastic cortex and the ventricle, typical in type-II FCD, is clearly visible with the FLAWS sequence (white dashed arrow). Image kindly provided by Prof. M. Guye (CRMBM-CEMEREM, CHU Timone, Marseille).*

12.4.2. *Brain tumors*

In a similar way, T_2*-weighted imaging plays an important role at 7 T in the characterization of brain tumors. It can help to delimit the tumor infiltration and the area of vascular proliferation, but it also provides information on the tumor's metabolism with an increased contrast related to higher oxygen consumption and the amount of deoxyhemoglobin (van der Kolk et al. 2013). Contrast and resolution of conventional anatomical imaging techniques can help refine the diagnosis with potential effects on the the patient's treatment (see Figure 12.9).

Finally, metabolic CEST imaging (sensitive to the concentration of proteins and providing information on the tumor's heterogeneity) and ^{23}Na or ^{17}O imaging (providing information on cell viability) can also help to guide the biopsy in regions that are the most representative of the tumor's aggressiveness and improve the precision and presurgical evaluation of vital brain areas before tumor ablation. They can also provide new markers for therapeutic monitoring, detection of IDH gene mutations, or early detection of responses to treatments (Regnery et al. 2018; Paech et al. 2020).

12.4.3. *Focal epilepsy*

Over the last decade, investigations have clearly shown the value of 7 T MRI in epilepsy cases (Opheim et al. 2021). 7 T MRI enables better identification of epileptogenic areas, brain cortex malformations and areas of focal cortical dysplasia (see Figure 12.10), and thus better patient treatment with direct implications for electrode implantation, surgery and prognostic regarding the occurrence of seizures.

12.4.4. *Multiple sclerosis*

7 T MRI is advantageous for diagnosing MS, an inflammatory disease of the brain and spinal cord characterized by the presence of lesions.

The lesions can arise around small veins and are then referred to as central vein signs (CVS). Note that 75% of the lesions exhibit these signs (Castellaro et al. 2020), with a specificity of 92% and a sensitivity of 95% in differential diagnosis. Since they are easily detectable on T_2*-weighted images with sub-millimetric spatial resolutions (see Figure 12.11(b)), 7 T imaging has become a remarkable tool for detecting these lesions (Bruschi et al. 2020). Susceptibility imaging is also very promising for detecting iron accumulation around the lesion contours; this deposition can be a sign of progressive tissue lesion (chronic lesion with pro-inflammatory microglia/macrophages), and thus become a prognostic marker (Dal-Bianco et al. 2017).

Thanks to its spatial resolution and contrast, 7 T MRI can also detect cortical lesions more precisely (see Figure 12.11(a)) when these were hardly visualizable before (small size, lower inflammation degree than white matter lesions, partial volume effects with cerebrospinal liquid) (Maranzano et al. 2019). These lesions, associated with handicap progression and cognitive deficiency, could represent an important biomarker for the evaluation of MS progression.

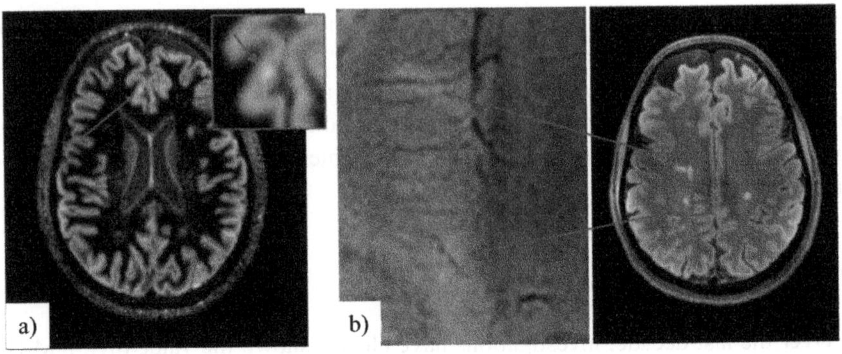

Figure 12.11. *7 T MRI of a patient reporting headaches without any medical history. First, 3 T MRI scans have revealed multiple FLAIR hypersignals of the supratentorial white matter. A 7 T scan has detected three more FLAIR hypersignals, one of them cortical (a). More than 40% of the lesions exhibit a central vein sign (b). These new elements support a probable multiple sclerosis diagnosis. Images kindly produced and provided by Prof. R. Guillevin (CHU Poitiers). For a color version of this figure, see www.iste.co.uk/ratiney-beuf/challenges.zip*

12.4.5. *Sodium imaging*

As mentioned before, thanks to higher sensitivity and the commercially available dedicated coils, 7 T scanners have made exotic scans more feasible. For example, ^{23}Na MRI, by measuring the tissue sodium concentration in vivo, provides unique opportunities for investigating tissue homeostasis and thus detecting early modifications related to pathological processes leading to neurodegeneration or accumulations that indicate neuronal dysfunction as observed in MS, Huntington's disease, or amyotrophic lateral sclerosis.

Sodium MRI usually focuses on measuring the total sodium concentration in the tissues but other approaches, such as multiple quantum filtering or bi-exponential analysis of the T_2 decay of the sodium (Figure 12.12), can highlight variations in the concentration or relaxation time which can represent specific physiopathological mechanisms (Thulborn 2018). It should be noted that extracting these parameters by characterizing the transverse decay of the NMR signal remains controversial (Burstein and Springer 2019).

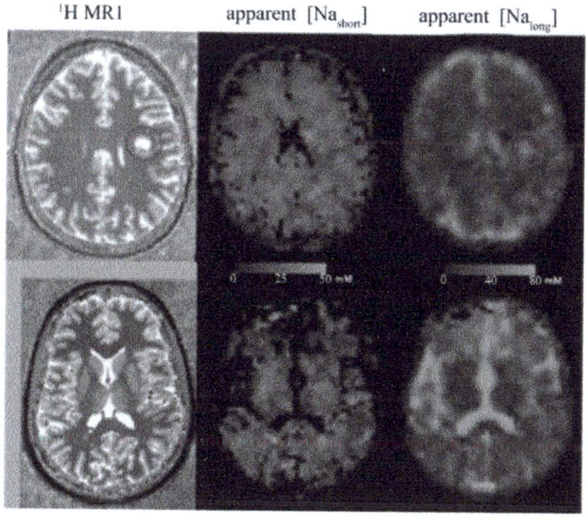

Figure 12.12. *Sodium MRI and "apparent" short and long concentrations derived from a bi-exponential analysis of the* T_2 *decay (Ridley et al. 2018). The figure shows two types of multiple sclerosis features: a lesion with variations of apparent sodium long-component concentration and another with changes in the short-component concentration, which can correspond to different physiopathological conditions. Images kindly shared by W. Zaaraoui and M. El Mendili (CRMBM-CEMEREM, Marseille). For a color version of this figure, see www.iste.co.uk/ratiney-beuf/challenges.zip*

12.4.6. *Creating new normalization spaces (templates)*

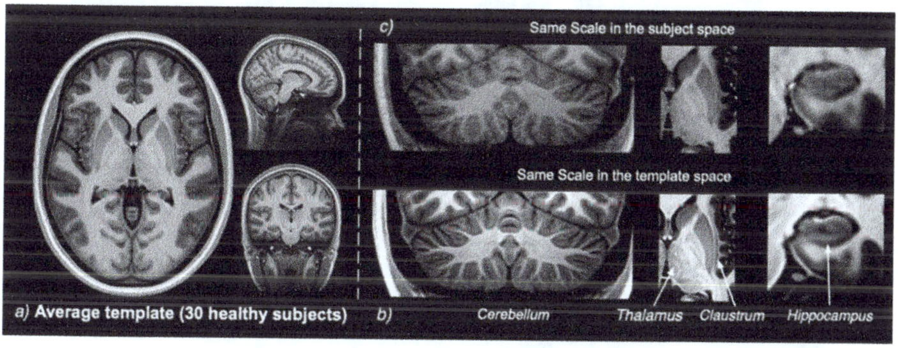

Figure 12.13. *(a) High-resolution* T_1*w MP2RAGE template (0.6 mm isotropic) showing high contrast and revealing (b) anatomical details in the cerebellum and basal ganglia, such as the thalamus, claustrum or hippocampus. These details are also visible for each subject at 7 T (c), being only hardly detectable at 3 T. Images kindly provided by A. Le Troter (CRMBM-CEMEREM, Marseille)*

In neuroscience, data analysis is often based on the co-registration of anatomical, structural, or functional data in a common space (e.g. Montreal Neurological Institute (MNI) reference or Talairach atlas). High-spatial-resolution imaging obtained at 7 T enables the creation of new normalization spaces (or templates, see Figure 12.13), making new structures or regions of interest (such as the claustrum or hippocampus) available, on which one or more imaging modalities from different subjects can be co-registered to facilitate group analysis.

12.4.7. *Imaging of the cartilage and muscle injuries*

Thanks to considerably improved spatial resolution, musculoskeletal and osteoarticular imaging have achieved significant advances with several applications (cartilage (see Figure 12.14(a)), spondylarthritis, tumor, muscle dystrophy, muscle injuries (see Figure 12.14(b)), etc.), both in morphological imaging and in quantitative imaging (mapping of T_1, T_2*, $T_1\rho$, sodium imaging, chemical exchange saturation transfer and spectroscopy) (Aringhieri et al. 2020). Besides better anatomical details of the involved structures, which are useful for diagnostic improvements (see Figure 12.14(c)), the biochemical and metabolic information that can now be obtained should help to better characterize tissue integrity in this domain.

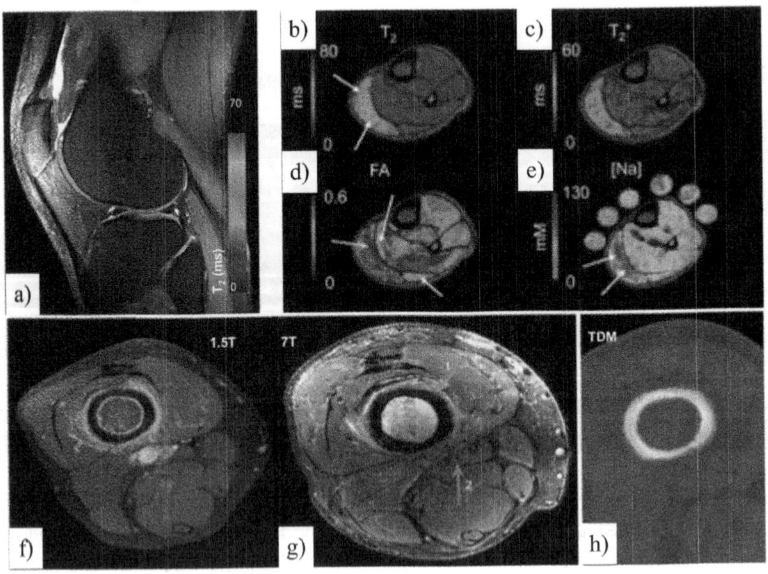

Figure 12.14. *Comparative value of 7T MRI in musculoskeletal imaging. For a color version of this figure, see www.iste.co.uk/ratiney-beuf/challenges.zip*

COMMENT ON FIGURE 12.14.– *(a) T_2 mapping of the knee cartilage of a healthy subject. 7 T MRI in a patient will allow visualizing reduced and/or damaged cartilage. (b–e) Maps of T_2/T_2*/diffusion (anisotropy fraction) and sodium concentration show and quantify local muscle injuries induced via electrical stimulation exercises (Fouré et al. 2019). (f–h) Imaging at 1.5 T, 7 T and tomodensitometric CT scan results in a patient with chondrosarcoma. 7 T MRI shows the cortical layers related to tumor growth (orange arrow) together with a fine visualization of the vessels. The achieved resolution (0.4 mm) helps evaluate the vascular aspects and plan future surgeries (Mattei et al. 2020). Images kindly shared by D. Bendahan (CRMBM-CEMEREM, Marseille).*

As mentioned previously, clinical routine applications focus on brain and musculoskeletal (knee) investigations. Nevertheless, 7 T imaging has opened many investigation possibilities, from clinical research ones to more fundamental applications. Other applications, such as abdominal imaging, still represent a challenge due to the non-uniformity of RF excitation and B_0 field and the constraints of energy deposition. However, novel opportunities are gradually unlocked thanks to the development of dedicated coils and fast techniques that can mitigate contrast inhomogeneities.

Finally, it should be noted that anatomical and quantitative imaging 7 T is mostly based on the same principles of 3 T sequences. Clearly, their parameters need to be adapted to optimize the obtained contrasts and markers, but this does not represent a major obstacle. Distortions due to susceptibility and B_0 field non-uniformity mentioned previously require more specific adjustments. The main challenges are related to the B_1^+ inhomogeneity and energy deposition (turbo spin echo sequences, magnetization transfer, etc.). These are hard to tackle with single-channel transmit coils in a reasonable scan time and we shall see in section 12.5 the perspectives which are offered by parallel transmission imaging.

12.5. Parallel transmission: technical solutions and imaging

Regarding the problems related to the often mentioned (in particular, in section 12.2.2) B_1^+ heterogeneities, different solutions can be implemented.

One passive solution requires the positioning of high dielectric constant (HDC) materials (Teeuwisse et al. 2012), called "pads", or metamaterials with equivalent properties (Dubois et al. 2018) in the form of patches, to be located near the areas requiring homogenization. The HDC materials behave as sources of secondary RF fields that modify the local RF distribution (Webb 2011). Nowadays, some dielectric pads have been approved for neurology applications and are widely used (e.g. $CaTiO_3$).

Another solution, an active one, employs parallel transmission (pTx) systems that can provide RF pulses separately for each channel of a multi-channel coil to create interferences among them (Padormo et al. 2016) (see Figure 12.15).

In its simplest version, called the "static RF shimming", for each channel, the amplitude and phase of the RF pulses with the same shape are simply modulated such that the sum of their B_1^+ fields is as homogeneous as possible. The achieved correction mainly depends on the number of available channels, but it remains limited (see Figure 12.15(b)).

A more elegant, as well as more complex solution is called the "dynamic RF shimming" (see Figure 12.15(c)). It is based on optimized RF pulses that enable the selection of a 2D (or even 3D) volume of interest (Décorps 2012). Such pulses can produce spatially selective excitation that can counteract the field distribution that is normally produced by the coil (Yip et al. 2005). Such implementation of this solution remains difficult to apply because it involves very long RF pulses. However, Grissom (Grissom et al. 2006) and Katscher (Katscher and Börnert 2006) have extended this approach by exploiting the parallel transmission to shorten the duration of the pulses. Alongside, other strategies have been introduced: customized pulses with shorter duration and more efficacy, such as "kt-points" (Cloos et al. 2012) or "SPINS" pulses (Malik et al. 2012), or, more recently, the "universal pulses" that do not require specific calibrations for each patient (Gras et al. 2017), making the technique almost ready for clinical use (currently, for brain applications only).

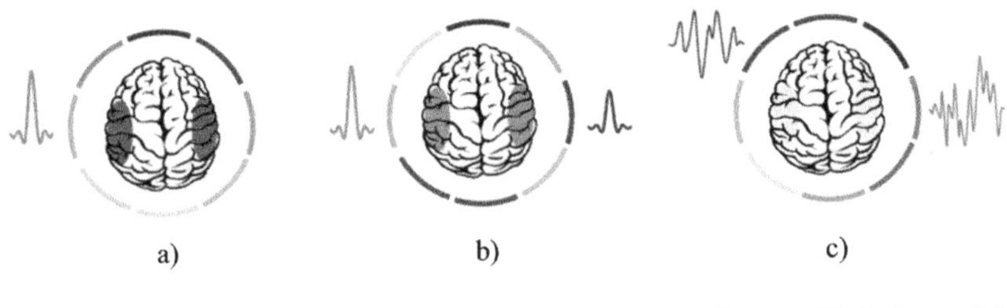

a) b) c)

Figure 12.15. *Each channel of a parallel transmit coil (here, with 8 channels) can be controlled independently. For a color version of this figure, see www.iste.co.uk/ratiney-beuf/challenges.zip*

COMMENT ON FIGURE 12.15.– *MRI scanners have many RF amplifiers that can be used in several ways: (a) as in a standard system, by mimicking a circular* *polarization mode with the same pulse incremented here by 45° for adjacent elements; (b) in static B_1^+ shimming mode, executing the same pulse but with different amplitudes and phases for each channel; or (c) in dynamic B_1^+ shimming mode, where different pulses are executed by each channel. The ability to correct for the spin excitation non-uniformities (represented here as temporal signal shadows) increases from left to right; the same is true for the complexity of pulse optimization executed by each channel (figure inspired by R. Tomi-Tricot and E. Poirion).*

An important aspect to highlight is that by using different pulses for each channel that interfere with each other to produce an RF field distribution according to the user's need, the local power dissipation can vary considerably from one imaging sequence to another. It becomes increasingly difficult to consider all of the scenarios and ensure that the imaging sequences can be executed without patient risks. Being too conservative can hinder the exploitation of the full potential of this approach, thus to ensure flexibility while preserving safety, it is necessary to calculate SAR_{local} for each case, ideally in real time, based on one or more models together with a lower safety margin. However, performing SAR_{local} calculations for a whole-body model in real time is not realistic with the computation resources available today. For this reason, the concept of virtual observation points (VOP) was introduced (Eichfelder and Gebhardt 2011) to calculate only a limited number of characteristic points and ensure safe and fast measurement of this value in real time, providing a systematically slightly overestimated estimation of SAR. This is a fast-growing new approach that has opened many possibilities for fully exploiting the potential of ultra-high field MRI.

12.6. Conclusion

In this chapter, we have highlighted the physical and methodological advantages and disadvantages related to ultra-high field imaging (see summary in Table 12.3), as well as the most common current uses. Mainly applied in the brain and knee, these applications have so far benefitted from improved spatial resolution and contrast to explore the physiopathological processes in more detail and improve the diagnosis, prognosis and treatment of some pathologies. The potential benefit of accelerated scans, on the other hand, has not yet been fully exploited.

This chapter has also described the domains of growing development stimulated by the challenges faced at ultra-high fields (non-uniformity of B_0 and B_1^+, SAR management and parallel transmit imaging).

	Advantages	Disadvantages
SNR ↗	Spatial resolution↗, Tacq↘, X-nuclei MRI sensitivity ↗, parallel imaging	
T_2* relaxation ↘	BOLD, SWI and QSM contrast imaging	Signal loss (gradient echo, etc.)
T_1 relaxation ↗	TOF, ASL and tagged imaging	Contrast loss, Tacq↗
Spectral broadening↗	Increased spectral discrimination (MRS, CEST)	Spectral localization, chemical shift ↗
Non-uniformity B_0 ↗		Larger MRS spectra, distortions (EPI) ↗ ↘ signal (dynamic fluctuations)
Non-uniformity B_1+ ↗		Spatial variation of the flip angle, ↘ signal, contrast loss/neutralization
SAR ↗		Limitation in number of slices, flip angle and TR
Technology	Short and actively shielded magnet, no helium waste (zero boil-off)	Few available RF coils, still requires technical support from the physicists
Neurology	Improvement of micro-anatomical and pathophysiological delimitations	Distortions at air-tissue interfaces (gradient echo), SAR limitations (TSE), RF imperfections
Whole body		Limited peak power, SAR restrictions, non-uniformities B_1+ and B_0
X-nuclei	^{23}Na and ^{31}P MRI/MRS spatial resolution ↗, ^{35}Cl and ^{19}K MRI feasibility, etc.	Optimal pulse often limited by SAR

Table 12.3. *Summary of main advantages and disadvantages of ultra-high field imaging*

Still expensive and much less available than routine clinical imaging scanners at 1.5 and 3 T, the 7 T scanners are currently dedicated to limited and very specific clinical applications in which the diagnosis or treatment can be improved. Open questions remain regarding exhaustive neuroradiological use of the new details and contrast anomalies observed in images acquired at 7 T. Optimal exploitation of these new opportunities should necessarily be accompanied by specific training of neuroradiologists.

To conclude, the investigations performed outside the brain, currently at a rather investigative or clinical research stage, have not been tackled in this chapter. However, they are growing and increasingly reported in several research studies in the MRI community. The same is true for activities on the development of higher-performance RF coils and imaging sequences with shorter scan times and lower SAR needs.

It is a safe bet that the landscape and applications of ultra-high fields will evolve very quickly in the following decade.

12.7. Acknowledgments

The authors thank Maxime Guye, Arnaud Le Troter, Wafaa Zaaraoui, David Bendahan, Rémy Guillevin, Nicolas Boulant, Vincent Gras, Franck Mauconduit, Alexis Amadon, Cécile Lerman, Lucie Hertz-Pannier, Michel Bottlaender and Éric Jouvent for providing clinical illustrations, and also Aurélien Massire and Thomas Troalen for making the technical data available.

12.8. References

Abosch, A., Yacoub, E., Ugurbil, K., Harel, N. (2010). An assessment of current brain targets for deep brain stimulation surgery with susceptibility-weighted imaging at 7 tesla. *Neurosurgery*, 67(6), 1745–1756.

Aringhieri, G., Zampa, V., Tosetti, M. (2020). Musculoskeletal MRI at 7 T: Do we need more or is it more than enough? *European Radiology Experimental*, 4(1), 48.

Bottomley, P.A., Hardy, C.J., Argersinger, R.E., Allen-Moore, G. (1987). A review of ^{1}H nuclear magnetic resonance relaxation in pathology: Are T_1 and T_2 diagnostic? *Medical Physics*, 14(1), 1–37.

Bruschi, N., Boffa, G., Inglese, M. (2020). Ultra-high-field 7-T MRI in multiple sclerosis and other demyelinating diseases: From pathology to clinical practice. *European Radiology Experimental*, 4(1), 59.

Burstein, D. and Springer, C.S. (2019). Sodium MRI revisited. *Magnetic Resonance in Medicine*, 82(2), 521–524.

Castellaro, M., Tamanti, A., Pisani, A.I., Pizzini, F.B., Crescenzo, F., Calabrese, M. (2020). The use of the central vein sign in the diagnosis of multiple sclerosis: A systematic review and meta-analysis. *Diagnostics*, 10(12), 1025.

Cloos, M.A., Boulant, N., Luong, M., Ferrand, G., Giacomini, E., Le Bihan, D., Amadon, A. (2012). kT-points: Short three-dimensional tailored RF pulses for flip-angle homogenization over an extended volume. *Magnetic Resonance in Medicine*, 67(1), 72–80.

Collins, C.M. and Wang, Z. (2011). Calculation of radiofrequency electromagnetic fields and their effects in MRI of human subjects. *Magnetic Resonance in Medicine*, 65(5), 1470–1482.

Cox, E.F. and Gowland, P.A. (2010). Simultaneous quantification of T_2 and T'_2 using a combined gradient echo-spin echo sequence at ultrahigh field. *Magnetic Resonance in Medicine*, 64(5), 1440–1445.

Dal-Bianco, A., Grabner, G., Kronnerwetter, C., Weber, M., Höftberger, R., Berger, T., Auff, E., Leutmezer, F., Trattnig, S., Lassmann, H. et al. (2017). Slow expansion of multiple sclerosis iron rim lesions: Pathology and 7 T magnetic resonance imaging. *Acta Neuropathologica*, 133(1), 25–42.

De Guio, F., Vignaud, A., Ropele, S., Duering, M., Duchesnay, E., Chabriat, H., Jouvent, E. (2014). Loss of venous integrity in cerebral small vessel disease: A 7-T MRI study in cerebral autosomal-dominant arteriopathy with subcortical infarcts and leukoencephalopathy (CADASIL). *Stroke*, 45(7), 2124–2126.

Décorps, M. (2012). *Imagerie de résonance magnétique*. EDP Sciences, Les Ulis.

Donadieu, M., Le Fur, Y., Confort-Gouny, S., Le Troter, A., Guye, M., Ranjeva, J.-P. (2016). Evidencing different neurochemical profiles between thalamic nuclei using high resolution 2D-PRESS semi-LASER 1H-MRSI at 7 T. *Magnetic Resonance Materials in Physics, Biology and Medicine*, 29(3), 491–501.

Dubois, M., Leroi, L., Raolison, Z., Abdeddaim, R., Antonakakis, T., de Rosny, J., Vignaud, A., Sabouroux, P., Georget, E., Larrat, B. et al. (2018). Kerker effect in ultrahigh-field magnetic resonance imaging. *Physical Review X*, 8(3), 031083.

Eichfelder, G. and Gebhardt, M. (2011). Local specific absorption rate control for parallel transmission by virtual observation points. *Magnetic Resonance in Medicine*, 66(5), 1468–1476.

Fagan, A.J., Bitz, A.K., Björkman-Burtscher, I.M., Collins, C.M., Kimbrell, V., Raaijmakers, A.J.E., ISMRM Safety Committee (2021). 7T MR safety. *Journal of Magnetic Resonance Imaging*, 53(2), 333–346.

Finn, E.S., Huber, L., Bandettini, P.A. (2020). Higher and deeper: Bringing layer fMRI to association cortex. *Progress in Neurobiology*, 207, 101930.

Fouré, A., Pini, L., Rappacchi, S., Ogier, A.C., Mattei, J.-C., Bydder, M., Guye, M., Bendahan, D. (2019). Ultrahigh-field multimodal MRI assessment of muscle damage. *Journal of Magnetic Resonance Imaging*, 49(3), 904–906.

Gras, V., Vignaud, A., Amadon, A., Le Bihan, D., Boulant, N. (2017). Universal pulses: A new concept for calibration-free parallel transmission. *Magnetic Resonance in Medicine*, 77(2), 635–643.

Grissom, W., Yip, C., Zhang, Z., Stenger, V.A., Fessler, J.A., Noll, D.C. (2006). Spatial domain method for the design of RF pulses in multicoil parallel excitation. *Magnetic Resonance in Medicine*, 56(3), 620–629.

Guérin, B., Villena, J.F., Polimeridis, A.G., Adalsteinsson, E., Daniel, L., White, J.K., Wald, L.L. (2017). The ultimate signal-to-noise ratio in realistic body models. *Magnetic Resonance in Medicine*, 78(5), 1969–1980.

Haacke, E.M., Xu, Y., Cheng, Y.-C.N., Reichenbach, J.R. (2004). Susceptibility weighted imaging (SWI). *Magnetic Resonance in Medicine*, 52(3), 612–618.

Haeberlin, M., Kasper, L., Barmet, C., Brunner, D.O., Dietrich, B.E., Gross, S., Wilm, B.J., Kozerke, S., Pruessmann, K.P. (2015). Real-time motion correction using gradient tones and head-mounted NMR field probes. *Magnetic Resonance in Medicine*, 74(3), 647–660.

Hagberg, G.E. and Scheffler, K. (2013). Effect of R_1 and R_2 relaxivity of gadolinium-based contrast agents on the T_1-weighted MR signal at increasing magnetic field strengths. *Contrast Media & Molecular Imaging*, 8(6), 456–465.

Henning, A. (2018). Proton and multinuclear magnetic resonance spectroscopy in the human brain at ultra-high field strength: A review. *NeuroImage*, 168, 181–198.

Hoff, M.N., McKinney, A., Shellock, F.G., Rassner, U., Gilk, T., Watson, R.E., Greenberg, T.D., Froelich, J., Kanal, E. (2019). Safety considerations of 7-T MRI in clinical practice. *Radiology*, 292(3), 509–518.

Hoult, D.I. and Phil, D. (2000). Sensitivity and power deposition in a high-field imaging experiment. *Journal of Magnetic Resonance Imaging*, 12(1), 46–67.

International Standard (IEC) (2010). International Electrotechnical Commission. Medical electrical equipment – Part 2–33: Particular requirements for the safety of magnetic resonance diagnostic devices.

Internationale Arbeitsorganisation, International Commission on Non-Ionizing Radiation Protection, Weltgesundheitsorganisation (eds) (2006). *Static Fields*. WHO, Geneva.

Kang, C.-K., Park, C.-A., Kim, K.-N., Hong, S.-M., Park, C.-W., Kim, Y.-B., Cho, Z.-H. (2010). Non-invasive visualization of basilar artery perforators with 7T MR angiography. *Journal of Magnetic Resonance Imaging*, 32(3), 544–550.

Katscher, U. and Börnert, P. (2006). Parallel RF transmission in MRI. *NMR in Biomedicine*, 19(3), 393–400.

Kogan, F., Hariharan, H., Reddy, R. (2013). Chemical Exchange Saturation Transfer (CEST) imaging: Description of technique and potential clinical applications. *Current Radiology Reports*, 1(2), 102–114.

van der Kolk, A.G., Hendrikse, J., Zwanenburg, J.J.M., Visser, F., Luijten, P.R. (2013). Clinical applications of 7T MRI in the brain. *European Journal of Radiology*, 82(5), 708–718.

Koopmans, P.J., Manniesing, R., Niessen, W.J., Viergever, M.A., Barth, M. (2008). MR venography of the human brain using susceptibility weighted imaging at very high field strength. *Magnetic Resonance Materials in Physics, Biology and Medicine*, 21(1), 149.

Kraff, O. and Quick, H.H. (2019). Radiofrequency coils for 7 tesla MRI. *Topics in Magnetic Resonance Imaging*, 28(3), 145–158.

Lauterbur, P.C. (1973). Image formation by induced local interactions: Examples employing nuclear magnetic resonance. *Nature*, 242(5394), 190–191.

Lévy, S., Roche, P.-H., Guye, M., Callot, V. (2021). Feasibility of human spinal cord perfusion mapping using dynamic susceptibility contrast imaging at 7T: Preliminary results and identified guidelines. *Magnetic Resonance in Medicine*, 85(3), 1183–1194.

Liu, Y., Gu, Y., Yu, X. (2017). Assessing tissue metabolism by phosphorous-31 magnetic resonance spectroscopy and imaging: A methodology review. *Quantitative Imaging in Medicine and Surgery*, 7(6), 707–726.

Malik, S.J., Keihaninejad, S., Hammers, A., Hajnal, J.V. (2012). Tailored excitation in 3D with spiral nonselective (SPINS) RF pulses. *Magnetic Resonance in Medicine*, 67(5), 1303–1315.

Maranzano, J., Dadar, M., Rudko, D.A., Nigris, D.D., Elliott, C., Gati, J.S., Morrow, S.A., Menon, R.S., Collins, D.L., Arnold, D.L., Narayanan, S. (2019). Comparison of multiple sclerosis cortical lesion types detected by multicontrast 3T and 7T MRI. *AJNR Am. J. Neuroradiol.*, 40(7), 1162–1169.

Marques, J.P., Kober, T., Krueger, G., van der Zwaag, W., Van de Moortele, P.-F., Gruetter, R. (2010). MP2RAGE, a self bias-field corrected sequence for improved segmentation and T_1-mapping at high field. *NeuroImage*, 49(2), 1271–1281.

Marrakchi-Kacem, L., Vignaud, A., Sein, J., Germain, J., Henry, T.R., Poupon, C., Hertz-Pannier, L., Lehéricy, S., Colliot, O., Van de Moortele, P.-F., Chupin, M. (2016). Robust imaging of hippocampal inner structure at 7T: In vivo acquisition protocol and methodological choices. *Magma (New York, N.Y.)*, 29(3), 475–489.

Mattei, J.-C., Foure, A., Rochwerger, A., Troter, A.L., Varoquaux, A., Chagnaud, C., Bouvier, C., Bendahan, D., Mattei, J.-C., Guye, M. et al. (2020). Are we heading to the future of musculoskeletal tumor imaging with ultra-high field 7T MRI? *Clinical Oncology and Research*, 1–8.

Mattern, H., Sciarra, A., Godenschweger, F., Stucht, D., Lüsebrink, F., Rose, G., Speck, O. (2018). Prospective motion correction enables highest resolution time-of-flight angiography at 7T. *Magnetic Resonance in Medicine*, 80(1), 248–258.

Moenninghoff, C., Kraff, O., Maderwald, S., Umutlu, L., Theysohn, J.M., Ringelstein, A., Wrede, K.H., Deuschl, C., Altmeppen, J., Ladd, M.E. et al. (2015). Diffuse axonal injury at ultra-high field MRI. *PLoS ONE*, 10(3), e0122329.

Monti, S., Cocozza, S., Borrelli, P., Straub, S., Ladd, M.E., Salvatore, M., Tedeschi, E., Palma, G. (2017). MAVEN: An algorithm for multi-parametric automated segmentation of brain veins from gradient echo acquisitions. *IEEE Transactions on Medical Imaging*, 36(5), 1054–1065.

von Morze, C., Xu, D., Purcell, D.D., Hess, C.P., Mukherjee, P., Saloner, D., Kelley, D.A.C., Vigneron, D.B. (2007). Intracranial time-of-flight MR angiography at 7T with comparison to 3T. *Journal of Magnetic Resonance Imaging*, 26(4), 900–904.

Ocali, O. and Atalar, E. (1998). Ultimate intrinsic signal-to-noise ratio in MRI. *Magnetic Resonance in Medicine*, 39(3), 462–473.

Opheim, G., van der Kolk, A., Markenroth Bloch, K., Colon, A.J., Davis, K.A., Henry, T.R., Jansen, J.F.A., Jones, S.E., Pan, J.W., Rössler, K. et al. (2021). 7T epilepsy task force consensus recommendations on the use of 7T MRI in clinical practice. *Neurology*, 96(7), 327–341.

van Osch, M.J.P. and Webb, A.G. (2014). Safety of ultra-high field MRI: What are the specific risks? *Current Radiology Reports*, 2(8), 61.

Padormo, F., Beqiri, A., Hajnal, J.V., Malik, S.J. (2016). Parallel transmission for ultrahigh-field imaging. *NMR in Biomedicine*, 29(9), 1145–1161.

Paech, D., Nagel, A.M., Schultheiss, M.N., Umathum, R., Regnery, S., Scherer, M., Wick, A., Platt, T., Wick, W., Bendszus, M. et al. (2020). Quantitative dynamic oxygen 17 MRI at 7.0 T for the cerebral oxygen metabolism in glioma. *Radiology*, 295(1), 181–189.

Park, C.-A., Kang, C.-K., Kim, Y.-B., Cho, Z.-H. (2018). Advances in MR angiography with 7T MRI: From microvascular imaging to functional angiography. *NeuroImage*, 168, 269–278.

Pohmann, R., Speck, O., Scheffler, K. (2016). Signal-to-noise ratio and MR tissue parameters in human brain imaging at 3, 7, and 9.4 tesla using current receive coil arrays. *Magnetic Resonance in Medicine*, 75(2), 801–809.

Price, D.L., De Wilde, J.P., Papadaki, A.M., Curran, J.S., Kitney, R.I. (2001). Investigation of acoustic noise on 15 MRI scanners from 0.2 T to 3 T. *Journal of Magnetic Resonance Imaging*, 13(2), 288–293.

Pruessmann, K.P., Weiger, M., Börnert, P., Boesiger, P. (2001). Advances in sensitivity encoding with arbitrary k-space trajectories. *Magnetic Resonance in Medicine*, 46(4), 638–651.

Quettier, L., Aubert, G., Belorgey, J., Berriaud, C., Bredy, P., Dilasser, G., Dubois, O., Gilgrass, G., Guihard, Q., Jannot, V. et al. (2020). Commissioning completion of the iseult whole body 11.7 T MRI system. *IEEE Transactions on Applied Superconductivity*, 30(4), 1–5.

Rauschenberg, J., Nagel, A.M., Ladd, S.C., Theysohn, J.M., Ladd, M.E., Möller, H.E., Trampel, R., Turner, R., Pohmann, R., Scheffler, K. et al. (2014). Multicenter study of subjective acceptance during magnetic resonance imaging at 7 and 9.4 T. *Investigative Radiology*, 49(5), 249–259.

Regnery, S., Adeberg, S., Dreher, C., Oberhollenzer, J., Meissner, J.-E., Goerke, S., Windschuh, J., Deike-Hofmann, K., Bickelhaupt, S., Zaiss, M. (2018). Chemical exchange saturation transfer MRI serves as predictor of early progression in glioblastoma patients. *Oncotarget*, 9(47), 28772–28783.

Ridley, B., Nagel, A.M., Bydder, M., Maarouf, A., Stellmann, J.-P., Gherib, S., Verneuil, J., Viout, P., Guye, M., Ranjeva, J.-P., Zaaraoui, W. (2018). Distribution of brain sodium long and short relaxation times and concentrations: A multi-echo ultra-high field 23Na MRI study. *Scientific Reports*, 8(1), 4357.

Robitaille, P.M., Abduljalil, A.M., Kangarlu, A., Zhang, X., Yu, Y., Burgess, R., Bair, S., Noa, P., Yang, L., Zhu, H. et al. (1998). Human magnetic resonance imaging at 8 T. *NMR in Biomedicine*, 11(6), 263–265.

de Rochefort, L., Liu, T., Kressler, B., Liu, J., Spincemaille, P., Lebon, V., Wu, J., Wang, Y. (2010). Quantitative susceptibility map reconstruction from MR phase data using bayesian regularization: Validation and application to brain imaging. *Magnetic Resonance in Medicine*, 63(1), 194–206.

Rodgers, C.T., Piechnik, S.K., Delabarre, L.J., Van de Moortele, P.-F., Snyder, C.J., Neubauer, S., Robson, M.D., Vaughan, J.T. (2013). Inversion recovery at 7 T in the human myocardium: Measurement of T_1, inversion efficiency and B_1+. *Magnetic Resonance in Medicine*, 70(4), 1038–1046.

Rooney, W.D., Johnson, G., Li, X., Cohen, E.R., Kim, S.-G., Ugurbil, K., Springer, C.S. (2007). Magnetic field and tissue dependencies of human brain longitudinal ^1H_2O relaxation in vivo. *Magnetic Resonance in Medicine*, 57(2), 308–318.

Schenck, J.F. (1996). The role of magnetic susceptibility in magnetic resonance imaging: MRI magnetic compatibility of the first and second kinds. *Medical Physics*, 23(6), 815–850.

Schenck, J.F. (2000). Safety of strong, static magnetic fields. *Journal of Magnetic Resonance Imaging*, 12(1), 2–19.

Schick, F. (2005). Whole-body MRI at high field: Technical limits and clinical potential. *European Radiology*, 15(5), 946–959.

Sengupta, S., Welch, E.B., Zhao, Y., Foxall, D., Starewicz, P., Anderson, A.W., Gore, J.C., Avison, M.J. (2011). Dynamic B_0 shimming at 7 T. *Magnetic Resonance Imaging*, 29(4), 483–496.

Singh, A., Haris, M., Cai, K., Kassey, V.B., Kogan, F., Reddy, D., Hariharan, H., Reddy, R. (2012). Chemical exchange saturation transfer magnetic resonance imaging of human knee cartilage at 3 T and 7 T. *Magnetic Resonance in Medicine*, 68(2), 588–594.

Stäb, D., Roessler, J., O'Brien, K., Hamilton-Craig, C., Barth, M. (2016). ECG triggering in ultra-high field cardiovascular MRI. *Tomography*, 2(3), 167–174.

Stockmann, J.P. and Wald, L.L. (2018). In vivo B_0 field shimming methods for MRI at 7T. *NeuroImage*, 168, 71–87.

Stout, J., Hozer, F., Coste, A., Mauconduit, F., Djebrani-Oussedik, N., Sarrazin, S., Poupon, J., Meyrel, M., Romanzetti, S., Etain, B. et al. (2020). Accumulation of lithium in the hippocampus of patients with bipolar disorder: A lithium-7 magnetic resonance imaging study at 7 tesla. *Biological Psychiatry*, 88(5), 426–433.

Stucht, D., Danishad, K.A., Schulze, P., Godenschweger, F., Zaitsev, M., Speck, O. (2015). Highest resolution in vivo human brain MRI using prospective motion correction. *PloS One*, 10(7), e0133921.

Teeuwisse, W.M., Webb, A.G., van Osch, M.J.P. (2010). Arterial spin labeling at ultra-high field: All that glitters is not gold. *International Journal of Imaging Systems and Technology*, 20(1), 62–70.

Teeuwisse, W.M., Brink, W.M., Webb, A.G. (2012). Quantitative assessment of the effects of high-permittivity pads in 7 tesla MRI of the brain. *Magnetic Resonance in Medicine*, 67(5), 1285–1293.

Thulborn, K.R. (2018). Quantitative sodium MR imaging: A review of its evolving role in medicine. *NeuroImage*, 168, 250–268.

Trattnig, S., Springer, E., Bogner, W., Hangel, G., Strasser, B., Dymerska, B., Cardoso, P.L., Robinson, S.D. (2018). Key clinical benefits of neuroimaging at 7T. *NeuroImage*, 168, 477–489.

Triantafyllou, C., Polimeni, J.R., Wald, L.L. (2011). Physiological noise and signal-to-noise ratio in fMRI with multi-channel array coils. *NeuroImage*, 55(2), 597–606.

Uğurbil, K. (2018). Imaging at ultrahigh magnetic fields: History, challenges, and solutions. *NeuroImage*, 168, 7–32.

Uludağ, K., Müller-Bierl, B., Uğurbil, K. (2009). An integrative model for neuronal activity-induced signal changes for gradient and spin echo functional imaging. *NeuroImage*, 48(1), 150–165.

Vannesjo, S.J., Wilm, B.J., Duerst, Y., Gross, S., Brunner, D.O., Dietrich, B.E., Schmid, T., Barmet, C., Pruessmann, K.P. (2015). Retrospective correction of physiological field fluctuations in high-field brain MRI using concurrent field monitoring. *Magnetic Resonance in Medicine*, 73(5), 1833–1843.

Vannesjo, S.J., Clare, S., Kasper, L., Tracey, I., Miller, K.L. (2019). A method for correcting breathing-induced field fluctuations in T_2*-weighted spinal cord imaging using a respiratory trace. *Magnetic Resonance in Medicine*, 81(6), 3745–3753.

Vaughan, J.T., Garwood, M., Collins, C.M., Liu, W., DelaBarre, L., Adriany, G., Andersen, P., Merkle, H., Goebel, R., Smith, M.B., Ugurbil, K. (2001). 7T vs. 4T: RF power, homogeneity, and signal-to-noise comparison in head images. *Magnetic Resonance in Medicine*, 46(1), 24–30.

Ward, K.M., Aletras, A.H., Balaban, R.S. (2000). A new class of contrast agents for MRI based on proton chemical exchange dependent saturation transfer (CEST). *J. Magn. Reson.*, 143(1), 79–87.

Webb, A.G. (2011). Dielectric materials in magnetic resonance. *Concepts in Magnetic Resonance Part A*, 38A(4), 148–184.

Wiesinger, F., Van de Moortele, P.-F., Adriany, G., De Zanche, N., Ugurbil, K., Pruessmann, K.P. (2004). Parallel imaging performance as a function of field strength – An experimental investigation using electrodynamic scaling. *Magnetic Resonance in Medicine*, 52(5), 953–964.

Winkler, S.A., Schmitt, F., Landes, H., DeBever, J., Wade, T., Alejski, A., Rutt, B.K. (2018). Gradient and shim technologies for ultra high field MRI. *NeuroImage*, 168, 59–70.

Yacoub, E. and Wald, L.L. (2018). Pushing the spatio-temporal limits of MRI and fMRI. *NeuroImage*, 164, 1–3.

Yip, C., Fessler, J.A., Noll, D.C. (2005). Iterative RF pulse design for multidimensional, small-tip-angle selective excitation. *Magnetic Resonance in Medicine*, 54(4), 908–917.

Zhang, X., Petersen, E.T., Ghariq, E., Vis, J.B.D., Webb, A.G., Teeuwisse, W.M., Hendrikse, J., van Osch, M.J.P. (2013). In vivo blood T_1 measurements at 1.5 T, 3 T, and 7 T. *Magnetic Resonance in Medicine*, 70(4), 1082–1086.

Zimmer, F., O'Brien, K., Bollmann, S., Pfeuffer, J., Heberlein, K., Barth, M. (2016). Pulsed arterial spin labelling at ultra-high field with a B_1+ -optimised adiabatic labelling pulse. *Magma (New York, N.Y.)*, 29(3), 463–473.

List of Authors

Emmanuel Luc BARBIER
GIN
Inserm
Université Grenoble Alpes
and
IRMaGe, CNRS
Inserm
CHUGA
Université Grenoble Alpes
France

Olivier BEUF
CREATIS, CNRS
Inserm
INSA Lyon
Université Claude Bernard Lyon 1
France

Fawzi BOUMEZBEUR
NeuroSpin
CEA
Gif-sur-Yvette
France

Virginie CALLOT
CRMBM, CNRS
Université Aix-Marseille
and
CEMEREM
AP-HM
Hôpital de la Timone
Marseille
France

Éléna CHABRAN
ICUBE, CNRS
Université de Strasbourg
France

Thomas CHRISTEN
GIN
Inserm
Université Grenoble Alpes
France

Nadège CORBIN
CRMSB, CNRS
Université de Bordeaux
France

Laetitia DEGIORGIS
ICUBE, CNRS
Université de Strasbourg
France

Guillaume DUHAMEL
CRMBM, CNRS
Université Aix-Marseille
and
CEMEREM
AP-HM
Hôpital de la Timone
Marseille
France

Julien FLAMENT
MIRCen
CEA
Fontenay-aux-Roses
France

Giulio GAMBAROTA
Laboratoire de biophysique
Université de Rennes
France

Philippe GARTEISER
Centre de recherche sur l'inflammation
Inserm
Paris
France

Olivier GIRARD
CRMBM, CNRS
Université Aix-Marseille
and
CEMEREM
AP-HM
Hôpital de la Timone
Marseille
France

Laura Adela HARSAN
ICUBE, CNRS
Université de Strasbourg
France

Frank KOBER
CRMBM, CNRS
Université Aix-Marseille
France

Aimé LABBÉ
BIOMAPS, CNRS
Inserm
CEA
Université Paris-Saclay
France

Denis LE BIHAN
NeuroSpin
CEA
Gif-sur-Yvette
France

Benjamin LEPORQ
CREATIS, CNRS
Inserm
INSA Lyon
Université Claude Bernard Lyon 1
France

Paulo LOUREIRO DE SOUSA
ICUBE, CNRS
Université de Strasbourg
France

Sylvain MIRAUX
CRMSB, CNRS
Université de Bordeaux
France

Valéry OZENNE
CRMSB, CNRS
Université de Bordeaux
France

Marie POIRIER-QUINOT
BIOMAPS, CNRS
Inserm
CEA
Université Paris-Saclay
France

Bruno QUESSON
CRMSB, CNRS
Université de Bordeaux
and
IHU Liryc
Université de Bordeaux
France

Hélène RATINEY
CREATIS, CNRS
Inserm
INSA Lyon
Université Claude Bernard Lyon 1
France

Émeline RIBOT
CRMSB, CNRS
Université de Bordeaux
France

Ludovic DE ROCHEFORT
CRMBM, CNRS
and
CEMEREM
AP-HM
Hôpital de la Timone
Marseille
France

Hervé SAINT-JALMES
LTSI
Inserm
Université de Rennes
France

Marion SOURTY
ICUBE, CNRS
Université de Strasbourg
France

Lucas SOUSTELLE
CRMBM, CNRS
Université Aix-Marseille
and
CEMEREM
AP-HM
Hôpital de la Timone
Marseille
France

Aurélien TROTIER
CRMSB, CNRS
Université de Bordeaux
France

Kevin TSE VE KOON
CREATIS, CNRS
Inserm
INSA Lyon
Université Claude Bernard Lyon 1
France

Jonathan VAPPOU
ICUBE, CNRS
Université de Strasbourg
France

Alexandre VIGNAUD
NeuroSpin
CEA
Gif-sur-Yvette
France

Index

B

C, D

E

F

G, H

I, K

L, M

N, O

T

U, V

W, Z

Printed and bound by CPI Group (UK) Ltd, Croydon, CR0 4YY

13/09/2026

14960998-0008